Current and Future Issues in Hemophilia Care

Current and Future Issues in Hemophilia Care

EDITED BY

EMÉRITO-CARLOS RODRÍGUEZ-MERCHÁN MD, PHD

Consultant Orthopedic Surgeon
Department of Orthopedic Surgery and Hemophilia Unit
La Paz University Hospital;
Associate Professor of Orthopaedic Surgery
School of Medicine
Autonomous University
Madrid, Spain

LEONARD A. VALENTINO MD

Professor of Pediatrics, Internal Medicine,
Immunology/Microbiology and Biochemistry
Director, Hemophilia and Thrombophilia Center
Rush University Medical Center
Chicago, IL, USA

WILEY-BLACKWELL

A John Wiley & Sons, Ltd., Publication

This edition first published 2011 © 2011 by John Wiley & Sons Ltd

Wiley-Blackwell is an imprint of John Wiley & Sons, formed by the merger of Wiley's global Scientific, Technical and Medical business with Blackwell Publishing.

Registered office: John Wiley & Sons, Ltd, The Atrium, Southern Gate, Chichester, West Sussex, PO19 8SQ, UK

Editorial offices: 9600 Garsington Road, Oxford, OX4 2DQ, UK

The Atrium, Southern Gate, Chichester, West Sussex, PO19 8SQ, UK

111 River Street, Hoboken, NJ 07030-5774, USA

For details of our global editorial offices, for customer services and for information about how to apply for permission to reuse the copyright material in this book please see our website at www.wiley.com/wiley-blackwell

Library of Congress Cataloging-in-Publication Data

Current and future issues in hemophilia care / edited by Emérito-Carlos Rodríguez-Merchán, Leonard A. Valentino.
     p. ; cm.
   Includes bibliographical references and index.
   ISBN-13: 978-0-470-67057-6 (hardcover : alk. paper)
   ISBN-10: 0-470-67057-6 (hardcover : alk. paper)
  1. Hemophilia. I. Rodríguez-Merchán, E. C. II. Valentino, Leonard A.
   [DNLM: 1. Hemophilia A–prevention & control.   2. Hemophilia A–therapy.   3. Blood Coagulation
Factors.   WH 325]
   RC642.C87 2011
   616.1′572–dc22

2011007517

A catalogue record for this book is available from the British Library.

This book is published in the following electronic formats: ePDF 9781119979371; Wiley Online Library 9781119979401; ePub 9781119979388; Mobi 9781119979395

Set in 9.25/12pt Minion by Aptara® Inc., New Delhi, India
Printed and bound in Great Britain by TJ International Ltd, Padstow, Cornwall

2   2011

Contents

Contents

Contributors

Lydia Abad-Franch MD
Specialist in Family Medicine
Hemostasis and Thrombosis Unit
La Fe University Hospital
Valencia, Spain

Louis M. Aledort MD
The Mary Weinfeld Professor of Clinical Research
in Hemophilia
Mount Sinai School of Medicine
New York, NY, USA

Carmen Altisent MD
Unitat d'Hemofília
Hospital Universitari Vall d'Hebron
Barcelona, Spain

Maria-Teresa Alvarez-Román MD
Consultant Hematologist
Hemostasis and Thrombosis Unit
La Paz University Hospital
Madrid, Spain

Jan Astermark MD, PhD
Associate Professor
Lund University;
Malmö Centre for Thrombosis and Haemostasis
Skåne University Hospital
Malmö, Sweden

Günter Auerswald MD
Klinikum Bremen-Mitte
Ambulanz für Thrombose und
Hämostasestörungen, Prof.-Hess Kinderklinik
Bremen, Germany

José A. Aznar MD
Head of Hemostasis and Thrombosis Unit
Department of Hematology and Hemotherapy
La Fe University Hospital
Valencia, Spain

Erik Berntorp MD, PhD
Professor of Hemophilia
Lund University;
Malmö Centre for Thrombosis and Haemostasis
Skåne University Hospital
Malmö, Sweden

Jan Blatny MD, PhD
Consultant Hematologist
Department of Pediatric Hematology
Center for Thrombosis and Hemostasis
Children's University Hospital Brno
Brno, Czech Republic

Lisa N. Boggio MS, MD
Assistant Professor of Medicine and Pediatrics
Division of Hematology and Oncology
Rush University Medical Center
Chicago, IL, USA

Ana R. Cid MD
Hematologist
Hemostasis and Thrombosis Unit
La Fe University Hospital
Valencia, Spain

Caroline Cromwell MD
Assistant Professor of Medicine
Division of Hematology/Oncology
Mount Sinai School of Medicine
New York, NY, USA

Donna M. DiMichele MD
Weill Cornell Medical College;
Deputy Director
Division of Blood Diseases and Resources
National Heart, Lung and Blood Institute
New York, NY, USA

Gerard Dolan MB ChB, FRCP,
FRCPath
Consultant Haematologist
Nottingham University Hospitals
Nottingham, UK

Kathelijn Fischer MD, PhD
Pediatric Hematologist and Clinical
Epidemiologist
Van Creveldkliniek, Department of Hematology,
and Julius Center for Health Sciences
and Primary Care
University Medical Center Utrecht
Utrecht, The Netherlands

Angela L. Forsyth PT, DPT
Physiotherapist
Penn Hemophilia and Thrombosis Program
Hospital of the University of Pennsylvania
Philadelphia, PA, USA

Paul L.F. Giangrande BSc, MD, FRCP,
FRCPath, FRCPCH
Consultant Haematologist and Director
Oxford Haemophilia and Thrombosis Centre
Churchill Hospital
Oxford, UK

Nicholas J. Goddard MB FRCS
Consultant Orthopaedic Surgeon
Department of Orthopaedic Surgery
Royal Free Hospital
London, UK

Alessandro Gringeri MD, MSc
Department of Medicine and Medical Specialities
Fondazione IRCCS Cà Granda – Ospedale
Maggiore Policlinico and University of Milan
Milan, Italy

Contributors

Narine Hakobyan PhD
Assistant Professor
Rush Hemophilia and Thrombophilia Center;
Department of Pediatrics
Rush Children's Hospital and Rush University
Medical Center
Chicago, IL, USA

Saturnino Haya MD
Hematologist
Hemostasis and Thrombosis Unit
Department of Hematology and Hemotherapy
La Fe University Hospital
Valencia, Spain

Christoph J. Hofbauer Dipl.-Ing. (FH)
Department of Immunology
TA BioTherapeutics
Baxter Innovation GmbH
Vienna, Austria

Frank M. Horling PhD
Manager Immunotoxicology
Department of Immunology
TA BioTherapeutics
Baxter Innovation GmbH
Vienna, Austria

Victor Jiménez -Yuste MD, PhD
Consultant Hematologist
Department of Hematology and Hemostasis Unit
La Paz University Hospital;
Associate Professor of Hematology
School of Medicine
Autonomous University
Madrid, Spain

Karin Kurnik MD
Klinikum Bremen-Mitte
Ambulanz für Thrombose und
Hämostasestörungen, Prof.-Hess Kinderklinik
Bremen, Germany

Christine A. Lee MA, MD, DSc, FRCP,
FRCPath, FRCOG ad eundem
Emeritus Professor of Haemophilia
University of London
London, UK

Marilyn J. Manco-Johnson MD
Director, Hemophilia and Thrombosis Center;
Professor of Pediatrics
University of Colorado Denver
Aurora, CO, USA

Mónica Martín-Salces MD
Consultant Hematologist
Hemostasis and Thrombosis Unit
La Paz University Hospital
Madrid, Spain

Carmen Martín-Hervás MD, PhD
Consultant Radiologist
Department of Musculo-Skeletal Radiology
La Paz University Hospital;
Associate Professor of Radiology
School of Medicine
Autonomous University
Madrid, Spain

Prasad Mathew MB, BS, DCH, FAAP
Professor of Pediatrics
Director, Ted R. Montoya Hemophilia Program
and Pediatric Hemostasis
University of New Mexico
Albuquerque, NM, USA

Alec Miners BSc (Hons), MSc, PhD
Lecturer in Health Economics
Faculty of Public Health and Policy
London School of Hygiene and Tropical Medicine
London, UK

Andrés Moret MS
Hemostasis and Thrombosis Unit
La Fe University Hospital
Valencia, Spain

Claude Negrier, MD, PhD
Professor
Hematology Division
Edouard Herriot University Hospital
Lyon, France

Johannes Oldenburg MD, PhD
Professor and Director
Institute of Experimental Hematology and
Transfusion Medicine
Haemophilia Center Bonn
University Clinic Bonn
Bonn, Germany

Anna Pavlova MD, PhD
Senior Lecturer
Institute of Experimental Hematology and
Transfusion Medicine
Haemophilia Center Bonn
University Clinic Bonn
Bonn, Germany

Pia Petrini MD
Associate Professor
Department of Pediatrics
Coagulation Unit
Karolinska University Hospital
Stockholm, Sweden

Felipe Querol MD, PhD, PT
Professor of Physiotherapy
Hemostasis and Thrombosis Unit
La Fe University Hospital
Valencia, Spain

Savita Rangarajan FRCP, FRCPath
Consultant Hematologist
Comprehensive Care Centre for Haemophilia
Haemostasis and Thrombosis
Basingstoke and North Hampshire NHS
Foundation Trust
Basingstoke, UK

Birgit M. Reipert PhD
Associate Professor
Director R&D
Department of Immunology
TA BioTherapeutics
Baxter Innovation GmbH
Vienna, Austria

Eduardo Remor PhD
Associate Professor
Department of Psychobiology and Health
Faculty of Psychology
Autonomous University
Madrid, Spain

**Emérito-Carlos
Rodríguez-Merchán** MD, PhD
Consultant Orthopedic Surgeon
Department of Orthopedic Surgery and
Hemophilia Unit
La Paz University Hospital;
Associate Professor of Orthopaedic Surgery
School of Medicine
Autonomous University
Madrid, Spain

Hans-Peter Schwarz MD, PhD
Professor
Vice President and Head TA BioTherapeutics
Baxter Innovation GmbH
Vienna, Austria

Mindy L. Simpson MD
Clinical Instructor of Pediatrics
Pediatric Hematology/Oncology
Rush University Medical Center
Chicago, IL, USA

Benny Sørensen MD, PhD
Director of HRU and Associate Professor
Aarhus University, Denmark;
Haemostasis Research Unit
Centre for Haemophilia and Thrombosis
Guy's and St Thomas' NHS Foundation Trust
London, UK

Katharina N. Steinitz Mag Rer Nat
Department of Immunology
TA BioTherapeutics
Baxter Innovation GmbH
Vienna, Austria

Jerome Teitel MD
Professor, University of Toronto
Division of Hematology and Oncology
St Michael's Hospital
Toronto, ON, Canada

H. Marijke van den Berg MD, PhD
Pediatric Hematologist
Meander Hospital, Amersfoort;
Department of Chemistry and Haematology
University Medical Center Utrecht
Utrecht, The Netherlands

Johanna G van der Bom MD, PhD
Associate Professor of Clinical Epidemiology
Department of Clinical Epidemiology and Jon J
van Rood Center for Clinical Transfusion Medicine
Leiden University Medical Center
Leiden, The Netherlands

Francisco Vidal PhD
Unitat de Diagnòstic i Teràpia Molecular
Banc de Sang i Teixits
Barcelona, Spain

Thynn Thynn Yee MD, FRCP
Consultant Hematologist
Katharine Dormandy Haemophilia Centre and
Thrombosis Unit
Royal Free Hospital
London, UK

Leonard A. Valentino MD
Professor of Pediatrics, Internal Medicine,
Immunology/Microbiology and Biochemistry
Director, Hemophilia and Thrombophilia Center
Rush University Medical Center
Chicago, IL, USA

Guy Young MD
Pediatric Hematology and Oncology
UCLA Health System
Los Angeles, CA, USA

Nichan Zourikian BSc, PT
Physiotherapist
Sainte-Justine Pediatric/Adult Comprehensive
Hemostasis Center and Quebec Reference Center
for Coagulation Inhibitors
Sainte-Justine University Hospital Center
Montreal, QC, Canada

Preface

Any text on hemophilia must acknowledge the roots of the disease. Hemophilia is an ancient bleeding disorder, first described in the 2nd century AD. Little attention was paid to this disease until the early 1900's when it was determined that Queen Victoria passed the gene down to several of her daughters, who carried the disease into several of the royal families of Europe. As such, the care of hemophilia has evolved from the time of Alexei, the son of Alexandra and Nicholas, Czar of Imperial Russia, to the current comprehensive model of care which has resulted in substantial decreases in morbidity and mortality and an improvement in the quality of life of patients with hemophilia. Many milestones mark the course of time for the disease but few so important as the discovery of cryoprecipitate in the 1960's which lead to development of advanced products to treat hemophilia including recombinant factor products essentially devoid of the risk of transmission of infectious diseases. These advancements laid the foundation for the development of treatment regimens designed to prevent bleeding and the complications of bleeding. Prophylaxis, initiated in young children, now has the potential to deliver patients into adolescence and adult life with normal joints, having nearly identical quality of life of their unaffected peers. This treatment comes at a price. The economic value of prophylaxis in hemophilia remains a matter of debate, especially in countries with limited resources available for healthcare. Adherence to prophylaxis and the transition to independence remains a major concern for providers of care. Management of patients at the ends of the age spectrum has attracted considerable attention. Key to optimal perinatal care and genetic counseling for carriers of hemophilia is an accurate molecular diagnosis and appropriate management of delivery to a healthy start to life of a boy with hemophilia.

This text attempts to address the current and future issues patients affected with the disease as well as the nurses, doctors and other care givers treating these patients must face in order to provide optimal care. In the first three chapters Cromwell and Aledort review the history of hemophilia, an appropriate starting place for any book such as this. Next Lee discusses the care of hemophilia in the modern world focusing on the worldwide improvements in diagnosis and care and the new problems of ageing with its associated co-morbidities. Finally the issues of inherited bleeding disorders in women are discussed. Mathew continues in this section to introduce the comprehensive care model but also draws attention to the necessities of funding in order to sustain the pinnacle of care that should be the goal of all nations and providers of hemophilia care in order to reduce morbidity and mortality and increase quality of life.

The next section delves into the day to day management issues that caregivers face with our patients. This begins with a discussion of prophylaxis in children by Manco-Johnson and moves to a review by Aznar and colleagues of the issues around changing from an on-demand regimen to prophylaxis. This is especially important in countries with limited resources. Miners deals with the economics of prophylaxis in the next chapter addressing the question, "Does prophylaxis with clotting factor represent value for money?" His conclusion, although not surprising, offers somewhat of a mandate to the bleeding disorders community and specifically to the manufacturers of clotting factor, to find ways to reduce the high cost of these life- and joint-saving biologicals. Jiménez-Yuste and colleagues address the difficult topic of prophylaxis for adult patients. Although many providers treating these patients feel there may be some benefit, the cost-effectiveness remains to be proven and represents a barrier to be overcome. As each of us has done (some better than others I suspect), we have transitioned from childhood to adulthood. This task is particularly problematic for patients with hemophilia as they face numerous obstacles, which, as Petrini discusses in the next chapter, "can have a significantly negative effect on morbidity and mortality in young adults." The utility and effectiveness of programs to specifically assist young people with hemophilia during this vulnerable time await evaluation and more importantly, validation. As a congenital disease, hemophilia begins in neonates, not all of which are symptomatic. However, sub-optimal care at this fragile time can result in a lifetime of challenges for the boy with hemophilia. Altisent and Vidal reviews the management of pregnant women who are carriers of hemophilia and appropriate molecular diagnosis. Finally, this section ends with a discussion by Rangarajan and Yee on managing the mature person with hemophilia. This population brings many new challenges to hemophilia clinics across the globe including insuring links between hemophilia care providers and those in the areas of geriatrics, oncology, cardiology and primary care in order to provide a comprehensive and coordinated approach to care.

The development of alloantibodies against factor VIII or factor IX which inhibit the function of infused clotting factor is the most common, serious complication that must be faced by this population. Inhibitor development is only recently beginning to be understood. Reipert and her colleagues, leading researchers in this area, provide the reader with a state of the art review of the immunology of inhibitor formation. Van der Bom, in the next chapter, discusses the epidemiology of inhibitor formation including the evidence behind a multitude of putative risk factors and explains a framework for interpretation of publications describing rates of inhibitor development including potential confounding variables. The novel approach of Auerswald and Kurnik to prevent, or at least reduce, the likelihood of inhibitor development is presented in the next chapter. This provocative (and as yet unproven) approach involves administration of small doses of clotting factor to patients in the absence of "danger signals" and will be not only a frequent topic for discussion at future meetings but will also be more importantly, the focus of several national and international clinical trials. Next, Van der Berg and Fischer present provocative data on their model to predict inhibitor formation in a specific patient. If validated, this model could change the management decisions and the treatment paradigms used, especially in very young children with severe hemophilia. As noted previously, inhibitor development is complex and Oldenburg and Pavlova discuss the genetic basis for inhibitor formation followed by a discussion of the non-genetic risk factors by Boggio and Simpson.

The next section focuses on the difficult area of management of patients with inhibitors to factor VIII or factor IX. Optimally, immune tolerance should be undertaken in an attempt to eradicate the inhibitor and return the patient to his prior non-inhibitor state allowing the use of factor VIII or IX as replacement therapy. Blatny and Mathew first discuss immune tolerance programs designed to achieve this goal focusing on the important questions including which regimen to use, when to initiate and abort immune tolerance therapy, which product to use and how to identify the ideal patient for immune tolerance as well as discussing the issues around venous access and the control of bleeding. This is followed by the review by Valentino and Young on the use of prophylaxis in inhibitor patients and then the presentation of treatment guidelines by Giangrande and Teitel. Despite what is considered optimal treatment of bleeding, as many as 20–30% of hemorrhages may not respond to bypassing therapy. Astermark discusses the discordancy observed in the treatment of bleeding

with bypassing agents and the factors which may play a role in these divergent responses. When bleeding is poorly controlled, such as that which occurs in patients with inhibitors, the joint is the main focus of morbidity. Valentino and Hakobyan discuss the experimental studies which shed light on the pathobiology of blood-induced joint disease. Berntorp then provides a review of the instruments available for the assessment of joint function and Martín-Hervás and Rodríguez-Merchán discuss imaging of the joints to better quantify not only the damage which occurs after bleeding but also to provide objective tools to assess the impact of new treatment modalities designed to reduced musculoskeletal morbidity including surgical interventions that are discussed by Rodríguez-Merchán and colleagues in the next chapter. Thrombosis is a major concern in patients undergoing orthopedic surgery and thromboprophyalxis in this population is reviewed by Dolan and colleagues next. Finally this section of inhibitor management concludes with a stimulating (and likely provocative) chapter on physiotherapy by Zourikian and Forsyth which focuses on the physiotherapy evaluation and intervention opportunities available during the acute bleeding episode.

The next section explores the new modalities that are on the horizon including a review of the new technologies in pre-clinical and clinical development for improvement in the pharmacokinetic profile of coagulation factors by Valentino and a discussion on gene therapy by Alvarez-Román and colleagues. The new developments in hemophilic arthropathy, including an assessment of the costs related to the occurrence of hemophilic arthropathy and management of arthropathy in elderly patients, are summarized by Rodríguez-Merchán and Valentino. In the next chapter, Sorensen and Negrier provide a rational for the use of an individualized "theranostic" approach utilizing global laboratory assays to tailor choices around the most suitable bypassing agent as well as to guide selection of effective dosages of bypassing agents. The last chapter in this section by Gringeri addresses the use of combination sequential therapy with bypassing agents, which have a synergistic effect *in vitro* and *in vivo*. Although this approach seems efficacious in children and in adults, care must be taken as adverse events are possible and this modality should be considered a salvage treatment due to its potential risks.

Finally, the management of the patient with hemophilia has as its goal the optimization of quality of life. Remor discusses the tools and instruments available to estimate quality of life and addresses the links of quality of life with health and well-being as well as the merits of the various disease-specific measures of quality of life.

Emérito-Carlos Rodriguez-Merchán
and Leonard A. Valentino

1 Introduction

1 History of Hemophilia

Caroline Cromwell and Louis M. Aledort

Mount Sinai School of Medicine, New York, NY, USA

Introduction

The word hemophilia is derived from the Greek words "*haima* – αἷμα: blood" and "*philia* – φιλος: love or tendency to". The history behind hemophilia is fascinating and complex. What is outlined here is a brief history of important events in development and discovery in this field.

History of hemophilia

Historical accounts are full of references to the disease. The first written description of hemophilia is found in the Babylonian Talmud, during the second century. In it is written "If she circumcised her first child and he died, and a second also died, she must not circumcise her third child" [1].What is fascinating is what is already understood and described from this decree. The familial nature was recognized. Rabbi Simon Ben Galaliel forbade a boy to be circumcised whose mother sisters' sons had died after circumcision. In the twelfth century the physician Moses Maimonides enforced this ruling for sons of women who had married twice, thus indicating a further understanding of the maternal inheritance of this disease [2,3].

In the United States in 1803, Otto described a family in which the males had prolonged bleeding after trauma. He noted that unaffected females pass on the disorder to a proportion of their sons, whom he described as "bleeders". In 1828 the disorder was coined "haemorrhaphilia", meaning, "love of hemorrhages" (Brinkhous *Handbook of Hemophilia*) which eventually evolved into the name hemophilia. During the nineteenth century there were continued publications describing this condition and varied family pedigrees were extensively documented.

The royal history of hemophilia is well known. Queen Victoria of England is one of the most well-known historical figures in hemophilia (Figure 1.1). She transmitted the disorder to her eighth son, Leopold, and two of her daughters were carriers. Leopold was known to have suffered from severe major bleeding episodes. He died at the age of 31 from a cerebral hemorrhage after trauma. Perhaps the most well-known descendant of Queen Victoria is Alexis, son of Tsar Nicholas II of Russia. Historically it is thought that Alexis's illness allowed for the undue influence of Rasputin. Rasputin was thought to have healing powers. Through Alexis he gained access and influence over the royal family, and this was thought to contribute in part to the eventual downfall of the empire. This fascinating history is well documented in R.K. Massie's 1968 book *Nicholas and Alexandra*.

The conclusions drawn by astute physicians and caring doctors during those early times were that (1) hemophilia caused excessive bleeding; (2) that predominantly males were affected; and (3) The disorder was passed down through females.

As one can imagine, many varied therapies were historically attempted in patients with hemophilia, from the administration of oxygen, injection of sodium citrate, to splenectomy to the use of egg white extract [4]. A more scientifically based approach was the use of coagulant snake venom by R.G. Macfarlane in the 1930s, with some success [5]. The first treatment of hemophilia occurred in 1840. Samuel Lang performed a blood transfusion to treat a hemophilia patient. It would be many years until the process of blood transfusion was developed. However by the early 1920s, it was understood that blood transfusions appeared to ameliorate bleeding by providing something that was missing in the hemophiliac patient's blood. In 1939, Kenneth Brinkhouse described something which he termed antihemophilic factor, now called factor VIII. His work was instrumental in the advancement of the understanding of hemophilia. In 1944, Edwin Cohn, a biochemist, developed a process known as fractionation, allowing

Current and Future Issues in Hemophilia Care, First Edition. Edited by Emérito-Carlos Rodríguez-Merchán and Leonard A. Valentino.

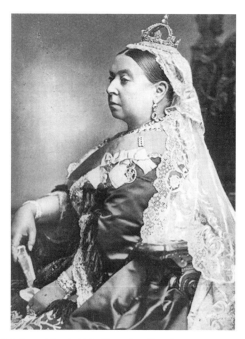

Figure 1.1 Queen Victoria 1887. (Reproduced from http://commons
.wikimedia.org/wiki/File:Queen_Victoria_1887.jpg. Accessed 4 March 2011.)

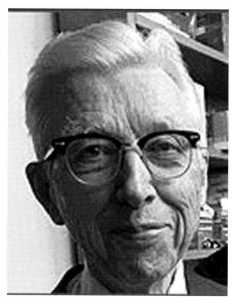

Figure 1.2 Kenneth Brinkhous. (Courtesy of UNC Chapel Hill.)

plasma to be separated into its different components. In 1952, Brinkhous developed the PTT test, which allowed for assessment of coagulation function. During this same time, it was discovered that there were two types of hemophilia. Previously it had been recognized that in certain cases the blood of two different hemophiliacs could be mixed, with correction of the clotting defect. Blood testing on Stephen Christmas, a child from Canada with hemophilia, revealed him to have a deficiency in factor IX as opposed to factor VIII. Factor IX deficiency became known as "Christmas" disease. Of great interest to note, recent investigation with novel DNA technologies have revealed the "royal disease" to be in fact, hemophilia B [6].

In 1964, Judith Graham developed cryoprecipitate. In the years that followed Kenneth Brinkhous (Figure 1.2) discovered how to purify factor VIII. Major changes in the treatment of hemophilia occurred during the 1970s. Large amounts of intermediate purity factor concentrates in lyophilized formulations became available. These concentrates were small volume, and easily injectable. This dramatically changed the face of treatment, as patients could receive treatment at home, either through self-administration or training of the caregiver. At the first sign of bleeding at home, these products could be administered, as opposed to wait for travel to a hospital. Hemophilia centers were able to focus on developing comprehensive care programs. These programs developed the concept of a team approach to care. The multi-faceted team was able to address all aspects of living with hemophilia, including the medical and psychosocial components. This was revolutionary at the time, and set the standard for the development of comprehensive care in other chronic illnesses. Orthopedic surgery became feasible in this patient population. Previously wheelchair-bound

patients could have reconstructive orthopedic surgery. Great steps were made towards allowing a hemophiliac to live a fully functional life, to work, to go to school and to live.

Ongoing discovery continued in the field of hemophilia treatment. In 1977, desmopressin was discovered, which became a mainstay of treatment for patients with mild hemophilia A and von Willebrand disease, although it was not licensed for this indication until the late 1980s in the United States. In the late 1970s, production of Factor VIII by pharmaceutical companies began on a large scale. Unfortunately transmission of hepatitis B and C was a devastating consequence for many patients treated with factor concentrates produced from pooled plasma. This heralded the era of HIV transmission. AIDS was first described in two patients with hemophilia in 1982. From the late 1970s to the mid-1980s, approximately half of the hemophilia population contracted HIV through blood products. In the ensuing years, heat treating which destroyed the HIV virus, became standard for production. It would still be many years until highly active retroviral therapy would be developed. Thousands of persons with hemophilia died of AIDS in the 1980s and 1990s. Further progress continued in the development of ways to inactivate blood-borne pathogens, such as implementation of the use of solvent detergent. These improvements in viral inactivation and viral screening have dramatically improved the safety of plasma derived products. There has been no transmission of HIV or hepatitis from plasma concentrates since 1987. Transmission of prions and subsequent variant Creutzfeldt–Jakob disease has been a concern since the discovery it could occur due to blood transfusion. However there has not been a case of transmission via plasma-derived products.

In 1984, the gene for factor VIII was located and cloned from human cells. This allowed for the development and production of recombinant factor VIII and eventually factor IX as well. Recombinant factor VIII was licensed by the US Food and Drug

Administration (FDA) in 1992. Since that time the use of recombinant factor has become the mainstay in North America and Western Europe. However in the last few years new data have challenged the trend towards use of recombinant factors. Two studies of previously untreated patients with hemophilia A suggest that the incidence of inhibitors is higher with recombinant factor VII than with plasma derived products. It is postulated that this may be due to the presence of other proteins in plasma derived products, such as von Willebrand factor. Further study is ongoing to address this important issue.

The development of inhibitors in the patient with hemophilia is a much dreaded, devastating consequence. Two bypassing agents are available for this patient population, one recombinant. Activated prothrombin complex concentrates (aPCC) have been used since the 1980s. The risk of thrombosis in association with their use is well-documented. The FDA licensed recombinant human coagulation factor VIIa (rFVIIa) on 25 March 1999, for bleeding in patients with hemophilia A or B and inhibitors to factors VIII or IX. In addition to great strides in treating bleeding patients with inhibitors, major research has occurred in the area of inhibitor eradication through immune tolerance induction. Two large international registries have documented that immune tolerance induction with large and frequent doses of factor VIII was effective in approximately 70% of patients [7,8]. More study regarding dosing and timing of factor VIII infusions are ongoing. However neither of these issues addresses the prevention of inhibitors through the maintenance of tolerance, which is the ultimate goal.

Primary prophylaxis is an ongoing area of research. Studies have demonstrated that while this method may be expensive, it is more efficacious than on demand treatment [9]. Various options currently exist for the dose and dose interval. While primary prophylaxis may be an option in wealthier countries, in many areas of the world it is financially impossible.

Conclusions

To have to now address the issues of the aging hemophiliac demonstrates the advances that have been made in the treatment of this disease [10]. The field of biologics is constantly evolving, and the goal is to continue to produce more effective and less immunogenic therapies. Strides must be made to address the need of the underserved international patient and access to care. The ultimate goal in coming years will be the cure of hemophilia through gene therapy. Promising studies in animal models continue to fuel scientific drive to apply such technology in patients. Through continued international collaboration in clinical research, through the drive and passion of physicians and patients, we hope these goals will be reached.

References

1. Katzenelson JL. Hemophilia; with special reference to the Talmud. Harofe Haivri Heb Med J. 1958;1:165–78.
2. Seligsohn U. Hemophilia and other clotting disorders. Isr J Med Sci. 1973 Sep–Oct;9(9):1338–40.
3. Kavakli K, Aledort LM. Circumcision and haemophilia: a perspective. Haemophilia. 1998 Jan;4(1):1–3.
4. Ingram GI. The history of haemophilia. J Clin Pathol. 1976 Jun;29(6):469–79.
5. Macfarlane RG. Russell's viper venom,1934–64. Br J Haematol. 1967 Jul;13(4):437–51.
6. Rogaev EI, Grigorenko AP, Faskhutdinova G, Kittler EL, Moliaka YK. Genotype analysis identifies the cause of the "royal disease". Science. 2009 Nov 6;326(5954):817.
7. Mariani G, Ghirardini A, Bellocco R. Immune tolerance in hemophilia-principal results from the International Registry. Report of the factor VIII and IX Subcommittee. Thromb Haemost. 1994 Jul;72(1):155–8.
8. DiMichele DM, Kroner BL. The North American Immune Tolerance Registry: practices, outcomes, outcome predictors. Thromb Haemost. 2002 Jan;87(1):52–7.
9. Manco-Johnson MJ, Abshire TC, Shapiro AD, Riske B, Hacker MR, Kilcoyne R, et al. Prophylaxis versus episodic treatment to prevent joint disease in boys with severe hemophilia. N Engl J Med. 2007 Aug 9;357(6):535–44.
10. Konkle BA, Kessler C, Aledort L, Andersen J, Fogarty P, Kouides P, et al. Emerging clinical concerns in the ageing haemophilia patient. Haemophilia. 2009 Nov;15(6):1197–209.

2 Hemophilia Care in the Modern World

Christine A. Lee

University of London, London, UK

Introduction

Hemophilia care in the modern world is described in the vision of the World Federation of Hemophilia (WFH) [1]. Their mission is to improve and sustain care to include all people with inherited bleeding disorders (IBDs). As they point out, this means those in the developing as well as the developed world, the young as well as the old, and both women and men.

Hemophilia care in the modern world has to embrace these challenges – the improved diagnosis and care around the world have introduced the new problems of an aging population with IBDs and co-morbidities; the benefit of primary prophylaxis is incontrovertible, but it needs to be tailored to the needs of young boys worldwide; the management of hemophilia requires the production of factor concentrates with prolonged efficacy and reduced immunogenicity; and the significance of IBDs in women has been increasingly recognized in the last two decades and these women now need to be identified and guided to clinical care.

Providing global care

The 2008 WFH Global Survey shows individuals from 72 countries worldwide with hemophilia, von Willebrand disease (VWD), rare factor deficiencies and inherited platelet disorders (Table 2.1). National hemophilia databases, including data on prevalence, treatment and outcome are essential for the care of hemophilia in the modern world. Such databases have been established in many countries including the UK, Italy, Germany, France, Spain, Australia, Canada, and the USA [2]. Advances in information technology open up many new possibilities [3].

Databases support three basic functions – healthcare planning, epidemiologic research, and pharmacovigilance. In developing countries where the clinical service provision for hemophilia is poorly developed, basic prevalence data may be useful for planning purposes. This is well-illustrated by the change over time of the relationship of economic capacity to the number of adults with hemophilia (Figure 2.1). Improving care can result in more children surviving into adulthood [1].

There are increasing attempts to harmonize databases – hemophilia is a rare disorder and effective research depends on international co-operation. This is well-illustrated by EUHASS: European Adverse Event System. Adverse events are now rare and hemophilia is a rare disease so any reporting system needs to be multinational for the frequencies of adverse events to be meaningful. EUHASS is a collaboration of 56 sentinel centers in 27

Table 2.1 Male and female patients by disorder from the 2008 World Federation of Hemophilia Global Survey. (Reproduced from Skinner MW. Building our global family – achieving treatment for all. Haemophilia 2010;16(suppl. 5):1–11.)

Disorder	Total	Male	Female
Hemophilia A	79 820	77 859	1817
Hemophilia B	16 976	16 318	651
Hemophilia type unknown	662	636	10
von Willebrand's disease	44 731	16 235	23 207
Factor I deficiency	806	319	396
Factor II deficiency	183	61	53
Factor V deficiency	817	348	363
Factor V + VIII deficiency	303	128	82
Factor VII deficiency	3608	1563	1630
Factor X deficiency	891	385	368
Factor XI deficiency	3484	1382	1690
Factor XIII deficiency	635	323	254
Bleeding disorders: type unknown	666	180	165
Platelet disorders: Glanzmann's thrombasthenia	977	294	310
Platelet disorders: Bernard Soulier syndrome	206	84	92
Platelet disorders: Other or unknown	3577	1211	1944

Current and Future Issues in Hemophilia Care, First Edition. Edited by Emérito-Carlos Rodríguez-Merchán and Leonard A. Valentino.

© 2011 John Wiley & Sons, Ltd. Published 2011 by Blackwell Publishing Ltd.

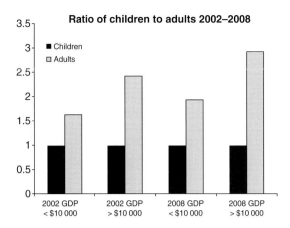

Figure 2.1 Change over time of relationship of economic capacity to number of adults with hemophilia. (Reproduced from Skinner MW. Building our global family – achieving treatment for all. Haemophilia 2010;16(suppl. 5): 1–10.)

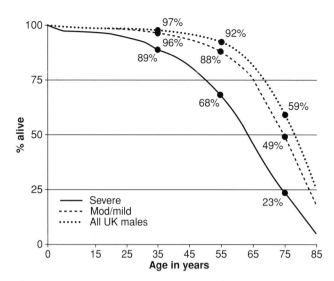

Figure 2.2 Survival in men in the UK who were not infected with HIV. (Reproduced from Darby SC, Kan SW, Spooner RJ et al. Mortality rates, life expectancy, and causes of death in people with haemophilia A or B in the United Kingdom who were not infected with HIV. Blood 2007;110:815–25.)

European countries. It collects anonymized data on new inhibitors (antibodies to FVIII or IX), allergic reactions, infections, thromboses, cancers and deaths. The system was developed in parallel with the European Principles of Hemophilia Care and aims to raise awareness of adverse events, collect data and improve safety [4].

An aging hemophilic population

In 1937 Carroll Birch reported the natural history of hemophilia without treatment – in a cohort of 113 patients 82 died before 15 years of age and only eight survived beyond the age of 40 years [5]. This contrasts with a study published in 2007 from the UK in people with hemophilia uninfected with HIV – a median life expectancy of 63 years for those with severe hemophilia and 75 years for those with non-severe hemophilia was found [6]. This approaches that for the normal male population (Figure 2.2). People with hemophilia worldwide have benefited from both the general factors contributing towards health improvement as well as those due to the advances in hemophilia care including the availability of safe, effective concentrate, comprehensive care programs, home treatment and prophylaxis. In the general population, up to 88% over the age of 65 years have one or more chronic medical condition. [7] Thus, particularly in the developed world, the elderly population of people with hemophilia will present the complex

co-morbidity of a tendency to bleed and the age-related problems of cardiovascular disease, neoplasia, renal and musculoskeletal problems. Studies are needed to explore these emerging health issues as there are currently few evidence based data of acute and chronic medical problems in older patients with hemophilia [8].

Prophylaxis

The pioneering work in prophylaxis was in the 1950s and 1960s in Sweden and the Netherlands. This has provided over two decades of follow-up data [9,10]. The two regimens differed in the age at start of treatment and the intensity of treatment. The Swedish regimen was associated with a significantly lower rate of joint bleeding but the FVIII consumption was two-fold higher. After nearly 20 years of follow-up the extent of hemophilic arthropathy measured by the radiologic scale was similar for the two regimens (Table 2.2).

The beneficial role of primary prophylaxis in young boys with hemophilia is now proven without doubt. It is unfortunate that the Cochrane Collaboration review in 2006 challenged the

	Dutch regimen ("intermediate-dose")	Swedish regimen ("high-dose")	*P*-value
Number of cases	42	18	<0.001
Age at start of prophylaxis (years)	4.6 (3.1–6.2)	1.2 (0.8–1.7)	<0.001
Number of joint bleeds per year	3.7 (1.7–5)	0.2 (0–0.3)	<0.001
Pettersson score	0 (0–5)	0	<0.001
Annual clotting factor use (IU kg^{-1} year^{-1})	2126 (1743–2755)	4616 (4105–5571)	<0.001

Table 2.2 Comparison of an intermediate dose to a high dose regimen: long-term follow-up results. (Reproduced from Fischer K, Astermark J, van der Bom JG et al. Prophylaxis treatment for severe haemophilia: comparison of an intermediate-dose to a high-dose regimen. Haemophilia 2002;8;753–60.)

Values are medians; values in parentheses are interquartile ranges [21].

evidence from the carefully conducted cohort studies [11]. In the USA definitive evidence was required from a randomized controlled trial that exposed young boys to the risk of life-threatening hemorrhage and unnecessary MRI scans [12].

There remain many questions for future research effort – how and when to initiate prophylaxis; the role of prophylaxis in the young adult; and the role of prophylaxis in other inherited bleeding disorders, particularly von Willebrand disease. Worldwide the greatest barrier to the implementation of prophylaxis is the high cost. It is therefore important that treatment is individualized to maintain the required protective plasma factor level [13].

Inhibitors

The effectiveness of modern hemophilia treatment is challenged by the development of inhibitory antibodies and this remains the greatest therapeutic challenge. A systematic review commissioned by the British Department of Health and conducted by the School of Health and Related Research, the University of Sheffield in 2003, showed a great variability of inhibitor prevalence and the prevalence of inhibitor development ranged from 10% to 44% (Table 2.3). It was recognized that that a lower incidence was found following treatment with a single plasma derived (pd) product than with multiple pdFVIII preparations or single recombinant preparations [14]. Concentrate immunogenicity is complicated for a number of reasons – the method of inhibitor testing, the varied study populations, the different risk factors such as ethnicity, type of gene mutation and age at first treatment. There is continued debate about the role of von Willebrand factor as an immunomodulator [15].

To answer the question on different immunogenicity an independent, international, multicenter, prospective, controlled, ran-domized, open-label clinical trial is being carried out on inhibitor frequency in previously untreated patients (PUPs) or minimally blood component-treated (MBCTPs) when exposed to plasma-derived, von Willebrand factor-containing factor VIII (VWF/FVIII) concentrates or to rFVIII concentrates. This is the SIPPET study [16,17]. The truly global nature of hemophilia research is reflected in this study – there will be 80 centers from 24 countries on four continents. Thus a quarter of a century following the quest for recombinant products to overcome the problem of the viral epidemics of HIV and hepatitis there could be a return to pd FVIII to overcome inhibitor development.

Future therapeutic strategies

The adoption of prophylaxis as the "gold standard" brings with it the challenges of the need for frequent intravenous injections in small boys and the difficulties of venous access. For these reasons there has been focus on the production of bioengineered clotting factors with a prolonged half-life [18].

Even though the ultimate "cure" of hemophilia through gene therapy remains elusive, considerable progress has been made [17]. Promising results have been obtained with adeno-associated viral (AAV) vector delivery to the liver for FIX, FVIII and FVIIa genes in animal models. The short half-life of FVIIa has been overcome by gene transfer with AAV vector via the portal vein in the hemophilic dog. This would provide improved treatment for inhibitor patients. Furthermore, for non-inhibitor patients it could provide an attractive alternative to hemostatic therapy thus preventing immunologic challenge with FVIII and possible inhibitor development [19].

Women with bleeding disorders

Although hemophilia affects men other inherited bleeding disorders including VWD, rare bleeding disorders and inherited platelet disorders affect women (Table 2.1). In developed countries the number of women reported with inherited bleeding disorders is growing rapidly – from 1991–2007 the number of female patients treated in US hemophilia treatment centers increased from 2365 to 9041 (Figure 2.3).

Bleeding disorders have a considerable impact on the health of women and their quality of life [20]. VWD is the most common inherited bleeding disorder worldwide with a prevalence of 1.3% [21]. Women experience early hemostatic challenge with menstruation and a systematic review of women with menorrhagia has shown a prevalence of VWD of 13% [22]. Outreach programs including Women Bleed Too in the UK, Project Red Flag in the US and the women's program of the Canadian Hemophilia Society have been established to both create awareness and to improve the quality of life and care for these women [23–25].

In many parts of the world, where first cousin marriage is common, the recessive rare bleeding disorders are a common cause of

Table 2.3 Prevalence of inhibitors in patients with severe hemophilia. (Reproduced from Wight J and Paisley S. The epidemiology of inhibitors in haemophilia A: a systematic review. Haemophilia 2003;9:418–35.)

Author, Date	Threshold FFVIII: C level for "severe"	Prevalence
Strauss 1969	0.5%	21% (16/77)
Rasi 1990	1%	17.3% (19/110)
Sultan 1992	1%	12.8% (198/1565)
Aronis 1995	1%	40% (19/49)
Izquierdo-Ramirez 1988	1%	44% (12/27)
Ghosh 2001	1%	hph8.2% (24/292)
Ikkala 1971	2%	16% (11/69)
Yee 1999	2%	10% (24/239)
Ören 1999	2%	41% (7/17)
Rizza 2001	2%	12.7% (196/1546)
Schwarzinger 1987	5%	17.5% (10/57)

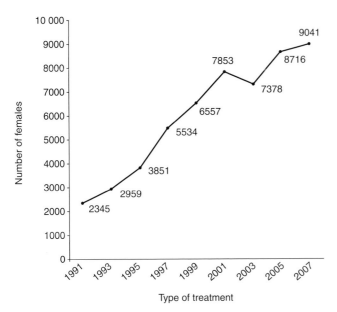

Figure 2.3 Females treated for bleeding disorders at federally funded treatment centers in the United States, 1991–2007. (Reproduced from Skinner MW. Building our global family – achieving treatment for all. Haemophilia 2010;16(suppl.5): 1–11.)

menorrhagia and bleeding in pregnancy. The WFH has realized the importance of this issue in the world and are encouraging innovative strategies and tools to reach these vulnerable populations where for the majority of women an inherited bleeding disorder remains a hidden condition to be suffered silently [1].

Conclusions

Within three-quarters of a century, the life expectancy for people with hemophilia has increased from less than 20 years to near 70 years in the developed parts of the world. Much of this achievement has been due to advances in clinical practice resulting from research in basic science. The challenge is to make these achievements possible in the developing world. Information technology allows for the development of databases, the most fundamental tool, after accurate diagnosis, for hemophilia care. The internet allows for the integration of such databases and as a resource to spread best practice. Worldwide, people with hemophilia can look forward to a bright future.

References

1. Skinner MW. Building our global family – achieving treatment for all. Haemophilia 2010;16(suppl. 5),110.
2. Hay CRM. National hemophilia databases. Textbook of Hemophilia, 2nd edition. Edited by Lee C, Berntorp E and Hoots K, 2010, Oxford: Blackwell Publishing.
3. Baker RI, Laurenson L, Winter M, et al. The impact of information technology on haemophilia care. Haemophilia 2004;10(Suppl. 4): 41–6.
4. EUHASS, European Haemophilia Safety Surveillance System http://www.ehass.org
5. Birch C, La F. Haemophilia, clinical and genetic aspects. Urbana: University of Illinois, 1937.
6. Darby SC, Kan SW, Spooner RJ, et al. Mortality rates, life expectancy, and causes of death in people with haemophilia A or B in the United Kingdom who were not infected with HIV Blood 2007;110: 815–25.
7. Hoffman C, Rice D, Sung HY. Persons with chronic conditions, their prevalence and costs. JAMA 1995;276:1473–9.
8. Dolan G. The challenge of an ageing haemophilic population. Haemophilia 2010;16(Suppl. 5),11–16.
9. Lofquist T, Nilsson IM, Berntorp, et al. Haemophilia prophylaxis in young patients – a long-term follow-up. J Int Med 1997;241: 395–400.
10. Fischer K, Astermark J, van der Bom JG, et al. Prophylaxis treatment for severe haemophilia: comparison of an intermediate-dose to a high-dose regimen. Haemophilia 2002;8;753–60.
11. Stobart K, Iorio A, Wu JK. Clotting factor concentrates given to prevent bleeding and bleeding-related complications in people with haemophilia A or B. Cochrane Database Syst Rev 2006;2:1–26.
12. Manco-Johnson MJ, Abshire TC, Shapiro AD, et al. Prophylaxis versus episodic treatment to prevent joint disease in boys with hemophilia. N Engl J Med 2007;357:535–44.
13. Blanchette VS. Prophylaxis in the haemophilia population. Haemophilia 2010;16(Suppl. 5),181–8.
14. Wight J, Paisley S. The epidemiology of inhibitors in haemophilia A: a systematic review. Haemophilia 2003;9:418–35.
15. Auerswald G, Spranger T, Brackmann HH. The role of plasma-derived factor VIII/von Willebrand factor concentrates in the treatment of hemophilia A patients. Haematologica 2003;88:EREP05.
16. SIPPET study http://www.clinicaltrials.gov, Study NCT 01064284; EUDRACT n. 2009-011186-88.
17. Batorova A, High K, Gringeri A. Special lectures in haemophilia management. Haemophilia 2010;16:(Suppl. 5),22–8.
18. Saenko EL, Pipe SW. Strategies towards a longer acting factor VIII. Haemophilia 2006;12:42–51.
19. Margaritis P, Roy E, Aljamali MN, et al. Successful treatment of canine haemophilia by continuous expression of canine FVIIa. Blood 2009;113;3682–9.
20. Shankar M, Chi C, Kadir RA. Review of quality of life: menorrhagia in women with or without inherited bleeding disorders. Haemophilia 2008;14:15–20.
21. Rodeghiero F, Castaman G, Dini E. Epidemiological investigation of the prevalence of von Willebrand's disease. Blood 1987;69:454–9.
22. Shankar M, Lee CA, Sabin CA, et al. von Willebrand disease in women with menorrhagia: a systematic review. BJOG 2004;111:734–40.
23. Kadir RA, Nazzaro AM, Winikoff R, et al. Advocacy for women with bleeding disorders. Chapter 13 In: Inherited Bleeding Disorders in Women. Edited by Lee CA, Kadir RA and Kouides P, 2009 Oxford: Wiley-Blackwell.
24. www.womenbleedtoo.org.uk
25. www.projectredflag.org

3 Comprehensive Care Model in Hemophilia

Prasad Mathew

University of New Mexico, Albuquerque, NM, USA

Introduction

Comprehensive care in hemophilia requires a multidisciplinary team approach provided through hemophilia treatment centers (HTC) involving the management of the patient and his family through continuous supervision of the medical and psychosocial aspects of the disease. This type of care addresses the physical, emotional, educational, financial and vocational needs of the patient, while keeping the patient and his family abreast of the latest developments in the field of hemophilia [1]. Hemophilia *cannot* be optimally managed in a general hematology department due to its complexity. This reality is recognized by the World Health Organization (WHO), the World Federation of Hemophilia (WFH), and all developed countries. In 1973, the National Hemophilia Foundation (NHF) in the United States launched a two-year campaign to establish a nationwide network of hemophilia diagnostic and treatment centers. The idea was based upon providing a range of services (diagnostic and therapeutic) for patients with hemophilia under one roof. Subsequently, in 1975, the US Congress legislated, through Section 1131 of the Public Health Service Act, the establishment and funding for a network of 22 hemophilia diagnostic and treatment centers [2]. Today there are about 141 federally funded treatment centers and programs across the country [3].

Comprehensive care philosophy

The mainstay and backbone of optimal hemophilia care is a comprehensive care approach. The goal of comprehensive care is to address acute management of bleeding episodes, long-term management of arthropathy and other significant complications, and to provide psychosocial support and education needed to manage this disorder [4]. It thus involves a core team consisting of a hematologist, nurse, social worker, physical therapist, an orthopedic surgeon, and laboratory staff, among others. With the advent of highly active anti-retroviral therapy for human immunodeficiency virus (HIV) infection and newer agents for treatment of hepatitis C virus (HCV) infection, infectious disease specialists and hepatologists now are often part of the treatment team. Risk reduction counseling, ongoing education of patients regarding their bleeding disorder management, and empowering them in being advocates for their care, are key activities of comprehensive care [4,5]. Management of adults, many of whom need treatment for HIV and/or HCV infections, arthropathy, and counseling for issues related to aging (falls, prostatic hypertrophy, cardiovascular disease, cancer risk, etc.) are also handled by the HTC staff [6,7]. The WFH defines the functions of a comprehensive care program as one that performs diagnostic tests necessary for the definitive diagnosis of hemophilia and other inherited bleeding disorders, manages bleeding episodes with appropriate treatment products and first aid, and educates patients and families regarding safety precautions for the prevention and early identification of bleeding episodes. Furthermore, in this model, there is development and frequent reviews of an individualized management plan for each individual patient, monitoring and management of complications resulting from hemophilia and its treatment, as well as promoting regular physical exercise to maintain muscle and joint health while providing rehabilitative services for restoring function following bleeding episodes. In addition, it provides genetic counseling and genetic diagnostic services for patients and family members, educates, advises, and counsels patients, family members, health care workers, educators, and employers to ensure that the patients' needs are met. It also conducts research to further knowledge and improve the management of bleeding disorders, often in collaboration with National and International hemophilia research centers [8].

Current and Future Issues in Hemophilia Care, First Edition. Edited by Emérito-Carlos Rodríguez-Merchán and Leonard A. Valentino.
© 2011 John Wiley & Sons, Ltd. Published 2011 by Blackwell Publishing Ltd.

Does the model work?

Comprehensive care results in significant improvement in the health of persons with hemophilia, with increased efficiency in delivering this care, while reducing the morbidity and mortality associated with this condition, and reducing use of healthcare resources [9,10]. In one of the earlier studies performed after the establishment of the initial 22 centers in the US, a five-year outcomes study showed that patients receiving care in a comprehensive care center experienced a decrease in the average number of days lost from work or school from 14.5 per year to 4.3 per year, and a decrease in the unemployment rate from 36% to 13%. This was accompanied by a decrease in the costs of care from about $15,800 per patient per year to $5932 per patient per year [11]. Today, the federally supported comprehensive HTCs are organized into 12 regions. Patients cared for in a comprehensive treatment center experience decreased morbidity and mortality, as well as a lower rate of unemployment, and reduced length of hospital stay and costs [12,13]. A Centers for Disease Control and Prevention (CDC) study of approximately 3000 people with hemophilia A and B, showed that those patients who visited an HTC were 30% less likely to die of hemophilia-related complications compared with those who did not receive care at an HTC, and were about 40% less likely to be hospitalized for bleeding complications [12,13].

As part of a comprehensive care set-up, HTCs in the US provide diagnostic services, treatment according to established treatment protocols, and follow recommendations provided through the Medical and Scientific Advisory committee (MASAC) of the National Hemophilia Foundation. In addition, they offer psychosocial and educational services, offer genetic counseling, refer patients for surgery as needed, consult for blood-borne disease prevention and treatment, and administer research and clinical trials to affected patients and their families [5]. Experience has shown that, through this approach, coalitions of patients, healthcare providers and governments can be built to achieve sustainable care. Clearly, with proper treatment, people with bleeding disorders can live nearly perfectly healthy lives, and history stands behind us to show that with research and constant striving to better the lives of people with bleeding disorders, one can achieve the vision that WFH has for the global bleeding disorder community, viz. the vision of "Treatment for All"; i.e. treatment will be available for all those with inherited bleeding disorders, regardless of where they live [14,15].

Improvements in care using HTCs

Epidemiological data show the benefits of improved hemophilia care through the years [16,17]. Hemophilia has moved from the status of a neglected and often fatal hereditary disorder to that of a defined group of disorders with a molecular basis for which safe and effective treatment is available. There are improved ad-

ministration techniques and dosing regimens, a shift from on-demand treatment to prophylaxis, successful treatment protocols for immune tolerance induction in patients with inhibitors and enhanced approaches to overall patient management [16,18,19]. Improvements also include the introduction of virus inactivation methods for plasma derived clotting factor concentrates and the development of recombinant factor VIII therapy, which has essentially eliminated the risk of infectious disease transmission. Recombinant factor concentrates are recommended as the treatment of choice by several national guidelines today. All these developments have resulted in increased health-related quality of life and life expectancy for hemophilia patients who are transitioning from childhood to adulthood with healthy joints and an overall excellent health status. As a result, the ageing hemophilia population will be afflicted with age-related musculoskeletal disease, cardiovascular disease and cancer, among other "usual" disorders men experience as they age that were not previously observed in this population [20]. With respect to this, the spectrum of hemophilia care will need to be extended to diseases of older ages with the need of including further disciplines in comprehensive hemophilia care programs, such as cardiology, nephrology, oncology, etc. [20,21]. Despite these advances, the short half-life of factor VIII, requiring re-administration every 2 or 3 days and the development of inhibitors remains a challenge [22,23].

Cutting edge care and research at an HTC

The strengths of the comprehensive treatment center model, and the benefits of being cared for in a comprehensive HTC, have clearly resulted in the historic decrease in the morbidity and mortality from bleeding disorders. These centers also have provided the framework for rapid dissemination of clinical and translational research advances into practice in the community. Participation in clinical trials provides patients access to promising state of the art investigational therapies, all carefully designed with the input from skilled experts and specialists in multiple disciplines, and critically reviewed before activation. Trials are conducted within the context of a rigorous framework of ongoing review, reporting and safety monitoring. Pooling of data and interim analyses provides for timely evaluation of outcomes and safety and promotes a rapid evolution in care [24].

Another benefit of receiving care as part of a comprehensive treatment center is that providers are part of a collective membership of providers of rare bleeding disorders – where expertise is shared and difficult diagnostic challenges are discussed among peers who know each other. This "membership" signifies meeting and maintaining certain standards of care deemed necessary to provide comprehensive multidisciplinary care [24]. The comprehensive centers in the US are also members of national organizations like the National Hemophilia foundation (NHF), the Hemophilia Federation of America, among others. The scientific arm of NHF, MASAC, provides guidelines and recommendations for standards of care on a variety of topics that involve care of patients with bleeding disorders. MASAC members meet on an annual basis and update recommendations and suggest new ones.

The burden in the US

The HTCs are a great example of the health care delivery system called for in the 2001 Institute of Medicine report to improve the quality of US health care [25]. However, numerous challenges exist, including inadequate reimbursement (the US health care reimbursement is on the basis of acute, not chronic care and third party payers do not routinely reimburse chronic care coordination), managed care (these plans often limit access to HTCs, and modify HTC treatment recommendations), static and/or decreasing federal grant funding, lack of specialists choosing a career in benign hematology, and reduced numbers of coagulation laboratories at US hospitals (many laboratories lack the expertise and experience to accurately process and interpret hemophilia diagnostic tests) [3]. Another challenge facing researchers and scientists in the US is lack of access to uniform data. The CDC had established the Universal Data Collection (UDC) system to address some of these issues, but this system will soon be closed in 2011. Efforts are under way to collect such data through the American Thrombosis and Hemostasis network (ATHN), which would provide a framework for a national data collection of information on patients with bleeding disorders.

340B – unique US-based program

The US Congress enacted section 340B to establish price controls to effectively limit the cost of drugs to certain Federal grantees (covered entities, including the HTCs). The Health Resources and Services Administration (HRSA) implemented this statutory mandate by establishing the 340B program, a unique program where HTCs are allowed to "sell" factor to generate revenue to supplement funds for the care provided through the comprehensive model. Funding for hemophilia care in the US is dwindling, which would greatly impact not only on the quality care provided but also on the availability of care through the HTCs. This government supported program is one way the HTCs are mitigating the economic burden of caring for these patients.

The background for this program is as follows: in 1990, Congress created the Medicaid rebate program in an effort to reduce the cost of expensive drugs available to state Medicaid agencies. The Medicaid rebate program requires drug companies to enter into a rebate agreement with the Secretary of the Department of Health and Human Services (HHS) as a precondition for coverage of their drugs by Medicaid. The rebate agreement specifies that, for each brand name outpatient drug covered under the Medicaid plan, the manufacturer of the drug must pay a rebate to Medicaid based on the manufacturer's "best price" for that drug. As a result of the Medicaid rebate law, many pharmaceutical companies had a disincentive to continue giving deep discounts on

drugs because they would have to pay larger rebates to Medicaid if they gave deeper discounts in the non-Medicaid market (establishing even better "best prices"). When manufacturers began raising their prices, the Medicaid savings achieved through the rebate program were offset by increased government spending on drugs purchased by other federal- and state-supported providers. To correct this situation, Congress, in November 1992, enacted Section 340B of the Public Health Service Act (created under Section 602 of the Veterans Health Care Act of 1992), which required pharmaceutical manufacturers participating in the Medicaid program to enter into a second agreement – called a pharmaceutical pricing agreement (PPA) – with the Secretary under which the manufacturer agreed to provide front-end discounts on covered outpatient drugs purchased by specified government-supported facilities, called "covered entities", that serve the nation's most vulnerable patient populations [26]. The benefits of these financial programs to the HTCs is continuous revenue to help fund the care of the nation's most vulnerable patients.

Conclusions

Comprehensive care for the bleeding disorder community in the US is provided through federal and state supported HTCs. Care provided through HTCs have improved the outcomes of these patients, decreasing morbidity and mortality and enhanced quality of life. Many of these patients now have life expectancy similar to the non-hemophilia population, which makes them now vulnerable to age-related co-morbidities that affect the general population. Funding challenges exist for the HTCs, and despite improved outcomes for these patients, the grim reality is that there are fewer physicians choosing to become coagulation specialists interested in the care of these patients creating an even greater demand.

References

1. Evatt BL. The natural evolution of hemophilia care: developing and sustaining comprehensive care globally. Haemophilia 2006;12(suppl 3):13–21.
2. PL 9463: The Public Health Service Act establishing the hemophilia diagnostic and treatment center program. No. 1131 of Public Law 9463. Washington, DC: Government Printing Office, 1975.
3. Baker JR, Crudder SO, Riske B, Bias V, Forsberg A. A model for a regional system of care to promote the health and well-being of people with rare chronic genetic disorders. Am J Public Health 2005;95:1910–16.
4. Bolton-Maggs PHB. Optimal hemophilia care versus the reality. Br J Haematol 2005;132:671–82.
5. Hoots WK. Comprehensive care for hemophilia and related disorders: why it matters. Curr Hematol Rep 2003;2:395–401.
6. Street A, Hill K, Sussex B, Warner M, Scully MF. Haemophilia and ageing. Haemophilia 2006;12:8–12.
7. Stephens S. Getting older: an intimate portrait of life after 50 for men with hemophilia. Hemaware 2006;11(6):35–41.

8. World Federation of Hemophilia: Benefits of comprehensive care for the treatment of bleeding disorders. http://www.wfh.org/2/docs/Publications/Diagnosis_and_Treatment/Guidelines_Mng_Hemophilia.pdf. Accessed October 20, 2010.

9. Mannucci PM. Modern treatment of hemophilia: from the shadows towards the light. Thromb Haemost 1993;70:17–23.

10. Mannucci PM, Tuddenham EG. The hemophilias – from royal genes to gene therapy. N Engl J Med 2001;344:1773–9.

11. Smith PS, Levine PH. The benefits of comprehensive care of hemophilia: a five year study of outcomes. Am J Public Health 1984;74:616–17.

12. Soucie JM, Nuss R, Evatt, B, Abdelhak A, Cowan L, Hill H, Kolakoski M, Wilber N, and the Hemophilia Surveillance System Project Investigators. Mortality among males with hemophilia: relations with source of medical care. Blood 2000;96:437–42.

13. Soucie JM, Symons J, Evatt B, Brettler D, Huszti H, Linden J, and the Hemophilia Surveillance System Project Investigators: Home-based factor infusion therapy and hospitalization for bleeding complications among males with hemophilia. Haemophilia 2001;7:198–206.

14. Skinner MW. Treatment for all: A vision for the future. Haemophilia. 2006 Jul;12 Suppl 3:169–73.

15. Evatt BL, Black C, Batorova A, et al. Comprehensive care for haemophilia around the world. Haemophilia 2004;10(suppl 4):9–13.

16. Mannucci PM, Tuddenham EG. The hemophilias – from royal genes to gene therapy. N Engl J Med 2001;344:1773–9.

17. Darby SC, Kan SW, Spooner RJ, et al. Mortality rates, life expectancy, and causes of death in people with hemophilia A or B in the United Kingdom who were not infected with HIV. Blood 2007;110:815–25.

18. Manco-Johnson MJ, Abshire TC, Shapiro AD, et al. Prophylaxis vs. episodic treatment to prevent joint disease in boys with severe haemophilia. N Engl J Med 2007;357:535–44.

19. Nilsson IM, Berntorp E, Lofqvist T, Pettersson H. Twenty-five years' experience of prophylactic treatment in severe haemophilia A and B. J Intern Med 1992;232:25–32.

20. Franchini M, Mannucci PM. Co-morbidities and quality of life in elderly persons with hemophilia. Br J Haematol 2010;148(4):522–33.

21. Mannucci PM, Schutgens RE, Santagostino E, Mauser-Bunschoten EP. How I treat age-related morbidities in elderly persons with hemophilia. Blood. 2009;114(26):5256–63.

22. Chalmers EA, Brown SA, Keeling D et al. Early factor VIII exposure and subsequent inhibitor development in children with severe haemophilia A. Haemophilia 2007;13:149–55.

23. Gouw SC, van der Bom JG, Auerswald G, et al. Recombinant vs. plasma-derived factor VIII products and the development of inhibitors in previously untreated patients with severe hemophilia A: the CANAL cohort study. Blood 2007;109:4693–7.

24. Murphy SB. Positive benefits of cooperative group membership: Being part of a networked rapid learning system. Pediatr Blood Cancer 2010;55:601–602.

25. Institute of Medicine. Crossing the Quality chasm: A new health system for the twenty first century. Washington, DC: National Academy Press; 2001.

26. http://www.hrsa.gov/opa. – accessed November 5, 2010.

2 General Topics

4 When Should We Switch from On-Demand to Prophylaxis Regimen?

José A. Aznar, Andrés Moret, Lydia Abad-Franch, Ana R. Cid, Saturnino Haya and Felipe Querol
La Fe University Hospital, Valencia, Spain

Introduction

Prophylaxis in hemophilia is the long-term continuous substitutive treatment that consists of regular intravenous administration of factor concentrate in order to prevent spontaneous hemorrhages and the development of hemophilic arthropathy [1]. In 1998, the European Paediatric Network for Hemophilia Management (PedNet) established the different prophylaxis procedures, which were subsequently reviewed in 2006 [2]. These procedures are complex and may be revised as they do not examine silent or subclinic hemarthroses.

Based on the studies from Aledort [3] and Manco-Johnson [4], we can simplify the different prophylactic regimens as:

• Primary prophylaxis: regular infusion of factor concentrates for more than 45 weeks a year, and started before any joint damage.
• Secondary prophylaxis: similar to primary prophylaxis, but started when joint damage already exists.

International recommendations

Since 1994, the World Health Organization (WHO) and the World Federation of Hemophilia (WFH) have recommended continuous prophylactic treatment [5]. In the same year, the Medical and Scientific Advisory Council (MASAC) of the National Hemophilia Foundation of the United States, after studying the Swedish experience in prophylaxis [6], recommended starting primary prophylaxis at an early age, 1–2 years, in children with severe hemophilia [7]. In 1994 Canada and in 1996 the Netherlands, proposed the same recommendation [6–8]. Later, in spite of the lack of controlled studies, prophylaxis was accepted by the scientific community as the standard treatment in severe hemophilic children in developed countries [9]. In 2001, the MASAC recommended prophylaxis as the best treatment choice in severe hemophilic patients of any age [10].

Early prophylaxis in children and its continuation in adolescents and adults

In 2007, Manco-Johnson et al. [4] published a prospective and multicenter randomized study in which, for the first time, scientific evidence of the efficacy of prophylaxis versus on-demand treatment in children with severe hemophilia A was established. This was valued using orthopedic, image and biological methods and confirmed what observational studies suggested some decades ago.

The results from the Swedish Cohort of children [6] focused the discussion on whether prophylaxis in severe hemophiliac children had to be started before the first hemarthrosis occurs. Later analysis of these studies suggested that primary prophylaxis should begin at an early age (≤ 2 years or ≤ 2 hemarthroses), although the start can be individualized upon the bleeding phenotypic pattern of each child [11,12]. Currently, there is an international consensus to consider primary prophylaxis started before the onset of joint damage as the treatment of choice in children with severe hemophilia A, at least in those countries with no restrictions in the use of factor VIII concentrates. However, it remains to be determined what is the optimal administration at the start of prophylaxis. Another reason to begin prophylaxis is the possible prevention of inhibitor development and hemorrhages that could threaten the patient's life [13].

In hemophilia B patients there is insufficient data to determine the optimal treatment, so it is necessary to perform prospective well-designed studies that can elucidate the optimal treatment strategy for these patients. In spite of this, prophylaxis in hemophilia B is practiced in developed countries [14].

Current and Future Issues in Hemophilia Care, First Edition. Edited by Emérito-Carlos Rodríguez-Merchán and Leonard A. Valentino.
© 2011 John Wiley & Sons, Ltd. Published 2011 by Blackwell Publishing Ltd.

The adherence to primary prophylaxis by children and parents is maximal until 12 years of age, as 90% of these patients show great adherence to the treatment. This percentage drastically falls to 54% in adolescents between 13 and 18 years of age [15] as these patients tend to overvalue the present and do not realize the prevention of future arthropathies as a relevant priority. Therefore, it is important to establish teamwork strategies (psychologists, parents, children and health professionals) to preserve the adherence to treatment in these critical phases of personal development, in order to assure a correct muscular–skeletal function when the hemophiliac patient reaches adult age.

Another area of debate regarding prophylactic treatment started at an early age is whether it can be discontinued when the patient reaches adult age. As Pipe and Valentino [16], the MASAC, the WHO and the WFH [8] recommend, whenever possible, prophylaxis should be continued over the patient's life, as traumatic bleeding risk does not disappear in adults, the severity of the hemophilia remains unchanged and the benefits of prophylaxis are the same in every stage of life [17]. A study in 22 European hemophilia centers revealed that 91% of the centers recommended long-term continuous treatment in those patients who started prophylaxis early [18]. However, there are also arguments favouring discontinuation of prophylaxis in adult patients, as adults are less active physically than children, which implies less traumatic risk. Moreover, animal experiments have shown that the cartilage in older joints is less susceptible to blood-induced damage than younger ones [19].

There are few publications about prophylaxis interruption in adults. Van Dijk et al. [20] studied 80 severe hemophilic patients born between 1970 and 1980, receiving prophylaxis in Denmark and the Netherlands. The mean age at the start of prophylaxis was 5.6 years in Denmark and 6 years in the Netherlands, and the mean follow-up was 19 years. At age of 26 years, 35% of the patients had changed to on-demand treatment having a mean of only three hemorrhages annually. Almost 4 years after the regimen switch, their joint status, evaluated radiographically and clinically, seemed to remain the same as before and was similar to the patients who continued on prophylaxis. However, Fischer [21] explained that the group from the Netherlands who interrupted their prophylaxis was composed of hemophiliacs who began prophylaxis later, received fewer doses of factor VIII concentrate and had a reduced incidence of hemarthroses, in other words, they were patients with a less severe bleeding phenotype. These factors may be useful to select suitable candidates to stop their prophylaxis. The lack of studies in this field suggests that prospective studies to evaluate which patients should withdraw from prophylaxis and which is the impact of this interruption are needed. Meanwhile, it could be an option to progressively reduce the frequency of prophylaxis until the equilibrium-point is reached, at which the patient does not show spontaneous hemorrhages capable of causing joint damage.

Summarizing, we highlight that nowadays there is a global consensus about the convenience of starting prophylaxis early in children with severe hemophilia A, although the initial regimen is still a matter of debate. In adolescence and adult age patients there is still controversy about maintaining prophylaxis or evaluating individually in each patient the switch from prophylaxis to an on-demand regimen. In any case, if changing to on-demand treatment causes repetitive hemarthroses, the patient should rapidly return to prophylaxis.

Secondary prophylaxis in adolescents and adults

Currently, we do not have enough data to evaluate the convenience of starting prophylaxis in those adolescents or adults who, after being treated on-demand, have developed an arthropathy. In any case, in developed countries without factor concentrate restrictions, the use of secondary prophylaxis increases every year.

A longitudinal study of Aledort [3] published in 1994, examined 477 severe hemophilia A patients under 25 years of age, and showed that secondary prophylaxis maintained during more than 45 weeks per year was associated with significantly less hemorrhagic episodes and a reduced incidence of arthropathy demonstrated radiographically and clinically. The number of hospital admissions was significantly reduced, as were school absences, and there was a favorable impact on psychosocial development. However, an increase in the dose of factor administered for prophylaxis was not significantly related to improvement in the clinical or radiological changes already present when prophylaxis was started.

Later, other studies ratified the benefits of the secondary prophylaxis. Miners in 1998 [22] observed a notable reduction of the bleeding frequency from 37 to 13 hemorrhages per year after changing from on-demand treatment to prophylaxis, although that meant a factor consumption three times higher. Aznar in 2000 [23] and Fischer in 2005 [24] concluded that secondary prophylaxis, when used long-term, prevents hemorrhages and delays joint damage, but does not completely avoid them. Tagliaferri in 2006 [25], also showed a decrease in bleeding frequency in 20 adolescent and adult patients, from 26.1 to 3.4 hemorrhages per year, after changing to prophylaxis.

Several studies to evaluate the impact of secondary prophylaxis have been performed. Coppola in 2005 [26], surveyed members of the Italian Association of Hemophilia Centers which included 84 severe hemophiliac patients who changed from on-demand treatment to prophylaxis in adolescence (n = 30) or in adult age (n = 54). Bleeding decreased by 70% after the treatment switch, with a moderate increase in factor VIII consumption and cost, combined with an improvement of the patient's quality of life, although the orthopedic score was not significantly better considering all the patients together.

In 2007, Richards [27] performed a survey of 21 physicians from 15 European countries who treat a total of 6365 patients with hemorrhagic diseases. Changes in the prophylactic treatment, permanent or temporary withdrawals, increases of dose or administration frequency and return to prophylaxis were evaluated for 218 patients between 16 and 24 years and for 251 patients above 50 years old with severe hemophilia A or hemophilia B. The authors point out that a significant number of adolescents and young children could interrupt or reduce the intensity of their prophylaxis; however, a percentage of these patients still required continuous prophylaxis and a notable percentage of older patients also required prophylaxis. The study concluded that there was an important disparity in the use and recommendations surrounding prophylaxis in adolescents, young patients and patients above 50 years old.

In 2009, Walsh and Valentino [28] carried out a survey in the United States, similar to the European one, to evaluate prophylaxis in hemophiliacs above 18 years old. Physicians caring for a total of 479 patients were studied. The conclusions were that starting, returning to or continuing prophylaxis in adults with hemophilia A is being carried out in the United States; it reduces bleeding frequency and can provide those patients some of the benefits observed in pediatric patients receiving prophylaxis. The results are promising and indicate that it is possible to reduce the development of arthropathy and to improve the quality of life in older patients with hemophilia.

On the other hand, Hay [29] argues that there are no convincing data which support a switch to prophylaxis in those adult patients who have been treated on-demand all their life and have an established arthropathy. Secondary prophylaxis would remain an option to treat individual problems, evaluated case by case, generally to prevent the development of a target joint or to postpone an orthopedic intervention.

It is necessary to carry out prospective, randomized and controlled studies in adolescents and adults with already developed arthropathy to establish the actual efficacy of prophylaxis versus on-demand treatment, and also to identify those patients who would not require prophylaxis.

A prospective and multicentric study recently published by Collins [30], compares the efficacy of on-demand and prophylactic treatments in 20 severe hemophilia A patients with ages between 30 and 45 years, who had a mean of two bleeding episodes monthly. The patients, before entering the study, had received more than 200 exposure days of factor VIII and did not develop inhibitors. The patients received treatment on-demand for 6 months, and afterwards were changed to prophylactic treatment (20–40 IU/Kg/three times weekly) for 7 months. The first prophylaxis month was considered as a run-in period to stabilize the prophylactic regimen. They measured the bleeding frequency, joint function (Gilbert scale) and the health-related quality of life (Haemo-QoL-A), and also several social-economical parameters and possible adverse events.

The comparison of both treatments showed that the incidence of hemarthroses during on-demand treatment was a mean of 15 episodes versus 0 during the prophylactic regimen. The joint status improved significantly during prophylaxis (18 points in the Gilbert score versus 25 for the on-demand period). Neither adverse events nor inhibitor development were reported. Another remarkable point was that 75% of the patients on prophylaxis showed factor VIII levels above 5% when measured 48 hours after administration and 57% showed more than 2% after 72 hours

post-infusion. This suggests that adults require lower factor doses than children to keep comparable levels of factor VIII in the blood, consistent with half-life studies [31].

Conclusions

There is global consensus to start prophylaxis in children with severe hemophilia A before joint damage appears. Continuing prophylaxis in adolescents who started it early as children is important to maintain the maximum adherence to treatment and continue the prophylaxis to at least adult age. Maintaining prophylaxis in adults who started it early must be evaluated individually based on the patient's bleeding pattern. If discontinued, it should be restarted soon if joint bleeding occurs after switching to an on-demand treatment, evaluating the optimal administration frequency, between 1 to 3 days weekly, to prevent hemarthroses. Starting secondary prophylaxis in adolescents and adults who already have joint alterations is an option. The results of the published works are encouraging, even though there is as yet no evidence which shows the efficacy of prophylaxis in these groups. This situation may resemble what occurred with primary prophylaxis before Manco-Johnson's publication, in other words, when we had the perception of the benefit of prophylaxis, but there was still no scientific evidence of its efficacy. This shows the importance of performing controlled studies in order to establish the efficacy of secondary prophylaxis in these patients.

References

1. Berntorp E. The treatment of haemophilia, including prophylaxis, constant infusion and DDAVP. Baillieres Clin Haematol. 1996;9:259–71.
2. Donadel-Claeyssens S. Current co-ordinated activities of the PEDNET (European Paediatric Network for Haemophilia Management). Haemophilia. 2006;12:124–7.
3. Aledort LM, Haschmeyer RH, Pettersson H. A longitudinal study of orthopaedic outcomes for severe factor-VIII-deficient haemophiliacs. The Orthopaedic Outcome Study Group. J Intern Med. 1994;236:391–9.
4. Manco-Johnson MJ, Abshire TC, Shapiro AD, et al. Prophylaxis versus episodic treatment to prevent joint disease in boys with severe hemophilia. N Engl J Med. 2007;357:535–44.
5. Lusher JM. Considerations for current and future management of haemophilia and its complications. Haemophilia. 1995;1:2–10.
6. Nilsson IM, Berntorp E, Lofqvist T, Pettersson H. Twenty-five years' experience of prophylactic treatment in severe haemophilia A and B. J Intern Med. 1992;232:25–32.
7. Berntorp E, Boulyjenkov V, Brettler D, et al. Modern treatment of haemophilia. Bull World Health Organ. 1995;73:691–701.
8. Skolnick AA. Hemophilia Foundation recommends prophylactic use of clotting factors. JAMA. 1994;272:1153–4.
9. Berntorp E, Astermark J, Bjorkman S, Blanchette VS, Fischer K, Giangrande PL, et al. Consensus perspectives on prophylactic

therapy for haemophilia: summary statement. Haemophilia. 2003;9(Suppl 1):1–4.

10. Valentino LA. Secondary prophylaxis therapy: what are the benefits, limitations and unknowns? Haemophilia. 2004;10:147–57.

11. Astermark J, Petrini P, Tengborn L, Schulman S, Ljung R, Berntorp E. Primary prophylaxis in severe haemophilia should be started at an early age but can be individualized. Br J Haematol. 1999;105:1109–13.

12. Fischer K, Van der Bom JG, Mauser-Bunschoten EP, et al. The effects of postponing prophylactic treatment on long-term outcome in patients with severe hemophilia. Blood. 2002;99:2337–41.

13. Morado M, Villar A, Jimenez-Yuste V, Quintana M, Hernandez Navarro F. Prophylactic treatment effects on inhibitor risk: experience in one centre. Haemophilia. 2005;11:79–83.

14. Aznar JA, Lucía F, Abad-Franch L, et al. Focusing on haemophilia B: prophylaxis in Spanish patients. Haemophilia 2010 DOI: 10.1111/j.1365-251632010.02412.x.

15. Petrini P, Seuser A. Haemophilia care in adolescents – compliance and lifestyle issues. Haemophilia. 2009;15(Suppl 1):15–9.

16. Pipe SW, Valentino LA. Optimizing outcomes for patients with severe haemophilia A. Haemophilia. 2007;13(Suppl 4):1–16;quiz 13, p. following 16.

17. Astermark J. When to start and when to stop primary prophylaxis in patients with severe haemophilia. Haemophilia. 2003;9(Suppl 1): 32–6. Discussion p. 37.

18. Chambost H, Ljung R. Changing pattern of care of boys with haemophilia in western European centres. Haemophilia. 2005;11: 92–9.

19. Hooiveld M, Roosendaal G, Vianen ME, et al. Immature articular cartilage is more susceptible to blood-induced damage than mature articular cartilage; an in vivo animal study. Arthritis Rheum. 2003;48:396–403.

20. Van Dijk K, Fischer K, Van de Bom JG, et al. Can long-term prophylaxis for severe haemophilia be stopped in adulthood? Results from Denmark and the Netherlands. Br J Haematol. 2005;130:107–12.

21. Fischer K, Van Der Bom JG, Prejs R, Mauser-Bunschoten EP, Roosendaal G, Grobbee DE, et al. Discontinuation of prophylactic therapy in severe haemophilia: incidence and effects on outcome. Haemophilia. 2001;7:544–50.

22. Miners AH, Sabin CA, Tolley KH, Lee CA. Assessing the effectiveness and cost-effectiveness of prophylaxis against bleeding in patients with severe haemophilia and severe von Willebrand's disease. J Intern Med. 1998;244:515–22.

23. Aznar JA, Magallon M, Querol F, et al. The orthopaedic status of severe haemophiliacs in Spain. Haemophilia 2000;6:170–76.

24. Fischer K, Van Dijk K, Van de Berg H. Late prophylaxis for severe hemophilia: effects of prophylaxis started in adulthood. J Thromb Haemost. 2005;3:0R205.

25. Tagliaferri A, Rivolta GF, Rossetti G, et al. Experience of secondary prophylaxis in 20 adolescent and adult Italian hemophiliacs. Thromb Haemost. 2006;96:542–3.

26. Coppola A, Cimino E, Macarone Palmieri N. Clinical and pharmacoeconomic impact of secondary prophylaxis in young-adults with severe hemophilia A. J Thromb Haemost. 2005;3:P1428.

27. Richards M, Altisent C, Batorova A, Chambost H, Dolan G, De Moerloose P, et al. Should prophylaxis be used in adolescent and adult patients with severe haemophilia? A European survey of practice and outcome data. Haemophilia. 2007;13:473–9.

28. Walsh CE, Valentino LA. Factor VIII prophylaxis for adult patients with severe haemophilia A: results of a US survey of attitudes and practices. Haemophilia. 2009;15:1014–21.

29. Hay CR. Prophylaxis in adults with haemophilia. Haemophilia. 2007; 13(Suppl 2):10–5.

30. Collins P, Faradji A, Morfini M, et al. Efficacy and safety on secondary prophylaxis vs. on demand sucrose-formulated recombinant factor VIII treatment in adults with severe hemophilia A: results from a 13-month cross over study. J Thromb Haemost. 2010;8: 83–9.

31. Björkman S, Folkesson A, Jónsson S. Pharmacokinetics and dose requirements of factor VIII over the age range 3–74 years. A population analysis based on 50 patients with long-term prophylactic treatment for haemophilia A. Eur J Clin Pharmacol. 2009;65: 989–98.

5 Prophylaxis in Children

Marilyn J. Manco-Johnson
University of Colorado, Aurora, CO, USA

Introduction

Prophylaxis refers to a type of substitution treatment strategy for hemophilia in which the deficient coagulation factor is replaced on a routine basis in the absence of bleeding. Substitution therapy in hemophilia A and B is currently limited by the relatively short half lives of the coagulation proteins and the requirement for an intravenous route of administration. In addition, prophylaxis does not restore a completely physiologic condition as protein catabolism and clearance commence immediately after injection, causing plasma concentrations to fluctuate between the peak concentration achieved in the hour following infusion and the trough level tolerated prior to the subsequent injection. Given these limitations, prophylaxis is still a remarkably effective therapy to prevent bleeding and the complications of bleeding in persons with hemophilia.

History of prophylaxis and current status in the United States

Prior to the discovery of cryoprecipitate by Judith Graham Poole in 1964, substitution therapy for factor VIII was not widely available [1]. By the later 1960s, early reports of prophylaxis were published from Sweden, Canada, the United States and the Netherlands [2–5]. Although availability and safety of factor concentrates limited broad application of prophylaxis to children, Inga Marie Nilsson continued to pioneer regular infusions of FVIII to prevent joint bleeding in young Swedish children with hemophilia [6]. In observational studies, Nilsson and her colleagues were able to demonstrate physical and radiologic evidence of improved joint outcome in children treated at a young age with prophylactic regimens [7]. Observational studies from hemophilia centers in

Sweden, Germany and The Netherlands were convergent in their suggestion that, to be effective, routine infusions must be started early in life, and that hemophilic arthropathy was not prevented in children who began prophylaxis at or beyond the age of 3 years [8–10]. In addition, initiation of prophylaxis after the onset of joint changes was determined to improve physical functioning and pain, but did not reverse or halt progressive arthritic changes [11]. However, despite data supporting the efficacy of prophylaxis in severe hemophilia, broad application of its use remained limited by cost, availability of sufficient safe factor replacement products, difficulties around venous access in small children and family stress incurred by regular home venipuncture [12].

To date there has been one prospective, controlled randomized clinical trial of prophylaxis in hemophilia A [13]. The Joint Outcome Study (JOS) randomized 65 young boys in the United States (US) with $\leq 2\%$ FVIII activity, less than 2.5 years of age, and with a history of two or fewer hemarthroses into any of the ankle, knee or elbow joints, to receive routine replacement infusions of FVIII at 25 IU/kg every other day, or to receive FVIII replacement only at the time of clinical bleeding. All treatment of bleeding events was clinically determined by the attending physician except for hemarthroses which were all treated with 40 IU/kg immediately upon symptomatic onset, and 20 IU/kg at 24 and 72 hours following the initial infusion. Participants on the episodic treatment arm were permitted to continue every other day infusions until complete resolution of pain and limitation in joint motion, up to four weeks. The primary endpoint was joint structure by magnetic resonance imaging (MRI) and plain X-ray. At study exit, at age six years, normal joint morphology, without evidence of bone or cartilage defects, was preserved in 93% of children on prophylaxis compared with 58% of children on episodic factor replacement (P = 0.02).

The US National Hemophilia Foundation (NHF) Medical and Scientific Advisory Council (MASAC) recommended "in view of

Current and Future Issues in Hemophilia Care, First Edition. Edited by Emérito-Carlos Rodríguez-Merchán and Leonard A. Valentino.
© 2011 John Wiley & Sons, Ltd. Published 2011 by Blackwell Publishing Ltd.

the demonstrated benefits of prophylaxis begun at a young age in persons with hemophilia A or B, prophylaxis (should) be considered optimal therapy for individuals with severe hemophilia A or B" [14]. In addition, the US Food and Drug Administration (FDA) reviewed the data from the JOS and granted an approval for use of Kogenate FS "to include routine prophylaxis to reduce the frequency of bleeding episodes and the risk of joint damage in children" [15].

The Centers for Disease Control and Prevention (CDC) Universal Data Collection (UDC) study collects surveillance data on more than 26,000 persons with bleeding disorders, including 8833 persons with severe factor A and B deficiency; in this database prophylaxis is defined as any routine replacement of clotting factor used at least once weekly. Using the CDC UDC data from 2009 it may be estimated that approximately three-fourths of children 2 through 18 years with severe hemophilia are currently treated on a continuous prophylactic regimen of any type, while 31% of adults with severe hemophilia report using continuous prophylaxis [16].

Current issues in prophylaxis

Dose and dose-frequency

Dosing for prophylaxis has been estimated using pharmacokinetic (PK) and non-pharmacokinetic approaches. Factor VIII has a half life of approximately 12 hours; factor IX has a half live of approximately 18 hours. In order to prevent bleeding events prophylaxis is usually required at intervals of 4 to 5 half-lives, resulting in a dose frequency of every two to three days for hemophilia A and every three to four days for hemophilia B.

Pharmacokinetic dosing

Using a PK approach, the maximal plasma concentration of replaced factor activity following infusion is dependent on the volume of distribution, which determines dose. Plasma clearance is the major determinant of duration of effect, which drives dose frequency. A curve of plasma disappearance of clotting factor activity following infusion may show a uniform decline (known as single compartment kinetics) or may show an initial rapid decline (called the distribution phase) followed by a slower decrease (called the elimination phase). In the latter case of 2-compartment kinetics, the terminal or elimination phase of clearance is generally calculated for PK studies. Dose and dose frequency are related as a higher initial peak will result in a longer time to a predetermined trough level, although rapidly diminishing returns are realized with progressively increased initial plasma factor activity. The first PK studies for factor VIII replacement were reported by Dr. Hirschman and colleagues at the US National Institute of Health in 1970 [17]. Based on this study, a prophylaxis dosing regimen of 25 IU/kg every other day was proposed to maintain a trough factor VIII level at 2% or greater; this was the schedule later adopted in Swedish hemophilia clinics. Factor PKs show some age-related trends with larger volume of distribution and accelerated clearance observed in populations of children under six years of age resulting in higher dose requirements in young children [18]. There is also considerable inter-individual variability with normal terminal half-life of factor VIII in adults ranging from 9.6 to 13.4 hours [18]. Longer terminal half-life results in higher trough levels on a standard dose schedule, such as every other day, and decreased time below a critical threshold level required to prevent spontaneous bleeding [19]. Rational use of PK data argues that daily dosing of factor VIII effectively prevents bleeding with dramatically reduced factor consumption [20]. However, significant education and reorientation of patient perspectives is necessary for widespread adoption of daily factor replacement.

Non-pharmacokinetic dosing

Despite the scientific logic of PK-based dosing for factor replacement, most treatment regimens are empiric and based upon prevention of clinically-evident bleeding events. In order to give patients a weekend "holiday", the PK-based alternate day dosing was altered to a Monday, Wednesday, Friday schedule. In fact, many patients with severe hemophilia, particularly older children and adults, find this schedule satisfactory with few breakthrough episodes of hemorrhage.

Once weekly infusions of factor VIII or IX were employed and found to decrease bleeding frequency in persons with severe hemophilia [21–23]. Weekly infusions were adopted as an initial prophylaxis regimen with progressive escalation on the Canadian Escalating Dose Prophylaxis Study, which used eligibility criteria identical to that of the JOS [24]. In this trial, an initial prophylaxis regimen of 50 U/kg once weekly was escalated, based on bleeding, to 30 U/kg twice weekly, and ultimately 25 U/kg every other day. The protocol allowed for escalation in the event of target joint hemorrhage defined as 3 or more hemorrhages into a single joint over three consecutive months, four hemorrhages at any site over three consecutive months, or five or more hemorrhages cumulatively into a single joint at any time during the study. Approximately 40% of subjects fulfilled criteria for target joint hemorrhage by 3.5 years, with 28% requiring alternate-day prophylaxis and 40% manifesting X-ray evidence of early bone and cartilage disease by 5 years; subjects on the Canadian escalation protocol consumed an average of 3656 IU FVIII/kg/year [24]. This compares with 7% rate of bone or cartilage damage by X-ray or MRI by age 6 years at a cost of 6000 IU/kg/year FVIII in the JOS [13].

Escalating prophylaxis, beginning with once weekly dosing, and increasing frequency based on a reduced threshold for bleeding rate, is currently employed for the initiation of prophylaxis in many hemophilia treatment centers in North American and Western Europe [25]. While most children require more frequent dosing, the regimen is often effective for several months in young infants beginning prophylaxis. The advantages of this strategy is that it allows time and opportunity for parents to learn venipuncture for home infusion, usually averts the need for an indwelling venous access device, and is well tolerated by most infants. Hemophilia centers in developing economies are beginning to explore the efficacy of very low dose prophylaxis to ameliorate bleeding and its consequences. While there are currently no data regarding the outcome of reduced dosing schedules, there is hope that low-dose prophylaxis can provide an entré into preventive strategies for hemophilia.

Reduced and individualized prophylaxis dosing schedules are again common in the older adolescent and young adult, following cessation of participation in team sports. Throughout childhood, activities are encouraged that promote weight-bearing impact without collision, such as walking and running, along with recommended daily requirements of vitamin D and calcium to promote healthy bone density. Starting at approximately 14 years of age, teen boys with hemophilia are encouraged to participate in regular supervised weight training to promote muscle strength and bulk. By attainment of an adult physique, a young man with hemophilia and no or minimal arthropathy is sometimes able to reduce prophylaxis frequency to every three to five days with minimal breakthrough bleeding. Two caveats must be kept in mind: (1) some children with a shortened factor half-life and frequent bleeding maintain a requirement for frequent replacement infusions as adults and should be maintained on a clinically effective dose schedule; and (2) strenuous or sustained activity, including manual labor, may require more frequent factor replacement. Adult prophylaxis is addressed in Chapter 6.

Route of administration

Prophylaxis is generally administered by peripheral intravenous route. Some infants and young children manifest a clinical requirement for frequency of administration that cannot be sustained using their peripheral veins. Several indwelling venous access devices and surgical fistulas have been applied to facilitate prophylaxis. Complications common to all devices include infection, thrombosis and mechanical failure. The uses and limitations of venous access devices have been reviewed and summarized [26,27]. When used, the goal for a venous access device is temporary usage while required, and removal as early as possible. However, irreversible arthropathy often develops rapidly following one or few significant episodes of hemarthroses in young children; hence, limitations of venous access should be addressed and should not be accepted as a routine limitation for the early initiation of prophylaxis.

Monitoring

All persons on prophylaxis should be monitored carefully. The most common monitoring technique is clinical assessment of bleeding frequency. The JOS determined MRI and/or X-ray evidence of arthropathy in six year-old boys with severe hemophilia A who had no history of clinical hemorrhage in the affected joint; however, arthropathy occurred only in those children who were not on prophylaxis [13]. While on prophylaxis, children manifested a median of 0.2 joint hemorrhages per year, and by the age of six years, none of the joints which had suffered one to four hemorrhages on prophylaxis showed bone or cartilage damage. A current follow-up of the children on the JOS will yield important information regarding the rates of damage incurred by children on prophylaxis throughout childhood until age 18 years.

The role of laboratory testing in monitoring prophylaxis is debated. Dr. Nilsson sought to maintain a trough factor level $\geq 1\%$ based on the clinical observation that individuals with moderate hemophilia had a low rate of spontaneous (i.e. non-traumatic) hemorrhages [7]. Petrini and colleagues challenged this premise with evidence that although 79% of boys in their clinic had a trough level determined at <1% FVIII activity, there was no difference in annual rate of joint hemorrhage related to detectable trough activity [25]. Following observations by Peters and colleagues [28] that inter-individual variation in the level of the von Willebrand protein, a plasma stabilizer of factor VIII, may modify the severity of hemophilia A, and the finding that children with severe hemophilia who carry the factor V Leiden mutation display slightly delayed onset of joint hemorrhage [29], interest was broadened beyond factor activity to other coagulation parameters [30–32]. Over the past several years investigators have applied global assays of hemostasis to the investigation of variability in response to prophylaxis [33]. It has been reported that thrombin generation over time following an infusion of factor VIII varies among individuals with severe hemophilia and shows only fair correlation with factor activity.

Currently, there are no accepted recommendations regarding the use of factor activity assays, global assessments of hemostasis, or testing of other coagulation protein levels in order to monitor prophylaxis. The currently ongoing investigations may serve a key role in helping to establish minimal effective dosing regimens, to elucidate the range of variability among individual patients and particularly to determine whether any one or more clinical or laboratory indicator predicts joint outcome of prophylaxis.

Age of initiation

To date, there is no universally accepted age for optimal initiation of prophylaxis to prevent joint damage. Some investigators recommend initiation of prophylaxis in persons with severe hemophilia prior to the first joint hemorrhage. This clinical event, however, varies widely and has been reported at a median of 24–30 months with a range from 6 months to almost 6 years [10,33,34]. Prophylaxis has also been shown to prevent other life-threatening hemorrhages, such as intracranial hemorrhage, which can occur in infants in the absence of joint hemorrhage [13,34].

Recently, epidemiologic data from the European study, "Concerted Action on Neutralizing Antibodies in Severe Hemophilia A (CANAL study)" suggested that early institution of prophylaxis was associated with a decreased risk for inhibitor formation [35]. The mechanism of this effect is postulated to occur through the prevention of bleeding, and subsequently, the reduction in episodes of intensive factor replacement therapy during a state of inflammation and heightened immune response which are likely to occur in the context of hemorrhage [36].

Currently, grade C evidence, "Expert Opinion" continues to hold that children with severe hemophilia A ought to begin prophylaxis at or prior to the age of two years or shortly after the first joint hemorrhage [37,38].

Benefits of continued primary and secondary prophylaxis in adolescents and young adults

Because prophylaxis dosing is based on weight, the cost of prophylaxis is least in the young child and increases with size. Persons with hemophilia who achieve adolescence and young adulthood following early initiation of prophylaxis with little or no joint damage, excellent muscle bulk and strength and normal range of motion are exploring schedules to reduce dose or dose frequency [39–41]. Secondary prophylaxis, defined as the initiation of routine replacement of deficient clotting factor after the onset of arthropathy, has been shown to reduce bleeding and to improve physical joint function and pain, although bone and cartilage defects persist and slowly progress [11,42,43]. Currently accepted indicators for assessment of efficacy of secondary prophylaxis include reduction in bleeding rate and improvement in: joint function, activity ability and performance, social participation, quality of life, and cost savings related to amelioration of progressive joint degeneration [44]. There are insufficient data to address the costs, risks and benefits of discontinuing secondary prophylaxis. Arthritic pain related to advanced arthropathy is unlikely to improve with secondary prophylaxis, and studies assessing the efficacy of secondary prophylaxis will need to separately address results in individuals with joint hemorrhage and synovitis who are likely to experience reduced pain and improved quality of life on prophylaxis from outcomes in persons with chronic disabling arthritic pain that will not be relieved by regular factor infusions.

Future issues

Currently, there is great enthusiasm around recently generated novel factor VIII and factor IX molecules with modifications engineered to prolong plasma half-life or to increase plasma procoagulant activity [45–48]. The promise of weekly or bi-weekly prophylaxis could become a reality at the conclusion of several clinical trials that are currently underway or soon to be initiated. In addition, the new generation of "designer molecules" includes molecular modifications that promise to improve the efficacy of prophylaxis in patients with high titer inhibitors, thus extending the benefits of prophylaxis to this currently underserved population [49]. Should there exist an intravenous therapy to prevent bleeding in hemophilia that can be administered at a reduced frequency, it is likely that many of the obstacles to prophylaxis will be overcome.

Conclusions

Prophylaxis is remarkably effective in prevention of arthropathy and other bleeding complications in children with severe hemophilia. For best results, prophylaxis must be started in the first year or two of life, prior to the development of any early joint disease, although efficacy has been shown following one or two promptly recognized and aggressively treated joint hemorrhages. Joint preservation has been proven using alternate day dosing at 25 IU/kg in a randomized clinical trial. Less frequent dosing, especially in infancy, appears to prevent clinically evident bleeding events, and is used in clinical practice. Individuals with early arthropathy, specifically with frequent episodes of joint hemorrhage and inflammatory synovitis benefit from institution of secondary prophylaxis, whereas chronic pain related to advanced-stage arthritis is unlikely to improve related to prophylaxis. The future holds a potential for more convenient, less frequent intravenous infusions of novel recombinant coagulation molecules with longer half-life and/or higher specific activity that should translate into broader application of prophylactic regimes in the treatment of severe hemophilia.

References

1. Pool JG, Hershgold EJ, Pappenhagen AR. High-potency antihaemophilic factor concentrate prepared from cryoglobulin precipitate, Nature 1964;203:312.
2. Ahlberg A. Haemophilia in Sweden. VII. Incidence, treatment and prophylaxis of arthropathy and other musculoskeletal manifestations of haemophilia A and B. Acta Orthop Scand 1965;77(suppl):3–132.
3. Robinson PM, Tittley P, Smiley RK. Prophylactic therapy in classical hemophilia: a preliminary report. Can Med Assoc J 1967;97:559–61.
4. Shanbrom E, Thelin GM. Experimental prophylaxis of severe hemophilia with a factor VIII concentrate. JAMA 1969;208:1853–6.
5. Van Creveld S. Prophylaxis of joint hemorrhages in hemophilia. Acta Haematol 1969;41:206–214.
6. Nilsson IM, Blombäck M, Ahlberg Ä. Our experience in Sweden with prophylaxis on haemophilia. The hemophiliac and his world. Bibl Haematol 1970;34:111–24.
7. Nilsson IM, Berntorp E, Lofqvist T, Pettersson H. Twenty-five years' experience of prophylactic treatment in severe haemophilia A and B. J Intern Med 1992;232:25–32.
8. Astermark J, Petrini P, Tegborn L, Shulman S, Ljung R, Berntorp E. Primary prophylaxis in severe haemophilia should be started at a young age but can be individualized. Br J Haematol 1999;105: 1109–13.
9. Kreuz W, Escuriola-Ettingshausen C, Funk M, Schmidt H, Kornhuber B. When should prophylactic treatment in patients with haemophilia A and B start? – The German experience. Haemophilia 1998;4:413–7.
10. Fischer K, van der Bom JG, Mauser-Bunschoten EP, Roosendaal G, Prejs R, de Kleijn P, Grobbee DE, van den Berg M. The effects of postponing prophylactic treatment on long-term outcome in patients with severe hemophilia. Blood 2002;99(7):2337–41.
11. Manco-Johnson MJ, Nuss R, Geraghty S, Funk S, Kilcoyne R. Results of secondary prophylaxis in children with severe hemophilia. Am J Hematol 1994;47:113–17.
12. Hacker MR, Geraghty S, Manco-Johnson M. Barriers to compliance with prophylaxis therapy in haemophilia. Haemophilia 2001;7(4):392–6.
13. Manco-Johnson MJ, Abshire TC, Shapiro AD, et al. Recombinant factor VIII for the prevention of joint disease in children with severe hemophilia: prophylaxis compared with episodic treatment. NEJM 2007;357:535–44.

14. MASAC Medical Bulletin #179, http://www.hemophilia.org/NHFWeb/MainPgs/MainNHF.aspx?menuid=57&contentid=1007, accessed November 15, 2010.

15. FDA package insert for Kogenate FS, http://www.fda.gov/BiologicsBlood/vaccines/BloodBloodProducts/ApprovedProducts/LicensedProductsBLAs/FractionatedPlasmaProducts/UCM089055.htm, accessed November 15, 2010.

16. CDC UDC website, https://www2a.cdc.gov/ncbddd/htcweb/UDC_Report/UDC_view1.asp?para1=NATION&para2=ALL&para3=&ScreenWidth=1280&ScreenHeight=1024, accessed November 16, 2010.

17. Hirschman RJ, Itscoitz SB, Shulman NR. Prophylactic treatment of factor VIII deficiency. Blood 1970;35:189–94.

18. Bjorkman S, Blanchette V, Fischer K, Oh M, Spotts G, Schroth P, Fritsch S, Patrone L, Ewenstein BM, for the Advate Clinical Program Group and Collins PW. Comparative pharmacokinetics of plasma- and albumin-free recombinant factor VIII in children and adults: the influence of blood sampling schedule on observed age-related differences and implications for dose tailoring. J Thromb Haemost 2010;8:730–6.

19. Collins PW, Blanchette VS, Fischer K, Björkman S, Oh M, Fritsch S, Schroth P, Spotts G, Astermark J, Ewenstein B; rAHF-PFM Study Group. Break-through bleeding in relation to predicted factor VIII levels in patients receiving prophylactic treatment for severe hemophilia A. J Thromb Haemost 2009;7:413–20.

20. Collins PW, Fischer K, Morfini M, Blanchette VS, Björkman S; on behalf of International Prophylaxis Study Group (IPSG) Pharmacokinetics Expert Working Group. Implications of coagulation factor VIII and IX pharmacokinetics in the prophylactic treatment of haemophilia. Haemophilia 2011;17(1):2–10.

21. Shanbrom E, Thelin GM. Experimental prophylaxis of severe hemophilia with a factor VIII concentrate. JAMA 1969;208:1853–6.

22. Kasper CK, Dietrich SL, Rapaport SI. Hemophilia prophylaxis with factor VIII concentrate. Arch Intern Med 1970;125:1004–9.

23. Aronstam A, Arblaster PG, Rainsford SG, et al. Prophylaxis in hemophilia: a double-blind controlled trial. Br J Haematol 1976;30:65–7.

24. Feldman BM, Pai M, Rivard GE, et al. Tailored prophylaxis in severe hemophilia A: interim results from the first 5 years of the Canadian Hemophilia Primary Prophylaxis Study. J Thromb Haemost 2006;4:1228–36.

25. Petrini P. What factors should influence the dosage and interval of prophylactic treatment in patients with severe haemophilia A and B? Haemophilia 2001;7:99–102.

26. Ewenstein BM, Valentino LA, Journeycake JM, et al. Consensus recommendations for use of central venous access devices in haemophilia. Haemophilia 2004;10:629–48.

27. Geraghty S, Kleinert D. Use and morbidity of venous access devices in patients with hemophilia. J Intraven Nurs 1998;21:70–5.

28. Fijnvandraat K, Peters M, ten Cate JW. Inter-individual variation in half-life of infused recombinant factor VIII is related to pre-infusion von Willebrand factor antigen levels. Br J Haematol 1995;91:474–6.

29. Kurnik K, Kreuz W, Horneff SW, et al. Effects of the factor V G1691A mutation and the factor II G20210A variant on the clinical expression of severe hemophilia A in children – results of a multicenter study. Haematologica 2007;92:982–5.

30. Barrowcliffe TW. Monitoring haemophilia severity and treatment: new or old laboratory tests? Haemophilia 2004;10:109–14.

31. Beltrán-Miranda CP, Khan A, Jaloma-Cruz AR, Laffan MA. Thrombin generation and phenotype correlation in haemophilia A. Haemophilia 2005;11:326–34.

32. Lewis SJ, Stephens E, Florou G, Macartney NJ, Hathaway LS, Knipping J, Collins PW. Measurement of global haemostasis in severe haemophilia A following factor VIII infusion. Br J Haematol 2007;138:775–82.

33. Van Dijk K, Fischer K, van der Bom JG, Grobbee DE, van den Berg HM. Variability in clinical phenotype of severe haemophilia: the role of the first joint bleed. Haemophilia 2005;11:438–43.

34. Kulkarni R, Soucie JM, Lusher J, et al.; Haemophilia Treatment Center Network Investigators. Sites of initial bleeding episodes, mode of delivery and age of diagnosis in babies with haemophilia diagnosed before the age of 2 years: a report from the Centers for Disease Control and Prevention (CDC) Universal Data Collection (UDC) project. Haemophilia 2009;15:1281–90.

35. Gouw SC, van der Bom JG, van den Berg HM, for the CANAL Study Group. Treatment-related risk factors of inhibitor development in previously untreated patients with hemophilia A: the CANAL cohort study. Blood 2007;109:4648–54.

36. Ter Avest PC, Fischer K, Mancuso ME, Santagostino E, Yuste VJ, ven den Berg HM on behalf of the CNAL study group. J Thromb Haemost 2008;6:2048–54.

37. Richards M, Williams M, Chalmers E, Liesner R, Collins P, Vidler V, Hanley J. A United Kingdom Haemophilia Centre Doctors' Organization guideline approved by the British Committee for Standards in Haematology: guideline on the use of prophylactic factor VIII concentrate in children and adults with severe haemophilia A. Brit J Haematol 2010;149:498–507.

38. Blanchette VS, Manco-Johnson M, Santagostino E, Ljung R. Optimizing factor prophylaxis for the haemophilia population: where do we stand? Haemophilia 2004;4:97–104.

39. Fischer K, van der Bom JG, Prejs R, Mauser-Bunschoten EP, Roosendaal G, Gorbbee DE, van den Berg HM. Discontinuation of prophylaxis in severe haemophilia: incidence and effects on outcome. Haemophilia 2001;7:544–50.

40. Van Dijk K, Fischer K, van der Bom J, Scheibel E, Ingerslev J, van den Berg H. Can long-term prophylaxis for severe haemophilia be stopped in adulthood? Results from Denmark and the Netherlands. Brit J Haematol 2005;130:107–12.

41. Richards M, Altisent C, Batorova A, et al. Should prophylaxis be used in adolescent and adult patients with severe haemophilia? A European survey of practice and outcome data. Haemophilia 2007;13:473–9.

42. Collins P, Faradji A, Morfini M, Enriquez MM, Schwartz L. Efficacy and safety of secondary prophylactic vs. on-demand sucrose-formulated recombinant factor VIII treatment in adults with severe Hemophilia A: results from a 13-month crossover study. J Thromb Haemost 2010;8:83–9.

43. Aledort L, Haschmeyer RH, Pettersson H. A longitudinal study of orthopaedic outcomes for severe factor-VIII-deficient haemophiliacs. J Intern Med 1994;236:391–9.

44. Globe D, Young NL, Von Mackensen S, Bullinger M, Wasserman J; Health related Quality Of Life Expert Working Group of the International Prophylaxis Study Group. Haemophilia 2009;15:843–52.

45. Mei B, Pan C, Jiang H, Tjandra H, et al. Rational design of a fully active, long-acting PEGylated factor VIII for hemophilia A treatment. Blood 2010;116:270–9.

46. Pipe SW. Go long! A touchdown for factor VIII? Blood 2010;116:153–4.

47. Saenko EL, Pipe SW. Strategies towards a longer acting factor VIII. Haemophilia 2006;12 Suppl 3:42–51.

48. Greene TK, Wang C, Hirsch JD, et al. In vivo efficacy of platelet-delivered, high specific activity factor VIII variants. Blood 2010; 116(26):6114–22.

49. Spira J, Plyushch O, Zozulya N, Yatuv R, Dayan I, Bleicher A, Robinson M, Baru M. Safety, pharmacokinetics and efficacy of factor VIIa formulated with PEGylated liposomes in haemophilia A patients with inhibitors to factor VIII – an open label, exploratory, cross-over, phase I/II study. Haemophilia 2010;16:910–8.

6 Prophylaxis in Adults with Hemophilia

Victor Jiménez-Yuste, Emérito-Carlos Rodríguez-Merchán, Maria-Teresa Alvarez-Román, and Mónica Martín-Salces

La Paz University Hospital, Madrid, Spain

Introduction

Joint hemorrhage is the most common manifestation of severe hemophilia and predisposes to arthropathy. The main goal of replacement therapy is to prevent this pathology. Although on-demand treatment can slow the progression of arthropathy, it does not seem to prevent it. Nevertheless, prophylaxis has been shown to be superior to episode-based, aggressive (enhanced) therapy in preventing joint damage in boys [1]. Based on the study of Manco-Johnson [1], primary prophylaxis is considered the standard of care for children in many countries [2] and the use of prophylaxis is becoming more common in adults.

There is a paucity of data on the benefits of prophylaxis for adult patients because most data on long-term outcomes of prophylactic treatment come from studies in pediatric patients [3,4]. Although the World Health Organization (WHO) recommends that prophylaxis be continued for the patient's lifetime [5], the optimal duration of prophylaxis has not been established, and hemophilic patients often discontinue prophylaxis as young adults [6] or switch to a more targeted form of prophylaxis, the question of whether prophylaxis is necessary or helpful in all adults with hemophilia remains unanswered.

Prophylaxis in children

The usefulness of primary prophylaxis in preventing joint disease comes from the studies of Nilsson and colleagues in Sweden. They observed that full-dose prophylaxis started in the first few years of life in boys with severe hemophilia could prevent recurrent joint bleeding and preserve an excellent musculoskeletal status after 25 years of follow-up [7,8]. The authors also observed that deterioration of a joint was often due to the progressive destruc-tion of joints in which bleeding had already occurred prior to the start of treatment. This observation indicated that prophylaxis should begin at a very early age, before the onset of joint bleeding. Their proposal regarding so-called primary prophylaxis has since been corroborated in many different reports [9,10]. After decades of observational studies, the prospective US Joint Outcome Study (JOS) confirmed the efficacy of prophylaxis in preventing bleeding episodes and joint damage in children with severe hemophilia A [1].

In consideration of these important findings in the pediatric population, the US National Hemophilia Foundation (NHF), the World Federation of Hemophilia (WFH) and the WHO recommended that prophylaxis be continued throughout a patient's lifetime. However, adolescence is characterized by simultaneous physical, psychological, social and hormonal changes that multiply the challenges faced by parents, health care providers and adolescents with hemophilia. Compliance with prophylactic factor replacement therapy frequently declines when patients pass from childhood to adolescence. The current generation of children and teenagers are not familiar with the long-term joint damage that classically occurs in patients with bleeding disorders. This ignorance and the tendency of teenagers to focus primarily on short term goals increase the likelihood that they do not perceive regular prophylactic replacement therapy as a high priority. However, most adolescents will accept prophylactic treatment prior to physical or social activities because short-term goals are more likely to be perceived as relevant [11].

Prophylaxis in adults

While patients with severe hemophilia still have a reduced life expectancy, their overall life expectancy is approaching that of the general male population [12,13]. With the introduction of prophylactic treatment regimens during childhood and, increasingly, continuation of some level of prophylactic treatment during adulthood, the general state of health among persons with hemophilia is also beginning to resemble that of the overall population.

However, despite the favorable results in the pediatric population, prophylaxis is administered by only about half of all people with severe hemophilia A participating in the Universal Data Collection (UDC) program [14].

In a very interesting analysis of the literature, Valentino reviewed prophylaxis in adults [14]. So few studies addressed the use of prophylaxis in adult hemophiliacs, with a series of methodological limitations (retrospective or non-controlled design, heterogeneity of patients, treatments and collected data, limited sample size and possible selection bias), that it has not been possible to establish evidence-based recommendations for prophylaxis in adults.

Hay [15] found that prophylaxis in adults offers a clinical benefit and the expenses of prophylaxis compared with on demand treatment may be balanced by days gained at work, decreased need for orthopedic surgery and improved quality of life (QoL). Another retrospective observational study conducted by Tagliaferri [16] at multiple hemophilia treatment centers in Italy, showed that the use of prophylaxis reduced the clinical orthopedic scores only in adolescents, but that adolescents and adults both experienced improvement in QoL compared with on demand therapy.

A survey of 21 European doctors about the use of prophylaxis in patients aged 16–24 years and adults over 50-year-old led by Richards et al. [17], found that 42% of 218 patients abandoned prophylaxis between the age of 16–24 years old, 30% permanently moved to on demand therapy and only 31% continued to receive prophylaxis. The results of a survey conducted in the US among HTCs and published by Walsh and Valentino [18], showed that, considering a total of 145 adult patients, prophylaxis prevents bleeding in adults with severe hemophilia A and that discontinuation of the prophylactic regimen is associated with increased bleeding episodes.

A recently published crossover prospective study [4] in adults documented a significantly reduced frequency of hemarthroses associated with secondary prophylaxis; although its results were limited by a very short follow-up (6 months), it did show a positive joint outcome and quality of life of primary/early secondary prophylaxis during adolescence and adulthood. The clinical needs emerging and the patients' prolonged life expectancy are challenging new issues for clinicians for the lack of evidence-based recommendations.

At present there are two ongoing clinical experiences and studies regarding prophylaxis in adult patients: The Trial to Evaluate the Effect of Secondary Prophylaxis With Recombinant FVIII (rFVIII) Therapy in Severe Hemophilia A Adult Subjects Compared to That of Episodic Treatment (SPINART; Clinical Trials.gov identifier: NCT00623480) and Prophylaxis vs. On-demand Therapy Through Economic Report (POTTER, NCT01159587).

SPINART was launched in March 2008. Patterned after the US JOS, the goal of this phase III study, which planned to enroll 80 participants aged 12–50 years, was to evaluate the effect of secondary prophylaxis on bleeding frequency (number of hemorrhages per year) and on joint damage (six index joints) compared with episodic treatment. The initial prophylactic regimen was rFVIII 25 IU/kg three times weekly. The dose was escalated in 5 IU/kg increments to a maximum of 35 IU/kg in patients who experience 12 or more bleeding episodes annually. MRI was to be used to evaluate joint structure of the index joints at baseline and after 3 years. The study was prematurely closed to subject enrollment on October 20, 2010.

The second trial is the Italian observational, multi-center, prospective POTTER study. This trial was launched in July 2004 (approximately 4 years before the SPINART study) [19] and enrolled, between July 2004 and September 2005, 58 patients aged 12–55 years from 11 Italian hemophilia centers. Its aim is to evaluate the efficacy (in terms of effects on bleeding, joint status and health-related quality of life [HRQoL]), safety, compliance and pharmaco-economic impact (through the evaluation of direct and indirect hemophilia-related costs) of long-term secondary prophylaxis compared to on-demand treatment in adolescent and adult severe hemophilia patients treated with rFVIII (Kogenate Bayer, Bayer Shering Pharma). The patients have been stratified according to treatment (prophylaxis 20–30 IU/kg two or three times per week vs. on-demand therapy) and age (12–25 years vs. 26–55 years). The study is closed and data analysis is planned after December 2010, when data of at least 5-year follow-up will be available for all patients. The final results of this trial, especially as regards the assessment of cost/benefit ratio, are much awaited as primary prophylaxis was introduced only recently on a large scale and there has been a reluctance for historical reasons from many physicians and patients to adopt late prophylaxis, even in the face of frequent joint bleeds [19].

The United Kingdom Hemophilia Center Doctors' Organization reviews management of this disease. In their meeting a guideline was proposed and approved by the British Committee for Standards in Hematology, for secondary prophylaxis in adults [20]. The recommendations of this group are: (1) Adolescent and adult patients with severe hemophilia should be encouraged to continue regular prophylaxis at least until they have reached physical maturity (Recommendation grade 2B). (2) In some individuals who have demonstrated a much milder phenotype, adapting formal prophylaxis to a more targeted policy may be considered but in such cases, there must be an agreed plan for monitoring and reintroducing prophylaxis if necessary (Recommendation grade 2C). (3) If significant hemarthroses occur after discontinuing prophylaxis, prophylaxis should be reinstituted to prevent joint damage and to maintain QOL, especially in situations in which bleeding interferes with education or employment (Recommendation grade 2C). (4) The dose and frequency of infusions should be adjusted, by the bleeding phenotype and, ideally, individual pharmacokinetics; the minimum amount of concentrate to prevent hemarthroses should be used irrespective of the trough levels (Recommendation grade 2C). (5) Pharmacokinetic studies may help dose adjustment and improve cost effectiveness. At a minimum, trough levels should be monitored, but more information can be obtained from half-life studies over a 48–72 h period (Recommendation grade 2C). (6) Patients on long-term prophylaxis should have their regimens critically reviewed at least every 6 months. If no break-through bleeds have occurred, a trial of dose reduction is appropriate, especially if the trough level >1 IU/dl (Recommendation grade 2D). (7) Short or long-term secondary prophylaxis should be considered in patients with advanced arthropathy if recurrent bleeding episodes significantly interfere with work or mobility (Recommendation grade 2C). (8) Long-term secondary prophylaxis is indicated following intracranial hemorrhage if no underlying cause can be corrected (Recommendation grade 2C – consensus opinion).

Conclusions

Data from both long-term prospective trials on adult prophylaxis will be available soon. The final results of the POTTER study and the rigorous data that the SPINART trial is collecting using a randomized design and the evaluation of joint status by MRI are expected to provide significant insights for addressing the numerous unresolved questions and evaluating the long-term outcome (i.e., joint status, QOL and economic impact) of secondary prophylaxis vs. episodic treatment in adult hemophiliacs.

Awaiting evidence-based recommendations on prophylaxis in adult patients, some question remain unresolved and have been well summarized by Valentino [14]: What are the benefits of secondary prophylaxis in a patient who has already developed a target joint? How can the transition from pediatric to adult care be facilitated so that patients continue to receive comprehensive hemophilia treatment throughout their lives? What are the risks and benefits of prophylaxis in and adults with cardiovascular risk factor? It is expected the two trials mentioned above will help to answer these questions.

References

1. Manco-Johnson MJ, Abshire TC, Shapiro AD, Riske B, Hacker MR, Kilcoyne R, et al. Prophylaxis versus episodic treatment to prevent joint disease in boys with severe hemophilia. N Engl J Med. 2007;357:535–44.
2. Chambost H, Ljung R. Changing pattern of care of boys with haemophilia in western European centres. Haemophilia. 2005;11:92–9.
3. Petrini P, Lindvall N, Egberg N, Blomback M. Prophylaxis with factor concentrates in preventing hemophilic arthropathy. Am J Pediatr Hematol Oncol. 1991;13:280–7.
4. Collins P, Faradji A, Morfini M, Enriquez MM, Schwartz L. Efficacy and safety of secondary prophylactic vs. on-demand sucrose-formulated recombinant factor VIII treatment in adults with severe hemophilia A: results from a 13-month crossover study. J Thromb Haemost. 2010;8:83–9.
5. Berntorp E, Boulyjenkov V, Brettler D, Chandy M, Jones P, Lee C, et al. Modern treatment of haemophilia. Bull World Health Organ. 1995;73:691–701.
6. Fischer K, Van Der Bom JG, Prejs R, Mauser-Bunschoten EP, Roosendaal G, Grobbee DE, et al. Discontinuation of prophylactic therapy in severe haemophilia: incidence and effects on outcome. Haemophilia. 2001;7:544–50.
7. Lofqvist T, Nilsson IM, Berntorp E, Pettersson H. Haemophilia prophylaxis in young patients–a long-term follow-up. J Intern Med. 1997;241:395–400.
8. Nilsson IM, Berntorp E, Lofqvist T, Pettersson H. Twenty-five years' experience of prophylactic treatment in severe haemophilia A and B. J Intern Med. 1992;232:25–32.
9. Berntorp E, Astermark J, Bjorkman S, Blanchette VS, Fischer K, Giangrande PL, et al. Consensus perspectives on prophylactic therapy for haemophilia: summary statement. Haemophilia. 2003;9 (Suppl 1):1–4.
10. Berntorp E. Prophylactic therapy for haemophilia: early experience. Haemophilia. 2003;9 (Suppl 1):5–9; discussion.
11. Petrini P, Seuser A. Haemophilia care in adolescents – compliance and lifestyle issues. Haemophilia. 2009;15 (Suppl 1):15–9.
12. Dolan G, Hermans C, Klamroth R, Madhok R, Schutgens RE, Spengler U. Challenges and controversies in haemophilia care in adulthood. Haemophilia. 2009;15 (Suppl 1):20–7.
13. Darby SC, Kan SW, Spooner RJ, Giangrande PL, Hill FG, Hay CR, et al. Mortality rates, life expectancy, and causes of death in people with hemophilia A or B in the United Kingdom who were not infected with HIV. Blood. 2007;110:815–25.
14. Valentino LA. Controversies regarding the prophylactic management of adults with severe haemophilia A. Haemophilia. 2009;15 (Suppl 2):5-18, quiz 9–22.
15. Hay CR. Prophylaxis in adults with haemophilia. Haemophilia. 2007;13 (Suppl 2):10–5.
16. Tagliaferri A, Franchini M, Coppola A, Rivolta GF, Santoro C, Rossetti G, et al. Effects of secondary prophylaxis started in adolescent and adult haemophiliacs. Haemophilia. 2008;14:945–51.
17. Richards M, Altisent C, Batorova A, Chambost H, Dolan G, de Moerloose P, et al. Should prophylaxis be used in adolescent and adult patients with severe haemophilia? An European survey of practice and outcome data. Haemophilia. 2007;13:473–9.
18. Walsh CE, Valentino LA. Factor VIII prophylaxis for adult patients with severe haemophilia A: results of a US survey of attitudes and practices. Haemophilia. 2009;15:1014–21.
19. Tagliaferri A. Awaiting evidence-based recommendations on prophylaxis in adult patients. Haemophilia. 2010;16:955–6.
20. Richards M, Williams M, Chalmers E, Liesner R, Collins P, Vidler V, et al. A United Kingdom Haemophilia Centre Doctors' Organization guideline approved by the British Committee for Standards in Haematology: guideline on the use of prophylactic factor VIII concentrate in children and adults with severe haemophilia A. Br J Haematol. 2010;149:498–507.

7 The Economics of Prophylaxis: Does Prophylaxis with Clotting Factor Represent Value for Money?

Alec Miners

London School of Hygiene and Tropical Medicine, London, UK

Introduction

The mainstay of treatment for people with severe (<1 iu/dl) hemophilia is replacement therapy with an appropriate clotting factor. Evidence suggests that the most clinically effective treatment is prophylaxis [1–3]. That is, treatment given to prevent bleeding episodes and associated complications in the first instance. Prophylaxis is usually defined as being "primary", initiated before the onset of serial bleeding, or "secondary" [4], when treatment is started sometime after this process has begun. The main alternative to prophylaxis is to treat people "on-demand", after a hemorrhage [5]. However, the clear clinical limitation of this approach is that bleeding and the associated sequelae are allowed to occur in this first place meaning it is associated with decreased levels of health-related quality-of-life and an increase in the rate of corrective surgical procedures [6,7].

Despite the lack of randomized controlled evidence, few would question that (primary) prophylaxis is the treatment of clinical choice. However, the main limitation of this approach is that it is costly to provide. Exact costs of treatment are difficult to estimate, because prices vary by country as to policies regarding infusion regimens, and treatment is largely determined by bodyweight – but a realistic estimate of a lifetime cost is in the region of £6 million per person [8].

Despite this, the provision of costly treatments is justified on economic grounds if they also generate proportional increases in (health) benefits. A health economic perspective emphasizes not only the cost of treatment, but also the return it yields, in this instance "health". Another way of saying this is that expenditures on costly treatments are justified if their provision represents 'value for money' or if they are considered to be "cost-effective" [9].

Economics

Economics as a discipline is concerned with the allocation of resources (land, labor and capital) given that demand for them outstrips their supply; resources are said to be finite and therefore scarce. It emphasizes the notion of "opportunity cost", that is, if one person receives resources (or a treatment) in effect, treatment is being denied to someone else. In a market situation, the interaction of those who demand health care and those who supply it, would determine how much of a good is purchased and at what price. Thus, in this instance, the market would be responsible for resource allocation. However, the provision of health care is rarely, if ever, left entirely to the market – governments usually intervene to some degree, typically for reasons of equity and because the provision of health care does not satisfy the criteria for markets to function efficiently and therefore to produce optimal results. In these instances, allocative decisions are no longer left to the market, instead some other method is required to estimate the costs and benefits of treatment in order for nominated decision makers to determine what to purchase [10].

Economic evaluations are designed to generate this information. A "full" evaluation compares the costs and benefits of two or more interventions, such as treatment on-demand and prophylaxis. There are a number of different forms of evaluation [9]. They are all similar with respect to the way that treatment costs are incorporated. However, they differ with respect to how health outcomes are measured and valued. In a cost-minimization analysis (CMA), health outcomes are assumed to be equivalent. Or at least, to use this form of analysis, there should be good evidence that competing technologies produce identical outcomes. When this condition is satisfied, the most cost-effective option is simply the least costly. In a cost-effectiveness analysis (CEA), health outcomes are measured but there is no attempt to place a value on them within the analysis itself. The chosen outcome measure is often disease specific, but can be more general such as "life-years gained". For example, existing CEAs of prophylaxis have typically used "(joint) hemorrhage prevented" as an outcome measure. The main limitation with CEAs is that they do not, or rarely, permit the cost-effectiveness of different treatments to be compared across different clinical settings because of the use of disease specific outcomes. Moreover, often treatments have an effect on more than one outcome. In this case of prophylaxis, this could be "bleeding frequency" but also say for example, "pain-free days". Thus this form of analysis is arguably limited. Having said this, it should be noted that at least one national health care reimbursement agency promotes the use of CEAs over other forms of analysis and also the concept of disease specific outcome measures [11].

Cost-utility analysis

Cost-utility analysis (CUAs) measure and value health benefits in terms of quality-adjusted life-year (QALYs). QALYs combine information on length of life with health-related quality-of-life, where the latter is expressed as a "utility". In many respects this form of analysis has come about because of limitations with the CEA approach [12]. A utility value of 0 is taken to be equivalent to death, whereas a value of 1 is taken to equal perfect health and represents a maximum value. All other states of health are measured on this scale, typically between 0 and 1, but negative values are also possible, indicating that a state of health is valued as being worse than death. One QALY is equivalent to 1 year in perfect health (1 year multiplied a utility value of 1).

The statistic that has been traditionally produced through a CUA, is referred to as an "incremental cost-effectiveness ratio" (ICER). An ICER is calculated by dividing differences in QALYs by differences in costs [9].

$$ICER = \frac{Cost\ B - Cost\ A}{QALYs\ B - QALYs\ A}$$

Where Costs/QALYs A and B represent the mean costs and QALYs associated with treatments A and B. The resulting statistic can be read as meaning it costs £x to gain one additional year of perfect health.

In theory all states of health, and all technologies can be valued using this QALY paradigm, meaning that their relative costs and benefits can be compared. The implication of this approach is that funds should be directed towards those technologies that are associated with relatively low ICERs (i.e. those that are most cost-effective) and away from those technologies that are relatively less cost-effective (i.e. are associated with relatively high ICERs).

CUAs are perhaps the most common form of published economic evaluation. However, not everyone agrees with the idea of condensing all aspects of "health" into a single index, and as a

form of analysis [13], it is limited to only incorporating issues that are strictly related to health – as QALYs are a product of evidence on mortality and morbidity. Cost benefit-analysis (CBA), on the other hand, measures and values benefits in terms of money. At first glance this might appear to be strange and possibly unethical – for example placing a monetary value on a person's life. However, if money is viewed merely as a means of exchange (and therefore relative value), perhaps such objections are lessened. The main advantage of a CBA is that it can consider non health issues such as process of care for example waiting times, privacy or even perhaps access related issues. However, while CBAs are perhaps the widest form of economic evaluation in terms of incorporating health and non-health benefits, the methods of application are relatively complex and studies have shown that different methods produce different results. Relatively few CBA can be found in the health literature, although in areas such as transport economics, they are common place [10].

Economic evaluation

There is no single standard template for performing an economic evaluation. However, there are arguably fairly well-accepted ideas with respect to good practice both in terms of design and the reporting of methods and results [10,14]. They include:
• A clear statement and description of the decision problem (the treatments to be compared, how they are used, who is to receive them, when treatment should be started and stopped etc).
• A relevant time horizon. Some would argue that all costs and benefits of treatment should be considered. In the context of prophylaxis this could be taken to mean a lifetime horizon [15]. However, there is a view that the relevant time horizon is the financial budget constraint faced by the decision maker [11].
• A clear description of the resources consumed and their associated unit costs.
• A clear statement of the perspective. For example, if the analysis was performed from a 'societal' perspective the analysis would include all health care and indirect costs such as time absent from work due to illness.
• A clear description of how the relative effectiveness of the treatments was estimated. Typically this evidence is taken/derived from RCT evidence, but in the case of treatments for hemophilia, this is not so straight forward.
• A clear description of the underlying framework. Economic evaluations are sometimes based on the results of RCTs, as they are considered to generate least biased estimates of treatment effect. However, it is common place for evaluations to be based on decision modeling techniques. There are many reasons why this might be the case, but in the context of hemophilia suitable RCTs will never exist and there is a need to extrapolate the results to the longer term [16].
• Presentation and discussion of a base case ICER.
• An assessment of the uncertainty surrounding the results, typically through a series of sensitivity analysis.

Economic evaluations of prophylaxis in severe hemophilia

A non-systematic review of the Medline, Embase and PubMed databases in September 2010 suggests that 9 economic evaluations of prophylaxis with clotting factor VIII or XI for the treatment of severe hemophilia have been published. The first study was published in 1996 and the most recent in 2009. Four studies used a CUA framework, three were CEAs, one was a CBA and one was a CMA (Table 7.1).

The results, taken at face value, are confusing from a policy perspective as they are very different and could lead to different conclusions. Everything from prophylaxis being "dominant" (that is, less costly and more effective) compared with treatment on demand to prophylaxis being associated with an ICER of over €1 million per additional QALY. It is difficult to say exactly where any threshold/acceptable ICER lies, but as something of a benchmark, it is worth noting that the UK's National Institute for Health and Clinical Excellence broadly considers any ICER per additional QALY above £20,000 to £30,000 to indicate that a treatment is not cost-effective and as a consequence should not be available to patients who require treatment on the National Health Service [15]. However, it is clear that such a broad array of results mean

that it is difficult to know whether prophylaxis is cost-effective or not.

To understand why the studies report such seemingly different results, each needs to be critically appraised. A formal critical appraisal has not been undertaken in this text, rather important elements of any economic evaluation have been focused upon (see Table 7.1).

The CMA by Bohn et al. [17] was based on data from the non-randomized Orthopaedic Outcomes Study [18]. It examined both health care costs such as clotting factor use and indirect costs such as time absent from paid employment. Individuals were stratified according to one of three treatment groups, according to how long they had received prophylaxis: 0–5 weeks (no prophylaxis), 6–45 weeks (partial prophylaxis) or greater than 46 (full-time prophylaxis) weeks per year respectively. The results from the analysis showed that the costs of clotting factor provision accounted for $USD30,800 PPY [per patient year], $USD79,600 PPY and $USD87,900 PPY for individuals receiving no, partial or fulltime prophylaxis respectively. Irrespective of the quality of the underlying clinical study, it is difficult interpret these results as they give no indication of "value" as no attempt was made to link differences in costs with differences in outcomes.

Three CEAs have been published in which health outcomes were expressed in terms of (joint) hemorrhages averted [19–21].

Table 7.1 Key study attributes

Author	Treatments	Evaluation form	Perspective	Time horizon	Discount rates	FVIII per iu	Base case ICER
Smith 1996 [20]	2^0 proph (?) vs. OD	CEA	Societal	Up to 50 years	Costs 5?% Benefits 0?%	$0.53	USD1,100–1,3800 per bleed averted
Szucs 1996 [21]	2^0 proph (?) vs. OD	CEA	Societal	1 year	N/A	N/S	DM 2,800 per averted joint bleed
Bohn 1998 [17]	1^0 and 2^0 proph (?) vs. OD	CMA	Societal	?	N/S	N/S	USD30,800 PPY OD, $USD79,600 PPY partial prophylaxis; $USD87,900 full-time prophylaxis
Miners 1998 [19]	2^0 proph vs. OD	CEA	Health care	9 years	Costs 6% Benefits 0%	N/S	£550 per bleed averted
Miners 2002 [8]	1^0 proph vs. OD	CUA	Societal	Lifetime	Costs 6% Benefits 1.5%	£0.325	£46,500 per QALY gained
Steen Carlsson 2004 [25]	Proph vs. OD	CBA	?	1 year (?)	N/A	?	Greater expected net benefit with prophylaxis than OD
Lippert 2005 [24]	2^0 proph (?) vs. OD	CUA	Health care	1 year	N/A	€0.7–0.9	Results range from OD being dominant to >€1 million per additional QALY for prophylaxis
Risebrough 2008 [23]	1^0 prop (different dosing schedules) vs. OD	CUA	Societal	5 years	Costs 3% benefits 3%	CAN $1.38	EscDose vs. OD demand $543,000 per QALY gained; Prophylaxis vs. EscDose >$1m per QALY gained
Miners 2009 [22]	1^0 prop vs. OD	CUA	Health care	Lifetime	Costs 3.5% Benefits 3.5%	£0.325	£38,500 per QALY gained

?, unclear; N/S, not stated, N/A, not applicable; 1^0 proph, primary prophylaxis; 2^0 proph, secondary prophylaxis; OD, on-demand; "Societal" indicates both health care costs and productivity losses; ICER; incremental cost-effectiveness ratio.

Given general good practice when conducting an economic evaluation, the study by Smith et al. is arguably the most complete as it attempts to consider the longer term (indeed lifetime) costs and health outcomes associated with prophylaxis. The studies by Szucs and Miners are arguably of poorer quality in comparison, particularly with respect to using shorter time horizons and the underlying clinical studies assessing treatment outcome. For example, the clinical study by Szucs is non-randomized and cross-sectional meaning it is difficult to link outcomes with specific treatments.

Irrespective of design, the results broadly suggest a maximum of USD1,400 to prevent an additional hemorrhage. However, in many respects this figure highlights the limitations with the CEA approach. That is, while it appears prophylaxis costs more than treatment on-demand, what society is willing to pay to prevent a hemorrhage (i.e. the threshold value) is known. Unless it is known with some degree of accuracy (is it USD1,000, USD10,000 or USD100,000?) the results remain largely uninterpretable from a policy perspective.

Three [8,22,23] of the four [24] CUAs were in some sense similar in design in so much that they are based on decision modeling techniques and consider a treatment for longer than a year treatment horizon. Although it should be noted that the 2009 UK-based evaluation by Miners is essentially an update of the 2002 publication.

The Risebrough et al. study reported the results a Canadian CUA of primary prophylaxis in children with severe (<2% iu) hemophilia A from a societal perspective. The evaluation was based on a Markov model with a time horizon of 6 years, from ages 1 to 6. Three different treatment regimens were evaluated: standard prophylaxis (25 iu/kg every other day), EscDose (prophylaxis with 50 iu/kg once a week, increasing to a maximum of 25 iu/kg every other day if patients continued to experience 3–4 bleeding episodes per quarter) and treatment on-demand (40 iu/kg upon presentation of bleeding and 20 iu/kg on days 1 and 3 after the hemorrhage). Future costs and QALYs were discounted at 3% per annum and the base case clotting factor cost was CAN $1.38. The models by Miners also used a Markov modeling approach to assess the cost-effectiveness of treating people with severe (<1 iu/dl) hemophilia A with primary prophylaxis for severe hemophilia A where treatment was designed to prevent clotting factor levels from falling below 1 iu/dl at all times. The base-case perspective was the UK NHS. The model covered the period from the start of treatment at an age of 1 year until the patient's death using a clotting factor. The model used data from a number of different sources, and where suitable data for certain parameters was absent it made a number of assumptions. Perhaps the most important of these assumptions was that patients treated with primary prophylaxis either experienced a level of health-related quality of life (HR-QoL) that was similar to the general UK population as a methods of estimating the long term outcomes of treatment in the absence of any other suitable data.

The fourth CUA [24] assessed the cost-effectiveness of (secondary) prophylaxis versus treatment on-demand for people with severe (<1 iu/dl) hemophilia A and B, over a 1-year time horizon, from a health care perspective. A combination of cross-sectional and 6 month retrospective data was collected from a number of European treatment centers Europe. Patients were classified as receiving prophylaxis if they had received treatment with prophylaxis 2–3 times per week for at least 6 months. Resource use data were collected retrospectively whereas utilities were estimated using the MOS SF-36 in a cross-sectional study. Few other methodological details are provided.

The CBA by Steen Carlsson is the only study to clearly conclude that prophylaxis is cost saving compared with treatment on-demand. The study concludes that per Swedish tax-payer, it costs €1.97 for treatment on-demand and €5.56 for prophylaxis, and compared to estimated willingness to pay estimates, both treatments results in positive net benefits (for on-demand €39–€1.97 and €65–€5.56 for prophylaxis). Moreover, that the overall net benefit is higher for prophylaxis compared with treatment on-demand. However, the robustness of this result is reliant on accepting that the utilized CBA methodology is sound. Traditionally in costs benefit analysis mean benefits are subtracted from mean costs. With positive net benefits indicating a treatment is "worthwhile". However, in this analysis the total costs attributable to treating all severe hemophilia patients (in Sweden) appear to have been divided by the national general population to calculate a "cost per taxpayer". Monetary benefits subtracted from this figure, on the other hand, were based on more standard willingness to pay techniques in so much that a mean willingness to pay per patient.

Why do the results differ so much?

It is difficult to be precise about why the results differ so markedly, but some likely reasons are listed below:
- The analyses use a variety of different economic forms and utilize different outcomes. Therefore it is debatable as to whether they should be compared together in the first instance.
- Even those analysis that do use identical forms (e.g. the CUAs) are based on very different structural frameworks (decision models) and derive their estimate of treatment effects from different sources.
- It is clear from the results that the ICER is very sensitive to small changes in the incremental benefits, meaning that small changes in this amount results in proportionally large changes to the ICER.
- Nearly all of the evaluations suggest that at least 90% of the total costs of treatment are attributable to the cost of clotting factor provision alone. Thus, the results are very sensitive to the underlying clotting factor cost, which vary remarkably across the studies (see Table 7.1).
- This also means that savings in indirect costs are unlikely to have much bearing on the cost-effective of treatment.
- The results are very sensitive to the rates which future health benefit are discounted, higher rates tend to result in less favorable ICERs in terms of promoting the use of prophylaxis.

- In all but a few studies, it is unclear how prophylaxis has been used. That is, frequency of treatment and size of each infusion. Moreover, in some studies it is even unclear whether treatment is primary or secondary. Thus, even if the studies were considered to be of good "technical" quality, it is unclear what has been evaluated.
- The results from the CEAs have been derived from relatively low quality clinical studies and because their results are expressed in terms of a cost per (joint) hemorrhage prevented, their results are difficult to interpret.
- Only the CBA clearly concludes prophylaxis is cost-effective compared with treatment on-demand, but the robustness of the underlying methodology is questionable.

Conclusions

All of the reviewed studies contain methodological weaknesses but some were considered to be weaker than others, especially those that relied purely on either cross-sectional or short-term retrospective data. Some differences between study results should rightly be expected as they implicitly or explicitly analyse different decision problems (e.g. primary compared with secondary prophylaxis, or different infusion schedules) and different (national) decision making bodies have different methodological requirements.

Only one study clearly concluded that prophylaxis was cost-effective compared with treatment on-demand, but the methods used to undertake the study are questionable. The results from the CUAs are variable, but even the most favorable results reported by Miners et al. suggest primary prophylaxis is unlikely to be cost-effective at conventional willingness to pay thresholds [15]. However, it is clear that reductions in the unit clotting factor dramatically improve the cost-effectiveness of treatment and future studies attempting to pin down exact differences between the modes of therapy in terms of health-related quality-of-life could result in dramatically different cost-effectiveness results.

References

1. Nilsson, I.M., et al., Prophylactic treatment of severe hemophilia A and B can prevent joint disability. Seminars in Hematology, 1994;31 (Suppl 2)(2): p. 5–9.
2. Nilsson, I.M., et al., Twenty-five years' experience of prophylactic treatment in severe haemophilia A and B. Journal of Internal Medicine, 1992;232(1): p. 25–32.
3. Manco-Johnson, M.J., et al., Prophylaxis versus Episodic Treatment to Prevent Joint Disease in Boys with Severe Hemophilia. N Engl J Med, 2007;357(6): p. 535–544.
4. Manco-Johnson, M.J., et al., Results of secondary prophylaxis in children with severe hemophilia. American Journal of Hematology, 1994;47(2): p. 113–117.
5. Allain, J.P., Dose requirement for replacement therapy in hemophilia A. Thrombosis & Haemostasis, 1979;42(3): p. 825–831.
6. Miners, A.H., et al., Assessing health-related quality-of-life in individuals with haemophilia. Haemophilia, 1999;5: p. 378–385.
7. Miners, A.H., et al., Primary prophylaxis for individuals with severe haemophilia: how many hospital visits could treatment prevent? Journal of Internal Medicine, 2000;247: p. 493–499.
8. Miners, A.H., et al., A cost-utility analysis of primary prophylaxis versus treatment on-demand for individuals with severe haemophilia. PharmacoEconomics, 2002;20(11): p. 759–774.
9. Drummond, M.F., et al., Methods for the economic evaluation of health care programmes. 3rd ed. 2005, Oxford: Oxford University Press, England.
10. Morris, S., N. Devlin, and D. Parkin, Economic analysis in health care. 2007, Chichester: John Wiley and Sons.
11. Institute for Quality and Efficiency in Health Care. General Methods for the Assessment of the Relation of Benefits to Costsv 1.0. 2009 [02/09/10]; Available from: http://www.iqwig.de/download/General_Methods_for_the_Assessment_of_the_Relation_of_Benefits_to_Costs.pdf.
12. Williams, A., Economics of coronary artery bypass grafting. British Medical Journal Clinical Research Ed, 1985;291(6491): p. 326–329.
13. Birch, S. and A. Gafni, Cost effectiveness/utility analyses. Do current decision rules lead us to where we want to be? Journal of Health Economics, 1992;11: p. 279–296.
14. Drummond, M.F. and T.O. Jefferson, Guidelines for authors and peer reviewers of economic submissions to the BMJ. The BMJ Economic Evaluation Working Party. BMJ, 1996;313(7052): p. 275–283.
15. National Institute for Health and Clinical Excellence. Guide to the methods of technology appraisal. 2008 [01/07/08]; Available from: http://www.nice.org.uk/niceMedia/pdf/TAP_Methods.pdf.
16. Buxton, M.J., et al., Modelling in economic evaluation: an unavoidable fact of life. Health Economics, 1997;6(3): p. 217–227.
17. Bohn, R.L., et al., Prophylactic use of factor VIII: an economic evaluation. Thrombosis & Haemostasis, 1998;79(5): p. 932–937.
18. Aledort, L.M., R.H. Haschmeyer, and H. Pettersson, A longitudinal study of orthopaedic outcomes for severe factor-VIII-deficient haemophiliacs. The Orthopaedic Outcome Study Group. Journal of Internal Medicine, 1994;236(4): p. 391–399.
19. Miners, A.H., et al., Assessing the effectiveness and cost-effectiveness of prophylaxis against bleeding in patients with severe haemophilia and severe von Willebrand's disease. Journal of Internal Medicine, 1998;244(6): p. 515–522.
20. Smith, P.S., et al., Episodic versus prophylactic infusions for hemophilia A: a cost-effectiveness analysis. Journal of Pediatrics, 1996;129(3): p. 424–431.
21. Szucs, T.D., A. Offner, and W. Schramm, Socioeconomic impact of haemophilia care: results of a pilot study. Haemophilia, 1996;2: p. 211–217.
22. Miners, A., Revisiting the cost-effectiveness of primary prophylaxis with clotting factor for the treatment of severe haemophilia A. Haemophilia, 2009;15(4): p. 881–887.
23. Risebrough, N.A., et al., Cost-utility analysis of Canadian tailored prophylaxis, primary prophylaxis and on-demand therapy in young children with severe haemophilia A. Haemophilia, 2008;14: p. 743–752.
24. Lippert, B., et al., Cost effectiveness of haemophilia treatment: A cross-national assessment. Blood Coagulation and Fibrinolysis, 2005;16(7): p. 477–485.
25. Steen Carlsson, K., et al., Willingness to pay for on-demand and prophylactic treatment for severe haemophilia in Sweden. Haemophilia, 2004;10(5): p. 527–541.

8 The Transition of Care for the Young Adult Hemophilia Patient

Pia Petrini

Karolinska University Hospital, Stockholm, Sweden

Introduction

Adolescence is a time of rapid physical, social and cognitive development which occurs during the transition from childhood to adulthood, usually between the ages of 10 and 24 years. Whereas the physical aspects of maturation are striking and well-characterized in early adolescence, it is not always appreciated that equally important changes are occurring in psychosocial domains throughout the adolescent and young adult years.

This is a challenging time for any teenager and even more so for those with a chronic disease. For them it is often harder to break family ties, harder to feel accepted by their peer group and to be realistic about their future.

An increasing number of young people with chronic illness or disability originating in childhood survive to adulthood and ultimately these young people need transition to adult care. Transition medicine is defined as the deliberate, coordinated process of moving a patient from pediatric-oriented health care to adult-oriented health care with the goal of optimizing the young adult's ability to assume adult roles and function.

Barriers to successful transition are unwillingness of pediatric-oriented providers and parents to "let go" of the young adults, and lack of training for adult-oriented providers to care for the non-adherent patient. Also, in many countries there are difficulties with funding and maintenance insurance for adult patients.

Recent efforts have focused on broadening the scope of health care transition from simply the transfer of care between pediatric and adult medicine to a guided educational and therapeutic process. Despite this, there is a paucity of data describing timing, barriers, and outcomes of transition.

Physical development at puberty

Puberty is a critical period of development. The physical changes of the boy precede and are necessary for the start of psychosocial maturation in adolescence. Psychosocial maturation is a slow process usually taking twice the time of physical development (Figure 8.1 [1]).

Male puberty is characterized by a huge variation between healthy individuals. The average time schedule of male pubertal development is entirely different from that of females. In girls puberty and growth spurt proceed and continue in a parallel fashion. On average boy puberty starts almost 2 years later and the maximum growth spurt in body height starts even later at mid-puberty, which is 3–3.5 years later than in girls (Figure 8.2). At this age (13–14 years) the developmental differences are the greatest between girls and boys and also between boys.

A delayed start of puberty is common in boys in contrast to girls. Duration of pubertal development may also vary from 2–5 years. Knowledge about variations in normal puberty in males is crucial to be able to give support during this demanding time when most boys are concerned about their current body image and peer acceptance.

Psychological maturation in adolescents

Psychological maturation in adolescents can be defined as a process of adaptation between the ages of 12 and 22 years. The developmental tasks of adolescence include emotional separation from parents and establishment of autonomy. Peers have a central role in building up the personality.

Current and Future Issues in Hemophilia Care, First Edition. Edited by Emérito-Carlos Rodríguez-Merchán and Leonard A. Valentino.
© 2011 John Wiley & Sons, Ltd. Published 2011 by Blackwell Publishing Ltd.

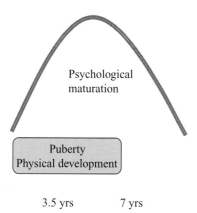

3.5 yrs   7 yrs

Figure 8.1 Schematic presentation of the average duration and interrelation of pubertal development and psychological maturation. (Reproduced with permission from Martti A. Siimes, Veikko Aalberg & Pia Petrini: Boys with haemophilia. Physical and psychosocial development at and after puberty. Nemo, 2006.)

A unique phenomenon of adolescence is the simultaneous psychosocial progression and regression (Figure 8.3). The phenomenon culminates during mid-puberty. During regression childlike features are again emphasized; the use of language changes and academic performance at school often deteriorates. Clashes with parents and other authority figures are common. In contrast basic intellectual abilities reach adult levels around age 16, long before the process of psychosocial maturation is completed.

Risk taking and novelty seeking are hallmarks of typical adolescent behavior. Adolescents seek new experiences and higher levels of rewarding stimulation, and often engage in risky behaviors, without considering future outcomes or consequences. Indeed, the risk of injury or death is higher during the adolescent period than in childhood or adulthood, and the incidence of depression, anxiety, drug use and addiction, and eating disorders increases [2].

Brain research has recently found that different parts of the brain mature at different times, resulting for several years in a functional imbalance between rational cognitive abilities and emotional forces on the one hand and less mature and less effective prefrontal executive functions on the other. The frontal lobes

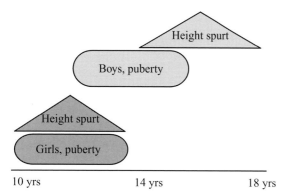

10 yrs   14 yrs   18 yrs

Figure 8.2 Timetable of puberty and growth spurt in height in an average girl and boy. (Reproduced with permission from Martti A. Siimes, Veikko Aalberg & Pia Petrini: Boys with haemophilia. Physical and psychosocial development at and after puberty. Nemo, 2006.)

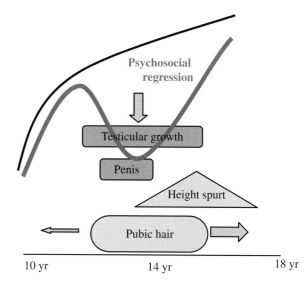

10 yr   14 yr   18 yr

Figure 8.3 Psychosocial development. (Reproduced with permission from Martti A. Siimes, Veikko Aalberg & Pia Petrini: Boys with haemophilia. Physical and psychosocial development at and after puberty. Nemo, 2006.)

where the control system is located reaches maturation at about 20 years of age, several years later than the rest of the brain [3].

Issues affecting adolescents and young adults with hemophilia

Teens with hemophilia face all of the usual challenges of adolescence, but their life-long bleeding disorder can result in additional issues. Most pediatric services will be very aware of the challenges adolescents bring and staff will have noticed a change from attentive child to provocative teenager. Before this time, from preschool years children should been spoken to directly about their treatment, and as they get older there is a greater emphasis and expectation that they will be knowledgeable about their condition and ideally take increasing responsibility for their own care. Parents also must be supported to gradually devolve to there child responsibilities for decision-making and for taking prescribed medications [4].

A Scandinavian survey in young men with severe and moderate hemophilia showed that the average age for a patient to take over responsibility for their treatment was 14 years, but 25% required parental assistance in hemophilia-related care until a mean age of 17.2 years. A majority (68%) treated bleeding immediately and 60% used extra infusions when needed. Thus one-third of them put themselves at risk for complications by an unwillingness to recognize the need for treatment. Over 40% had at some time failed to follow the treatment regimen [10].

A global survey from 147 hemophilia treatment centers showed a significant decrease in perceived level of adherence to prophylaxis from 90% being very high or high in children up to 12 years of age to 54% in adolescents 13–18 years (Figure 8.4 [11]). Poor compliance with hemophilia therapy during adolescence in combination

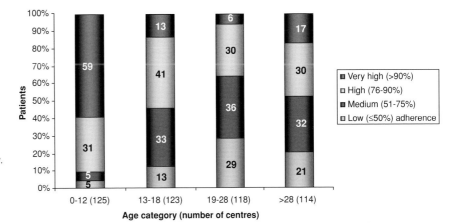

Figure 8.4 Adherence to prophylaxis by age category. Estimated by nurses in a global survey of 147 centers. (Reproduced from Geraghty S, et al. Practice pattern in haemophilia A therapy – global progress towards optimal care. Haemophilia, 2006;12(1):75–81.)

with risky behaviors, may result in serious and recurrent bleeding episodes with impact on future outcomes. The teenager may for the first time question their medical regimen and be ashamed of the diagnosis.

Normal adolescent development is characterized by experimentation, inconstant behavior and a sense of invincibility. Thus long-term health outcomes promoted by clinical staff can have very little relevance when young people are more concerned about their current body image and peer acceptance. It is hardly surprising that adherence reaches its lowest point in adolescence.

Teenagers may not perceive prevention of potential future joint disease as a high priority, but tend to focus on the present. As short-term goals are more likely to be perceived as relevant, substitution therapy to prevent bleeding episodes that interfere with daily activities is often are more acceptable by the maturing adolescent. Even daily infusions of factor concentrate can be accepted by young men who wish to participate in regular and frequent sporting activities [9]. This treatment regimen has been shown to be cost-effective. Physical activity should be encouraged for all adolescents. Participation in sporting activities has been shown to result in positive self-esteem and enhance social adaptation. Better coordination and strength can reduce joint bleeding in persons with hemophilia [12,17]. The increasing problem with obesity in the young generation may increase the problems with arthropathy in adults with hemophilia [13].

During these adolescent years, prophylactic treatment is individualized to patients' bleeding pattern and lifestyle. Caregivers can support adherence by education, encouragement, and by providing positive feedback to the patient. The perception that treatment is a normal part of life is shown to increase adherence to therapy in adolescents [18].

Transition from pediatric to adult-orientated care for adolescents

Arranging efficient and caring transfer for adolescents from pediatric to adult care is one of the great challenges facing physicians caring for pediatric patients with hemophilia. The transfer

of young people, particularly those with special health care needs, from child to adult services requires specific attention. Health transition is one part of the wider transition from dependent child to independent adult. The greatest barrier to effective transition arises from the inability of pediatric professionals and parents to "let go" and trust the independence of the adolescent and the skills of the adult services. Obstacles to successful transition may also arise from adolescents themselves, or their parents, if they feel excluded from all decision-making in the new setting. Transition is a process not an event. Caregivers in the pediatric center must be able to take the time to communicate and listen in a nonjudgemental way and respect privacy and confidentiality [5,6,14].

Young people should be helped to take responsibility for medications from as early an age as possible, and should be seen by themselves during clinic visits during their teenage years (with parents invited to join the session later). A schedule of likely timing and events should be given to young people in early adolescence. Transition guidelines such as those published by the Medical and Scientific Advisory Committee (MASAC) of the National Hemophilia Foundation can be very helpful (Table 8.1). Support from peers with hemophilia during camps and meetings are of utter importance and the Internet can be used for information and communication [8,15].

Transition programs are necessary even when pediatric and adult services are in the same hospital, as geographical closeness often does not translate into a close professional relationship. A joint pediatric–adult clinic is very useful to introduce adolescents to adult physicians and to hand over clinical issues. Joint clinics between pediatric and adult health-care teams can improve the transfer and help young people to communicate with the new team [7].

Poor transition processes can have a significantly negative effect on morbidity and mortality in young adults. Patients may be "lost in transition". For example, Kipps et al. described that attendance of young people at four diabetes services averaged 94% before transfer to an adult clinic, but fell to 57% 2 years after transfer [16]. Adult hemophilia care teams usually have a high level of medical expertise but may be unprepared for the non-adherence with treatment seen in adolescents. Particularly in diseases such as hemophilia, young people with few complications may get little

Table 8.1 Example of checklist items from Medical and Scientific Advisory Committee (MASAC) Guidelines for Transition of People with Bleeding Disorders: Transition guidelines for 16–18 year olds In the category of 'Self Advocacy and Self Esteem'.

Transition Guidelines for 6–18 year olds for self-advocacy and self-esteem

Goals and objectives	Strategies
Young adult expresses medical, physical and social needs to others	Discuss bleeding disorder/impact on daily living and plans fo future
	Young adult should demonstrate knowledge of physical abilities
	Self-infusion, documentation and interaction with staff expected
Young adult will be able to advocate and negotiate for health care	Ensure young adult has *skills* to negotiate needs (travel letter, E.R. care, P.T. referral)
Young adult understands rights and responsibilities for health care	Discuss what is expected of the young adult and what can be expected from the health care staff
	Continue discussion re: problems with peers or awkward situations (i.e. infusions at school)
Young adult seeks information/services to ensure ongoing health	Discuss educational support (regional, NHF, WFH, Internet)
Young adult understands utilization of the adult health care system	Discuss plans for transition to adult care (primary care/bleeding disorder care). Provide written material as needed
	HTC staff should facilitate introductory visit Paediatric staff support may be offered for the first few months of transition

(Reproduced from Breakey VR, et al. Towards comprehensive care in transition for young people with haemophilia. Haemophilia 2010;1–10.)

attention from the adult team, who focus their time on older patients with more complications. Appropriate time has to be given to the young patient and his parents to build confidence between them and the new team.

There are several ways of effecting this transfer of care. None of them is proven to be better than any other, but the transfer should always be planned and expected by the patient and the parents.

Future work will include research evaluating models of adolescent support, evaluating and refining the transition checklist and ensuring that the time is right for each individual. International research on adherence and results from different treatment strategies on both sides of the transition gap has to be promoted.

Conclusions

Adolescence is a time of major physical and psychological changes. Young teenagers need to move towards independence and for

people with hemophilia this includes achieving self-management, maintaining adherence to therapy and coping with the impact of hemophilia on lifestyle. The combination of lack of compliance and the risk taking lifestyle typical during these years may result in severe and even life-threatening bleeding symptoms. The challenges faced by the adolescent should be addressed in the years before transition. Arranging efficient end caring transfer for young people with hemophila is one of the great challenges in the coming century. Evidence-based guidelines for transition and transfer need to be developed, and best practice needs to be shared.

References

1. Siimes MA, Aalberg V, Petrini P. Boys with Haemophilia: Physical and Psychosocial Development in Adolescence. Helsinki, Finland: Nemo Publishers, 2006.
2. Eaton DK, et al. Youth risk behaviour surveillance – US 2009 – MMWR Surveill Summ 2010 4;59:1–142.
3. Steinberg L. Risk taking in adolescence. New perspectives from brain and behavioural science. Curr Dir Psychol. Sci 2007;16(2): 55–9.
4. Kennedy A, et al. Young people with chronic illness; the approach to transition. Intern Med J 2007;37:555–60.
5. Watson A.R. Problems and pitfalls of transition from paediatric to adult renal care Pediatr Nephrol 2005;20:113–17.
6. Bryon M. Transition from paediatric to adult care: psychological principles. J Roy Soc Med 2001;94(Suppl 40):5–7.
7. Tuchman LK. Cystic fibrosis and transition to adult medical care. Pediatrics 2010;125:566–73.
8. Breakey VR, et al. Towards comprehensive care in transition for young people with haemophilia. Haemophilia 2010;16:848–57.
9. Petrini P, et al. Haemophilia care in adolescence – compliance and lifestyle issues. Haemophilia 2009:15(Suppl 1):15–9.
10. Lindvall K, et al. Compliance with treatment and understanding of own disease in patients with severe and moderate haemophilia. Haemophilia 2006;12;47–51.
11. Geraghty S, et al. Practice pattern in haemophilia A therapy – global progress towards optimal care. Haemophilia 2006;12:75–81.
12. Mulder K, et al. Risks and benefits of sports and fitness activities for people with haemophilia. Haemophilia 2004;10(Suppl 4): 161–3.
13. Hofstede FG, et al. Obesity: a new disaster for haemophilic patients? A nationwide survey. Haemophilia 2008;14:1035–8.
14. Mennito SH, et al. Transition medicine: a review of current theory and practice. Southern Med J 2010;103(4).
15. Viner R. Barriers and good practice in transition from paediatric to adult care. J Roy Soc Med 2001:94(Suppl. 40):2–4.
16. Kipps S, et al. Current methods of transfer of young people with type 1 diabetes to adult services. Diabet Med 2002;19:649–54.
17. Gomis M, et al. Exercise and sport in the treatment of haemophilic patients: a systematic review. Haemophilia 2009;15(1):43–54.
18. Kyngas H. Patient education: perspective of adolescents with a chronic disease. J Clin Nurs 2003;12:744–51.

9 Perinatal Clinical Care and Molecular Diagnosis in Hemophilia

Carmen Altisent[1] and Francisco Vidal[2]

[1]Hospital Universitari Vall d'Hebron, Barcelona, Spain
[2]Banc de Sang i Teixits, Barcelona, Spain

Introduction

Hemophilia A (HA) and B (HB) are X-linked congenital coagulopathies occurring in one of every 10,000 and 35,000 male births, respectively. Newborns with hemophilia can present several associated bleeding complications; hence, a well-monitored delivery and accurate follow-up in the perinatal period are essential for managing this condition. Familial cases can be diagnosed at birth or prenatally (Figure 9.1). Molecular testing enables a reliable prenatal diagnosis and precise genetic counseling, which help to prevent clinical complications in the perinatal period. However, one-third of cases do not have a family history of the disease (sporadic cases), and the diagnosis can only be made after birth, usually before the age of 1 year in severe forms. Over the last years, genetic counseling based on molecular study has contributed to reducing the ratio of familial versus sporadic cases, particularly in severe hemophilia. Thus, it is a rising challenge to provide neonatologists with adequate tools for early diagnosis and management of sporadic cases. Genetic counseling is an essential element of comprehensive hemophilia care that can avert various clinical complications of the disease, which often originate in the perinatal period.

The genetic basis and inheritance of hemophilia

A wide range of gene mutations can lead to an absence of functional coagulation factors VIII (FVIII) or IX (FIX), including gross gene deletions or rearrangements, insertions, and nonsense and missense mutations [1]. Among them, intron 22 inversion is an extremely recurrent mutation causing FVIII gene (F8) disruption that accounts for 40% to 50% of severe HA cases [2]. Another recurrent inversion involving intron 1 occurs in about 1–5% of patients with severe HA [3,4]. Apart from these, the most frequent mutations in both genes essentially consist of point mutations. More than 800 different single base pair substitutions within F8 and nearly 1000 within the FIX gene (F9) have been reported and listed in online locus specific mutation databases [5,6]. Large deletions and insertions, splice junction changes, and small rearrangements complete the spectrum of mutations responsible for hemophilia. Because of this enormous mutational heterogeneity, identification of the defect requires analysis of all the essential regions of the gene.

Molecular diagnosis of hemophilia

Molecular diagnosis of hemophilia is based on studies of the genetic material, mainly genomic DNA. The complexity and large size of the genes involved, especially F8, and the high rate of new mutations considerably complicates these studies. Investigation in F8 and F9 has allowed the development and application of increasingly more comprehensive and informative molecular analysis techniques.

In patients with severe HA, it is essential to first test for the presence of intron 22 and intron 1 inversions. Southern blotting, originally used to detect the intron 22 inversion [2], has now largely been replaced with the faster, single-tube, long PCR method (or modifications of the method) described by Liu et al. [7]. When inversions are ruled out, other mutations implicated in HA or HB can be investigated by several molecular analysis methods [8] that vary in sensitivity and simplicity, and in the information provided: (1) linkage analysis techniques or indirect techniques, based on a number of polymorphic markers, allow identification and follow-up of the chromosome that carries the defective gene; (2) mutation screening techniques, based on physical or chemical properties, enable differentiation between an amplified control

Current and Future Issues in Hemophilia Care, First Edition. Edited by Emérito-Carlos Rodríguez-Merchán and Leonard A. Valentino.
© 2011 John Wiley & Sons, Ltd. Published 2011 by Blackwell Publishing Ltd.

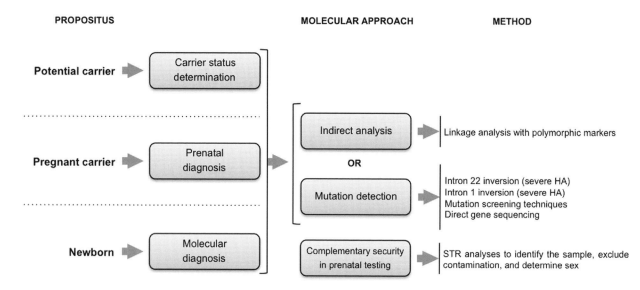

PROPOSITUS   MOLECULAR APPROACH   METHOD

Figure 9.1 Scheme for molecular diagnosis methods at different times of perinatal period in hemophilia.

DNA fragment and an identical fragment carrying a mutation; and (3) direct DNA sequencing, in which the gene associated with the pathology is analyzed by determining the nucleotide sequence. This is conceptually the simplest approach, and it is increasingly being used as the reference technique for molecular diagnosis of a number of hereditary diseases.

Molecular diagnosis of hemophilia is still performed using indirect techniques. Nevertheless, limitations such as uninformative families and sporadic cases without a prior family history (approximately one-third of HA patients) are discouraging many laboratories from continuing to use indirect approaches. The multiple benefits derived from identifying the mutation favor the development of methods to detect the gene defect. One such benefit is betterment of carrier and prenatal studies in terms of accuracy and safety.

Genetic diagnosis of carriers

Because there is currently no available method to correct the genetic defect, hemophilia is a lifelong condition. In families affected by hemophilia, it is important to identify women at risk of being carriers, so that they will be aware of their genetic status and reproductive options through appropriate genetic counseling before they become pregnant. The first step to determining carrier status is by conducting a family tree with reliable clinical data from affected males. Because hemophilia legacy is linked to the X-chromosome, it is possible to differentiate, in the first instance, between obligate carriers and possible carriers. Accurate carrier diagnosis is now possible by DNA analysis (Figure 9.1), and at-risk women should be tested. To perform correct molecular diagnosis of carriers, it is advisable to begin studying a hemophiliac member of the family. When there are no affected family members, it is possible to perform molecular diagnosis of an obligate female

carrier, although this approach does not always yield conclusive results. Direct diagnosis includes investigation to determine the mutation responsible for the family coagulopathy [9,10].

The diagnosis of carriers in sporadic cases of hemophilia requires some additional specific considerations. The mutation must be tracked back through the parents and, if necessary, through the maternal grandparents to identify the individual in whom it originated. When the son has a true de novo mutation (somatic mosaicism), future brothers will not be hemophilic. However, in most cases, the mother carries the mutation, which was generated in the gametes of the maternal grandfather (although he did not have hemophilia) and inherited by the mother [11]. There is a 50% risk of the mother transmitting the defective gene. The mutation could also occur as an alteration in the mother's gametes, such that one or more oocytes contain the mutation (germinal mosaicism). There is some risk that this will occur more than once, but it is virtually impossible to determine the exact risk in these cases. In this situation, a conservative approach should be used in counseling and management.

Prenatal diagnosis

Prenatal diagnosis enables recommendations to be established for delivery and treatment of newborns with hemophilia. Molecular testing is feasible in carrier pregnancies when the mutation has been identified in a family member or linkage has been established in the family [12]. Genomic DNA for prenatal diagnosis can be obtained from amniotic fluid (AF) at approximately 15 to 18 weeks' gestation or chorionic villus samples (CVS) at approximately 10 to 12 weeks' gestation. The potential presence of maternal cells in AF or in CVS poses a significant pre-analytical risk for prenatal misdiagnosis that could result in inappropriate termination of a pregnancy [13]. Thus, a rigorous protocol should also include a battery of short tandem repeat (STR) polymorphism analyses to identify the sample, exclude contamination, and determine sex [13].

Alternative and complementary prenatal testing procedures

Percutaneous umbilical blood sampling (PUBS), also known as cordocentesis, is applied when the mutation responsible for hemophilia is unknown and linkage is uninformative. Prenatal diagnosis is possible using a fetal blood sample obtained by PUBS at approximately 18 to 21 weeks' gestation to assay clotting factor activity [14].

Preimplantation genetic diagnosis (PGD) is an emerging alternative to prenatal diagnosis for persons at risk of transmitting an inherited disease to their offspring. Embryos obtained through in vitro fertilization are tested for the genetic anomaly concerning the couple prior to being placed in the mother's womb; hence the risk of conceiving an affected child is greatly reduced. Although sex selection using FISH or PCR is the usual procedure applied in PGD for hemophilia, precise detection of the mutation would allow selection of mutation-free embryos regardless of gender [15].

Recommended mode of delivery

The related literature contains many controversial issues regarding the approaches to use at delivery of newborns with a known hemophilia risk. Medical guidelines usually recommend avoiding traumatic maneuvers (forceps or vacuum) and using vaginal delivery as the initial approach, unless there are specific obstetric contraindications.

In a recent review, Ljung recommends that the optimal delivery mode for infants with hemophilia is vaginal delivery, since the risk of serious bleeding in the affected neonate is small in a normal vaginal delivery [16]. Conversely, James and Hoots [17] advocate caesarean delivery as the optimal mode because the outcome of labor cannot be predicted. Planned vaginal delivery carries a risk of abnormal labor and operative vaginal delivery, both of which predispose to intracranial hemorrhage (ICH).

The incidence of ICH in the general population is very low, with rates in primiparous women of 1/860 deliveries involving forceps extraction and 1/664 deliveries by vacuum extraction, as well as in 1/907 cesareans indicated at the time of delivery, 1/2750 scheduled cesareans, and 1/1900 spontaneous vaginal deliveries [18]. These low rates contrast with those found in a study by Heibel et al. [19], who performed cranial ultrasound 3 days after delivery of 1000 consecutive neonates with no signs of distress and found 35 cases of perinatal ICH and 34 potential bleeding sequelae.

Cranial ultrasound is useful for screening ICH, but is not the best method for diagnosing subdural or subarachnoid hematoma; computed tomography scan (CT) or magnetic resonance imaging (MRI) are indicated in these cases. Whitby et al. performed a

prospective MRI study including 111 asymptomatic term babies to assess the incidence of subdural hematomas in relation to obstetric factors [20]. Nine babies had subdural hemorrhage and three of them were from normal vaginal deliveries. Since MRI was done within 48 h of delivery, the authors suggested that some acute subdural hemorrhages may have gone undetected because they are difficult to recognize on early MRI. A subsequent MRI at the age of 4 weeks showed complete resolution of subdural hemorrhage in all babies. Another MRI study in 88 asymptomatic neonates (65 vaginal delivery and 23 cesarean delivery) between the age of 1 and 5 weeks, analyzed ICH and its relationship with obstetric and neonatal risk factors [21]. Seventeen neonates had ICH and all had been delivered vaginally, yielding a 26% prevalence of ICH in vaginal births. Seven patients had two or more types of hemorrhages.

There is no consensus regarding imaging studies in newborns with hemophilia. In a questionnaire survey conducted in 45 hemophilia centers in the United Kingdom, 41% of responders always performed neonatal cranial ultrasound, 38% only when there were special conditions during delivery (prolonged or by forceps), and 21% only when there were clinical signs suggestive of bleeding [22]. Considering the available data as a whole, it seems reasonable to recommend routine screening by cranial imaging in all newborns with hemophilia, regardless of the mode of delivery.

Neonatal manifestations of hemophilia

About 15% to 33% of newborns with hemophilia present bleeding complications. The incidence of ICH is 3.58% to 12% and the mortality rate is 0.6% to 21.9%. Recent studies estimate the percentage of ICH at 3.5% to 4% in countries with optimal treatment conditions, a figure still considered high compared to the normal population, in which it is estimated at 0.03% in low-risk deliveries (cesarean) and 0.1% in high-risk deliveries (vacuum) [23].

In a literature review of 66 articles published between 1949 and 1999, Kulkarni described the neonatal complications occurring in 349 children with hemophilia [24]. The skull was the most common site of bleeding (intracranial in 27% and extracranial in 14% of cases). Bleeding occurred after circumcision in 30% of cases, after venipuncture in 16%, and after umbilical puncture in 6%. Bleeding in a gastrointestinal organ or joint was reported in less than 3%. In a second literature review covering the period of 1964 to 1996, Kulkarni and Lusher [25] reported 109 cases of intracranial (65%) and extracranial (35%) hemorrhage. The clinical symptoms included anemia, hypotension, shock, and lethargy. However, only patients with ICH had neurological deficits (15%) and late neurological sequelae (38%). This review also confirmed that these complications can occur regardless of the severity of hemophilia.

Subgaleal hematomas are an uncommon type of extracranial hemorrhage, generally associated with the use of a vacuum extractor. Blood loss can be significant and cause hypovolemic shock and cerebral compression. Kilani and Wetmore [26] estimated a

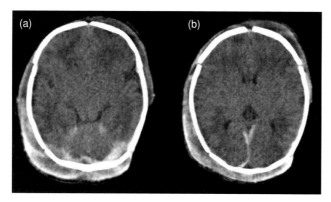

Figure 9.2 CT scan of sporadic hemophilic newborn (vacuum delivery) showing a large subgaleal hematoma and a subdural hematoma in: (a) posterior cranial fossa; and (b) posterior falx.

mortality of 11.8% in 34 neonates with subgaleal hematoma; 91.2% had undergone assisted delivery with vacuum or forceps and many cases were associated with ICH (Figure 9.2). In a literature review of 123 neonates with subgaleal hematoma [27], the estimated mortality was 22.8%; 64% were in assisted births, but also occurred in spontaneous vaginal delivery and cesarean delivery.

The presence of an important extracranial hemorrhage (cephalohematoma or subgaleal hematoma) in the absence of traumatic maneuvers should raise the suspicion of a possible coagulopathy.

Prophylaxis in the neonate

The consequences of ICH have suggested the need to administer low doses of coagulation factor to all neonates with a prenatal diagnosis of hemophilia [28]. There are no data in the literature to evaluate the pros and cons of prophylactic treatment in newborns with hemophilia. Kulkarni et al. reported the results of a prospective surveillance in babies with hemophilia [29]. In this USA cohort (580 neonates and toddlers), approximately 8% of newborns with severe hemophilia received factor concentrate within 24 hours of birth; more than half were prophylactic administration. The doubt about whether early treatment may increase the risk of inhibitor development [30] has led to a more expectant management approach in potentially high-risk situations. The multicenter retrospective CANAL study investigated 366 patients and the findings suggests that age at first exposition is associated with inhibitor development, but that this association is explained by intensity of treatment [31].

Management of the hemophilic newborn

Certain measures are needed to reduce the risk of hemorrhage in the neonate with hemophilia: cord blood should be obtained to determine clotting factors, especially if a prenatal diagnosis was

not established, heel prick and venipuncture should be carried out with great care and be followed by local application of pressure, and oral vitamin K should be administrated.

Concerning prophylactic treatment in newborns, a single low dose of clotting factor (<50 IU/kg) may not represent an increased risk of inhibitor development and is indicated in clinically suspected severe bleeding. In cases of suspected ICH, administration of clotting factor is recommended before diagnostic imaging, and CT or MRI are the modalities of choice in subdural and subarachnoid hemorrhage. In neonates with diagnosed ICH, prophylactic treatment should be started as soon as possible to avoid recurrence. Lastly, coagulation studies must be performed in all newborns with ICH and no family history of hemophilia, in order to detect sporadic cases.

Conclusions

Perinatal clinical care in hemophilia includes perinatal diagnosis, the approaches to use at delivery, prophylaxis in the neonate and the management of the hemophilic newborn. Molecular diagnosis in hemophilia is based in studies of the genetic material, mainly genomic DNA. The benefits derived from identifying the mutation favor the development of methods to detect the gene defect.

References

1. Graw J, Brackmann HH, Oldenburg J, Schneppenheim R, Spannagl M, Schwaab R. Haemophilia A: from mutation analysis to new therapies. Nat Rev Genet. 2005;6(6):488–501.
2. Lakich D, Kazazian HHJ, Antonarakis SE, Gitschier J. Inversions disrupting the factor VIII gene are a common cause of severe haemophilia A. Nat Genet. 1993;5(3):236–41.
3. Mantilla-Capacho JM, Beltran-Miranda CP, Luna-Zaizar H, et al. Frequency of intron 1 and 22 inversions of Factor VIII gene in Mexican patients with severe hemophilia A. Am J Hematol. 2007;82(4):283–7.
4. Cumming AM. The factor VIII gene intron 1 inversion mutation: prevalence in severe hemophilia A patients in the UK. J Thromb Haemost. 2004;2(1):205–6.
5. Kemball-Cook G, Tuddenham EG. The Factor VIII Mutation Database on the World Wide Web: the haemophilia A mutation, search, test and resource site. HAMSTeRS update (version 3.0). Nucleic Acids Res. 1997;25(1):128–32.
6. Giannelli F, Green PM, Sommer SS, Poon MC, Ludwig M, Schwaab R, et al. Haemophilia B: database of point mutations and short additions and deletions, 7th edn. Nucleic Acids Res. 1997;25(1):133–5.
7. Liu Q, Nozari G, Sommer SS. Single-tube polymerase chain reaction for rapid diagnosis of the inversion hotspot of mutation in hemophilia A. Blood. 1998;92(4):1458–9.
8. Goodeve A. Molecular genetic testing of hemophilia A. Semin Thromb Hemost. 2008;34(6):491–501.
9. Vidal F, Farssac E, Altisent C, Puig L, Gallardo D. Rapid hemophilia A molecular diagnosis by a simple DNA sequencing procedure: identification of 14 novel mutations. Thromb Haemost. 2001;85(4):580–3.

10. Vidal F, Farssac E, Altisent C, Puig L, Gallardo D. Factor IX gene sequencing by a simple and sensitive 15-hour procedure for haemophilia B diagnosis: identification of two novel mutations. Br J Haematol. 2000;111(2):549–51.

11. Kasper CK, Buzin CH. Mosaics and haemophilia. Haemophilia. 2009;15(6):1181–6.

12. Ghosh K, Shetty S, Tulsiani M. Evolution of prenatal diagnostic techniques from phenotypic diagnosis to gene arrays: its likely impact on prenatal diagnosis of hemophilia. Clin Appl Thromb Hemost. 2009;15(3):277–82.

13. Schrijver I, Cherny SC, Zehnder JL. Testing for maternal cell contamination in prenatal samples: a comprehensive survey of current diagnostic practices in 35 molecular diagnostic laboratories. J Mol Diagn. 2007;9(3):394–400.

14. Boulot P, Deschamps F, Lefort G, Sarda P, Mares P, Hedon B, et al. Pure fetal blood samples obtained by cordocentesis: technical aspects of 322 cases. Prenat Diagn. 1990;10(2):93–100.

15. Sanchez-Garcia JF, Gallardo D, Navarro J, Marquez C, Gris JM, Sanchez MA, et al. A versatile strategy for preimplantation genetic diagnosis of haemophilia A based on F8-gene sequencing. Thromb Haemost. 2006;96(6):839–45.

16. Ljung R. The optimal mode of delivery for the haemophilia carrier expecting an affected infant is vaginal delivery. Haemophilia. 2010;16(3):415–9.

17. James AH, Hoots K. The optimal mode of delivery for the haemophilia carrier expecting an affected infant is caesarean delivery. Haemophilia. 2010;16(3):420–4.

18. Towner D, Castro MA, Eby-Wilkens E, Gilbert WM. Effect of mode of delivery in nulliparous women on neonatal intracranial injury. N Engl J Med. 1999;341(23):1709–14.

19. Heibel M, Heber R, Bechinger D, Kornhuber HH. Early diagnosis of perinatal cerebral lesions in apparently normal full-term newborns by ultrasound of the brain. Neuroradiology. 1993;35(2):85–91.

20. Whitby EH, Griffiths PD, Rutter S, Smith MF, Sprigg A, Ohadike P, et al. Frequency and natural history of subdural haemorrhages in babies and relation to obstetric factors. Lancet. 2004;363(9412):846–51.

21. Looney CB, Smith JK, Merck LH, Wolfe HM, Chescheir NC, Hamer RM, et al. Intracranial hemorrhage in asymptomatic neonates: prevalence on MR images and relationship to obstetric and neonatal risk factors. Radiology. 2007;242(2):535–41.

22. Chalmers EA, Williams MD, Richards M, Brown SA, Liesner R, Thomas A, et al. Management of neonates with inherited bleeding disorders – a survey of current UK practice. Haemophilia. 2005;11(2):186–7.

23. Ljung RC. Intracranial haemorrhage in haemophilia A and B. Br J Haematol. 2008;140(4):378–84.

24. Kulkarni R, Lusher J. Perinatal management of newborns with haemophilia. Br J Haematol. 2001;112(2):264–74.

25. Kulkarni R, Lusher JM. Intracranial and extracranial hemorrhages in newborns with hemophilia: a review of the literature. J Pediatr Hematol Oncol. 1999;21(4):289–95.

26. Kilani RA, Wetmore J. Neonatal subgaleal hematoma: presentation and outcome – radiological findings and factors associated with mortality. Am J Perinatol. 2006;23(1):41–8.

27. Plauche WC. Subgaleal hematoma. A complication of instrumental delivery. JAMA. 1980;244(14):1597–8.

28. Rodriguez V, Schmidt KA, Slaby JA, Pruthi RK. Intracranial haemorrhage as initial presentation of severe haemophilia B: case report and review of Mayo Clinic Comprehensive Hemophilia Center experience. Haemophilia. 2005;11(1):73–7.

29. Kulkarni R, Soucie JM, Lusher J, Presley R, Shapiro A, Gill J, et al. Sites of initial bleeding episodes, mode of delivery and age of diagnosis in babies with haemophilia diagnosed before the age of 2 years: a report from The Centers for Disease Control and Prevention's (CDC) Universal Data Collection (UDC) project. Haemophilia. 2009;15(6):1281–90.

30. Lorenzo JI, Lopez A, Altisent C, Aznar JA. Incidence of factor VIII inhibitors in severe haemophilia: the importance of patient age. Br J Haematol. 2001;113(3):600–3.

31. Gouw SC, van der Bom JG, Marijke van den Berg H. Treatment-related risk factors of inhibitor development in previously untreated patients with hemophilia A: the CANAL cohort study. Blood. 2007;109(11):4648–54.

10 Managing the Mature Person with Hemophilia

Savita Rangarajan[1] and Thynn Thynn Yee[2]

[1]Basingstoke and North Hampshire NHS Foundation Trust, Basingstoke, UK
[2]Royal Free Hospital, London, UK

Introduction

A mature person is not defined by age and in hemophilia terms; this person can be defined as one who is responsible for the management of their life and health. Well established regimes with clotting factor concentrates (CFC) have shifted the mature hemophilia patients' life expectancy from less than 30 years to over 70 years [1,2]. More men with hemophilia are now becoming parents than in the era prior to effective replacement therapy and the emergence of acquired immunodeficiency syndrome (AIDS), resulting in an increase number of female carriers. As a consequence, a higher number of individuals with hemophilia could be born with increasing workload for the clinicians at both ends of the age spectrum.

As persons with hemophilia continue to age it will become increasingly important for hemophilia physicians to proactively assess and prevent some of the age associated morbidities such as coronary heart disease (CHD), stroke and falls. The service needs of elderly patients should take into account non preventable health issues such as cognitive and/or visual impairment which could hamper the independence of a hemophilia patient in self-infusion to treat themselves with CFC. Immobility, social isolation and depression may further reduce the quality of life (QoL) in these patients. Provision of adequate community nurses, physiotherapists and occupational therapists should be part of the strategic planning for future models of care for this cohort who are already burdened with arthropathy, chronic human immunodeficiency virus (HIV) and hepatitis C virus (HCV) infections.

There are well-established guidelines of care for the younger patients, but it is necessary to have models of care that meet the needs of the aging hemophilia population as well. This chapter aims at describing the current challenges faced by hemophilia physicians and highlights the future service needs of this group of patients.

Complications due to hemophilia or its treatment

Joint damage consequent to bleeding into joints is a characteristic feature of hemophilia. Initiation of primary prophylaxis in children has significantly reduced arthropathy and related morbidity. This is not the case for the surviving mature patient who missed out on primary prophylaxis and is therefore burdened with significant hemophilic arthropathy and age associated osteoarthritis eventually requiring joint replacement surgery [3].

Premature arthritis occurs, not only in patients affected with severe disease, but in those with moderate hemophilia and increases with age in a linear fashion [4]. The focus of management of arthropathy aims at a reduction or cessation of acute joint hemorrhages by introducing tailored secondary prophylaxis with CFC in previously "on demand" treated patients. Secondary prophylaxis at this stage does not prevent further joint deterioration but by reducing the numbers of acute hemorrhages, preventing acute pain, and joint immobilization and therefore improves QoL [5].

Pain relief, another key component for improving QoL is managed with medications such as paracetamol (it chronic use is cautioned in patients with liver disease), cyclo-oxygenase-2 (COX-2) inhibitors such as Celecoxib which does not increase bleeding risk and narcotics including codeine- and morphine-containing drugs [6]. Some patients may benefit from referral to a pain management clinic if the above strategies fail. Pre-emptive physiotherapy and hydrotherapy sessions may also improve joint stability and balance and should be offered to all patients.

Despite the above conservative measures, in many cases surgery is required with appropriate CFC either by bolus dosing or continuous infusion to maintain trough values at >60 u/dl in the first week and >25 u/dl in the following week after major orthopaedic surgery [6]. Many of these surgical procedures may be

Current and Future Issues in Hemophilia Care, First Edition. Edited by Emérito-Carlos Rodríguez-Merchán and Leonard A. Valentino.
© 2011 John Wiley & Sons, Ltd. Published 2011 by Blackwell Publishing Ltd.

revision operations and the risk of bleeding is higher. Interestingly, ankle joint involvement in hemophilia is now increasingly recognized and surgical management, by way of partial arthroscopic arthrodesis or ankle replacement, is being undertaken. Medicinal thromboprophylaxis should be considered for older patients undergoing major orthopedic surgery, as there is no evidence that patients with congenital coagulation defects are less prone to venous thromboembolism [7].

In patients with longstanding inhibitors who have multiple joints affected with athropathy and continuing joint bleeding, consideration should be given to prophylaxis with bypassing agents [8,9], as is the case in patients without inhibitors who receive CFC prophylaxis in order to improve QoL. In the past, much needed surgery in inhibitor patients was not undertaken because of lack of confidence in achieving hemostasis using bypassing agents and the associated exorbitant costs of the drugs. However, recent literature indicates that surgery can be safely performed in comprehensive care settings using either of the two available bypassing agents in a cost effective manner [10,11]. There are concerns however regarding the use of bypassing agents in elderly patients considered at increased risk of thrombotic complications. It is believed that if the bypassing agents are given according to established guidelines, this risk is negligible [12,13].

New inhibitor development usually occurs within first 50 exposures to CFC in severe hemophilia patients, but is a recognized complication in patients with mild and moderate hemophilia at advanced ages following intensive factor therapy for surgery or invasive procedures [14,15]. The inhibitory antibodies are directed against patient's own factor VIII, thus converting them into a severe hemophilia phenotype. The pattern of bleeding is akin to that observed in acquired hemophilia with large subcutaneous hematomas and muscle bleeding but rarely, joint bleeding. Management of bleeding in the presence of inhibitors is with bypassing agents. It is important to closely check for inhibitor development when mild or moderate hemophilia patients undergo surgery or are given intensive factor replacement.

Patients treated with plasma derived CFC between 1978 and 1986 were exposed to HIV infection [16], and many patients succumbed to AIDS. With the introduction of highly active antiretroviral therapy (HAART), the life expectancy has dramatically improved and the incidence of lymphomas and other HIV-related malignancies have decreased significantly. These patients can now look forward to enjoying a full lifespan, having children and integrating fully into society. Long-term therapy with HAART, however, is associated with side effects such as hyerlipidemia, lipodystrophy, renal insufficiency, osteopenia and hepatotoxicity. It is important to identify and manage these complications early to prevent long-term morbidity. Increased bleeding frequency is noted in patients receiving protease inhibitors (PI) and prophylaxis with CFC has to be introduced appropriately [17].

Currently available treatment for chronic HCV infection is with combination therapy consisting of pegylated interferon and oral ribavirin, with success rates between 40–50% for genotype 1 and 4 and up to 90% for genotype 2 and 3 [18]. The side effects of combination therapy include weight loss, alopecia, depression and hematological toxicity which may not be tolerated by older patients leading to dose reduction, and potentially, loss of efficacy. Co-infection with HIV accelerates the progression of liver disease and may render treatment difficult due to drug interactions and increasing intolerability. Many of the mature patients who failed to eradicate the HCV virus go on to develop cirrhosis [3,19]. Patients with chronic viremia and liver cirrhosis should be monitored for development of hepatocellular carcinoma (HCC) by ultrasound examination and alpha-fetoprotein levels every 6 months [20]. Referral for a liver transplant is mandatory in the event of early detection of HCC or a decompensation of liver function. It is also hoped that the new antiviral agents such as HCV-specific protease inhibitors will soon be available for treatment and may safely clear the virus in a higher proportion of elderly patients [21].

Renal insufficiency in mature hemophilia patients is multifactorial and is often due to frequent hematuria associated with renal structural abnormalities [22] and the resulting clot formation is worsened by concomitant use of antifibrinolytic therapy. The presence of viral infections (HIV and HCV) and exposure to nephrotoxic antiviral therapy (HAART) increases the incidence of renal insufficiency over time [23]. Anti-inflammatory medications (although not recommended in these patients) consumed for chronic arthropathic pain may also contribute to this. Chronic renal failure increases the incidence of hypertension and is a risk factor for cardiovascular disease and cerebral hemorrhage [3].

Osteoporosis is now known to be present in a significant proportion of mature hemophilia patients [24]. The presence of osteoporosis increases the risk of fractures and fracture related morbidity in elderly patients after falls due to imbalance which in itself is not uncommon. The severity of osteoporosis is directly proportional to the number and severity of arthropathic joints [24]. The causes of osteoporosis in this cohort include reduced mobility of joints, lack of activity, repeated joint hemorrhage (due to lack of adequate CFC in the past) all resulting in reduced bone loading. Additional factors include HCV infection, antiretroviral HIV medications, low body mass index due to muscle wasting, and poor nutrition. Physical activity, physiotherapy, and calcium and vitamin D supplements are recommended [25].

Impact of co-morbidities of aging on hemophilia

Hemophilia is reported to have a direct protective effect on the development of coronary heart disease attributable to the hypocoagulable state of the individuals [26]. Nevertheless, hemophilia patients may have the common cardiovascular risk factors such as arterial hypertension, smoking, dyslipidemias, diabetes mellitus and obesity. Recent literature shows an increase in the prevalence of ischemic heart disease (IHD) in hemophilia patients age 60 years and older [27] and an increasing number of deaths in hemophilia patients as a result of IHD [1]. Comprehensive clinical evaluations for older adults with hemophilia should now include an assessment for and prevention of these risk factors. Patients need to be

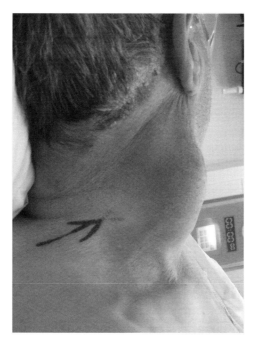

Figure 10.1 Development of a hematoma (arrow) in a mild hemophilia B patient on aspirin after carotid endarterectomy for carotid stenosis leading to stroke.

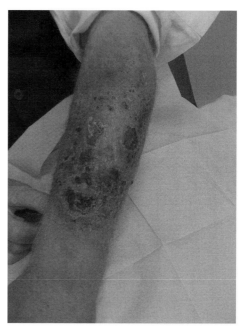

Figure 10.2 Extensive soft tissue hematoma after a fall in an elderly mild hemophiliac. The patient required intensive replacement therapy and rehabilitation.

educated and counseled on the benefits of living a healthy lifestyle as some older individuals still firmly believe that they are protected from IHD.

Chronic infections such as HIV, HCV and hepatitis B virus (HBV), seen in a subgroup of adult hemophilia patients can alter the complex inflammatory process of atherosclerosis and coronary heart disease and recent guidelines support for earlier initiation of antiretroviral therapy in HIV-infected individuals [28]. Specific antiretroviral agents currently linked to a higher risk of coronary heart disease should be avoided, particularly in patients with risk factors for IHD. This is best done in a setting of joint clinics staffed by experts in the treatment of hemophilia, heart disease and infectious diseases. Polypharmacy can lead to drug interactions between antiretroviral agents and medications for the common co-morbidities. Antiplatelet therapy for prevention of progression of atherosclerosis in hemophilia patients will need to be supported by regular infusions of CFC as these agents can lead to increased bleeding tendency. Figure 10.1 shows the development of a hematoma in a patient with mild hemophilia B treated with aspirin after carotid endarterectomy for carotid stenosis leading to stroke. This clearly illustrates some of the clinical challenges within the aging hemophilia population.

Use of anticoagulants is on the rise in patients with inherited bleeding disorders for prevention of venous thromboses at the time of intense replacement therapy with CFCs in the setting of surgery or trauma [29] and in atrial fibrillation. Clotting factor support is necessary to achieve adequate hemostasis in these situations.

There is a high prevalence of falls occurring in around 30% of individuals aged 65 years and over. This can lead to fractures in hemophilia patients as they are at risk for osteoporosis as outlined earlier. Elderly patients with hemophilia can also sustain extensive soft tissue hematomas after falls (Figure 10.2), requiring intensive replacement therapy and rehabilitation. Falls can lead to loss of confidence, immobility and psychological problems. Prevention of falls requires an interdisciplinary and a multifactorial approach of health-care professionals towards the patient. Vitamin D and calcium supplementation have been shown to be a simple intervention that can be incorporated into strategies for postural rehabilitation and primary and secondary fall prevention [30].

The use of HAART has prevented the progression of HIV infection to AIDS and therefore, the frequency of HIV related malignancies has declined in the hemophilia population. The most prevalent cancer in the older hemophilia patients currently is HCC on the background of chronic HCV infection. Surveillance programs for liver, colonic and prostate cancer should be in place and simple screening procedure such as routine colonoscopy can be more complex in the hemophilia as one needs to consider the inherent risk of bleeding. Currently there is little communication or cooperation between the fields of hemophilia, geriatrics and other specialities such as cardiology, oncology and urology. Improved interdisciplinary communication would facilitate care that is framed within the current service agreements.

Conclusions

Clinicians need to be ready to take appropriate care as more individuals with hemophilia are becoming older adults. Clinicians must be able to handle the many challenges related not only to hemophilia but also to general co-morbidities associated with aging. Communication and networking will be central for success of future models of care that will be able to provide for aging patients complex healthcare needs. Establishing links between interested specialized centers will help develop a core of expertise with links between hemophilia, geriatrics, oncology, cardiology and primary care ensuring a coordinated approach An important first step that needs to be taken towards the development of a strategic, focused and collaborative approach to the management of hemophilia in older people is to gain evidence-based guidance through national and international clinical trials and in the absence of trial data, through interdisciplinary workshops to provide expert opinion-based guidance.

References

1. Plug I, Van Der Bom JG, Peters M, Mauser-Bunschoten EP, De Goede-Bolder A, Heijnen L, et al. Mortality and causes of death in patients with hemophilia, 1992–2001: a prospective cohort study. J. Thromb. Haemost. 2006 Mar;4(3):510–516.

2. Darby SC, Kan SW, Spooner RJ, Giangrande PL, Hill FG, Hay CR, et al. Mortality rates, life expectancy, and causes of death in people with hemophilia A or B in the United Kingdom who were not infected with HIV. Blood 2007 Aug 1;110(3):815–825.

3. Siboni SM, Mannucci PM, Gringeri A, Franchini M, Tagliaferri A, Ferretti M, et al. Health status and quality of life of elderly persons with severe hemophilia born before the advent of modern replacement therapy. J. Thromb. Haemost. 2009 May;7(5):780–786.

4. Smit C, Rosendaal FR, Varekamp I, Brocker-Vriends A, Van Dijck H, Suurmeijer TP, et al. Physical condition, longevity, and social performance of Dutch haemophiliacs, 1972–85. BMJ 1989 Jan 28;298(6668):235–238.

5. Tagliaferri A, Franchini M, Coppola A, Rivolta GF, Santoro C, Rossetti G, et al. Effects of secondary prophylaxis started in adolescent and adult haemophiliacs. Haemophilia 2008 Sep;14(5):945–951.

6. Mannucci PM, Schutgens RE, Santagostino E, Mauser-Bunschoten EP. How I treat age-related morbidities in elderly persons with hemophilia. Blood 2009 Dec 17;114(26):5256–5263.

7. Hermans C, Hammer F, Lobet S, Lambert C. Subclinical deep venous thrombosis observed in 10% of hemophilic patients undergoing major orthopedic surgery. J. Thromb. Haemost. 2010 May;8(5):1138–1140.

8. Perry D, Berntorp E, Tait C, Dolan G, Holme PA, Laffan M, et al. FEIBA prophylaxis in haemophilia patients: a clinical update and treatment recommendations. Haemophilia 2010 Jan;16(1):80–89.

9. Konkle BA, Ebbesen LS, Erhardtsen E, Bianco RP, Lissitchkov T, Rusen L, et al. Randomized, prospective clinical trial of recombinant factor VIIa for secondary prophylaxis in hemophilia patients with inhibitors. J. Thromb. Haemost. 2007 Sep;5(9):1904–1913.

10. Giangrande PL, Wilde JT, Madan B, Ludlam CA, Tuddenham EG, Goddard NJ, et al. Consensus protocol for the use of recombinant activated factor VII [eptacog alfa (activated); NovoSeven] in elective orthopaedic surgery in haemophilic patients with inhibitors. Haemophilia 2009 Mar;15(2):501–508.

11. Rangarajan S, Yee TT, Wilde J. Experience of four UK comprehensive care centres using FEIBA for surgeries in patients with inhibitors. Haemophilia 2011 Jan;17(1):28–34.

12. Leebeek FW, Kappers-Klunne MC, Jie KS. Effective and safe use of recombinant factor VIIa (NovoSeven) in elderly mild haemophilia A patients with high-titre antibodies against factor VIII. Haemophilia 2004 May;10(3):250–253.

13. Franchini M, Lippi G. Acquired factor VIII inhibitors. Blood 2008 Jul 15;112(2):250–255.

14. Hay CR. Factor VIII inhibitors in mild and moderate-severity haemophilia A. Haemophilia 1998 Jul;4(4):558–563.

15. Wight J, Paisley S. The epidemiology of inhibitors in haemophilia A: a systematic review. Haemophilia 2003 Jul;9(4):418–435.

16. Ragni MV, Tegtmeier GE, Levy JA, Kaminsky LS, Lewis JH, Spero JA, et al. AIDS retrovirus antibodies in hemophiliacs treated with factor VIII or factor IX concentrates, cryoprecipitate, or fresh frozen plasma: prevalence, seroconversion rate, and clinical correlations. Blood 1986 Mar;67(3):592–595.

17. Wilde JT, Lee CA, Collins P, Giangrande PL, Winter M, Shiach CR. Increased bleeding associated with protease inhibitor therapy in HIV-positive patients with bleeding disorders. Br. J. Haematol. 1999 Dec;107(3):556–559.

18. Manns MP, McHutchison JG, Gordon SC, Rustgi VK, Shiffman M, Reindollar R, et al. Peginterferon alfa-2b plus ribavirin compared with interferon alfa-2b plus ribavirin for initial treatment of chronic hepatitis C: a randomised trial. Lancet 2001 Sep 22;358(9286): 958–965.

19. Posthouwer D, Yee TT, Makris M, Fischer K, Griffioen A, Van Veen JJ, et al. Antiviral therapy for chronic hepatitis C in patients with inherited bleeding disorders: an international, multicenter cohort study. J. Thromb. Haemost. 2007 Aug;5(8):1624–1629.

20. Thabut D, Le Calvez S, Thibault V, Massard J, Munteanu M, Di Martino V, et al. Hepatitis C in 6,865 patients 65 yr or older: a severe and neglected curable disease? Am. J. Gastroenterol. 2006 Jun;101(6):1260–1267.

21. Hezode C, Forestier N, Dusheiko G, Ferenci P, Pol S, Goeser T, et al. Telaprevir and peginterferon with or without ribavirin for chronic HCV infection. N. Engl. J. Med. 2009 Apr 30;360(18):1839–1850.

22. Prentice CR, Lindsay RM, Barr RD, Forbes CD, Kennedy AC, McNicol GP, et al. Renal complications in haemophilia and Christmas disease. Q. J. Med. 1971 Jan;40(157):47–61.

23. Kulkarni R, Soucie JM, Evatt B, Hemophilia Surveillance System Project Investigators. Renal disease among males with haemophilia. Haemophilia 2003 Nov;9(6):703–710.

24. Wallny TA, Scholz DT, Oldenburg J, Nicolay C, Ezziddin S, Pennekamp PH, et al. Osteoporosis in haemophilia – an underestimated comorbidity? Haemophilia 2007 Jan;13(1):79–84.

25. Kovacs CS. Hemophilia, low bone mass, and osteopenia/osteoporosis. Transfus. Apher. Sci. 2008 Feb;38(1):33–40.

26. Rosendaal FR, Briet E, Stibbe J, van Herpen G, Leuven JA, Hofman A, et al. Haemophilia protects against ischaemic heart disease: a study of risk factors. Br. J. Haematol. 1990 Aug;75(4):525–530.

27. Kulkarni R, Soucie JM, Evatt BL, Hemophilia Surveillance System Project Investigators. Prevalence and risk factors for heart

disease among males with hemophilia. Am. J. Hematol. 2005 May;79(1):36–42.

28. Panel on Clinical Practices for treatment of HIV Infection convened by the Department of Health and Human Services (DHHS): Guidelines for the use of Antiretroviral Agents in HIV-1 Infected Adults and Adolescents.10 January 2011. http://www.aidsinfo.nih.gov/ContentFiles/AdultandAdolescentGL.pdf.

29. Ritchie B, Woodman RC, Poon MC. Deep venous thrombosis in hemophilia A. Am. J. Med. 1992 Dec;93(6):699–700.

30. Annweiler C, Montero-Odasso M, Schott AM, Berrut G, Fantino B, Beauchet O. Fall prevention and vitamin D in the elderly: an overview of the key role of the non-bone effects. J. Neuroeng. Rehabil. 2010 Oct 11;7: 50.

11 Quality of Life in Hemophilia

Eduardo Remor

Autonomous University, Madrid, Spain

Introduction

In the past years a paradigm shift has occurred in monitoring and evaluating population health. Not only the changes in morbidity or extension of the lifespan but also, the way in which individuals experience their health, has gained importance as an outcome criterion [1]. As soon as perceived health emerges as a relevant outcome, the interest on patient-centered outcome research flourished and expanded the assessment to other domains of the human life. This development introduced us to the concept of health-related quality of life (HRQoL).

Although functional status, perceived health, quality of life, and HRQoL are often used interchangeably, these terms have subtle but important differences with respect to dimensionality, perspective and scope. In terms of health outcomes measures, researchers may use several different indicators. For example, wellbeing, HRQoL, and perceived health outcomes will have certain overlap; however they are not the same. We may distribute these concepts along a continuum where some are more psychologically subjective (e.g. wellbeing), and at the opposite end are the more physical or somatic outcomes (e.g. perceived health). All these outcomes are affected by the living conditions and socioeconomic status, the personality characteristics of the individual and the disease and its treatment in the case of non-healthy subjects.

To use a more precise terminology, *quality of life* (QoL) is understood as a general concept that implies an evaluation of the impact of all aspects of life on general wellbeing. Because this term QoL implies an evaluation of non-health-related aspects of life, it is too broad to be considered appropriate for a medical product claim or to assess effectiveness of medical treatments [2]. So, the use of HRQoL outcome as another measure of clinical effectiveness of medical treatments or to support labeling and promotional claims is more appropriate.

What does health-related quality of life mean?

HRQoL is defined as the subjective assessment of the impact of disease and treatment across the physical, psychological, social and somatic domains of functioning and wellbeing. As the definition implies, it is a subjective experience, and this is a crucial aspect of HRQoL. This means that only the patient may inform about their view and experience related to the disease, without the interpretation of the patient's response by a physician or anyone else. In addition, according to Bullinger's definition [3], HRQoL is a multidimensional construct pertaining to the physical, emotional, mental, social and behavioral components of wellbeing and function, as perceived by the patients and/or observers. The idea of observers is included here, because sometimes the patient is not able to inform about their experience, for example, young children, a cognitive impaired person, or someone with severe psychiatric illness. Therefore, the perception of a parent or caregiver becomes important.

Common dimensions of the HRQoL evaluation include physical health, bodily pain, functional status, emotional or affective functioning, social functioning and mental health. Sometimes these domains are summarized in a physical and psychological or mental component (e.g. MOS-SF-36). Some authors [2] have suggested that a minimum of three domains – physical, psychological and social – are essential to any assessment of HRQoL.

Importance of the evaluation of health-related quality of life

Several publications stress on the importance of the assessment of HRQoL as an additional health outcome. So, HRQoL is now

Current and Future Issues in Hemophilia Care, First Edition. Edited by Emérito-Carlos Rodríguez-Merchán and Leonard A. Valentino.
© 2011 John Wiley & Sons, Ltd. Published 2011 by Blackwell Publishing Ltd.

Table 11.1 Studies assessing HRQoL with disease-specific measures in hemophilia

Year	Authors	Country	Participants	Sample (n)	Measure
2000	Bullinger et al. [6]	6 European countries	Children/adolescents and parents	58*	Haemo-QoL
2004	v. Mackensen et al. [7]	6 European countries	Children/adolescents and parents	339#	Haemo-QoL
2004	Young et al. [8]	Canada	Children/adolescents and parents	50**	CHO-KLAT
2004	Arranz et al. [9]	Spain	Adults	73**	Hemofilia-QoL
				35*	(version 1.0)
2005	Remor et al. [5]	8 Latin-American countries	Adults	50**	Hemolatin-QoL
2005	Remor et al. [10]	Spain	Adults	121#	A36 Hemofilia-QoL
2005	v. Mackensen et al. [11]	Italy	Adults	233#	Hemo-A-QoL
2006	Gueróis et al. [12]	France	Children/adolescents and parents, adults	70**	QUAL HEMO
2008	Rentz et al. [13]	Germany, Spain, USA, Canada	Adults	221#	Haemo-QoL-A

*Pilot testing, psychometric; **Development study; #Psychometric field study. CHO-KLAT (Canadian Haemophilia Outcomes – Kids Life Assessment Tool); Haemo-QoL (Children's Haemophilia Quality-of-life questionnaire); Haemo-QoL-A (Adults Haemophilia Quality-of-life questionnaire) A36 Hemofilia-QoL (Adults Haemophilia Quality of Life questionnaire); HemoLatin-QoL (Adults Haemophilia Quality of Life questionnaire); Hemo-A-QoL (Hemophilia QoL questionnaire for adults).

increasingly used as a measure of health status in national health surveys and one of the major descriptors and outcome criteria discussed in the health care systems in recent years [2]. The purpose of the HRQoL evaluation is to go beyond the presence and severity of symptoms of disease or side effects of treatment, examining how patients perceive and experience these manifestations in their daily lives. So, measurement of HRQoL may be essential to a full understanding of how successful particular treatments or interventions are likely to be in the recipient's terms. It enables health-care providers to compare interventions for the same disease and across different diseases. Where good cross-cultural measures are available then they may facilitate comparison of outcomes from international clinical trials. For those individuals diagnosed with a chronic condition where cure is not attainable and therapy may be prolonged, HRQoL is the essential outcome, also.

Thus, the objectives of HRQoL research depend on the type of study perspective. For example, an epidemiological study has as its objective the description of the wellbeing, health status and disease-related function. The clinical or pharmacological study will focus on the evaluation of treatment effects, and the public health or health economics study will include an analysis of quality and cost of care. So, the instruments to assess the QoL should be chosen taking into account the perspective of the study.

What types of measurement of the HRQoL are available? The most frequently form of measurement is the questionnaire or patient reported outcomes (PRO) measures, however a few structured interviews, or utility measures (for health economics approach) are available as well. The characteristics of the HRQoL instruments may be classified as generic vs. disease-specific, one-dimensional vs. multidimensional, self-rated vs. other-rated (proxy), in person vs. distance (web/phone/mail) and paper vs. electronic (web, digital devices).

Quality of life assessment in hemophilia

Several studies have been published addressing quality of life issues in people with hemophilia, most of which employed generic measures for the QoL assessment. A review of studies assessing HRQoL with generic measures (e.g., SF-36, EQ-5D or CHQ-CF/PF) have been published earlier [4,5]. Table 11.1 provides an update overview of the studies using a disease-specific measure (data is presented in chronological order).

A few studies [3,4,7,9] have warned about the possible limitations that generic instruments pose for the evaluation of specific concerns of hemophilia patients. For the adequate assessment of HRQoL and following the tendency in other medicine fields, different working groups have started the development of disease-specific measures to assess QoL in people living with hemophilia in different regions of the world. These new, more recent measures for children and adults were specially developed and validated for the adequate assessment of HRQoL in people living with hemophilia, and are comprehensive and multidimensional.

Choosing a hemophilia PRO measure

Nowadays several hemophilia PRO measures are available (Tables 11.1 and 11.2). When a HRQoL measure is to be chosen, study- and instrument-related aspects have to be taken into account. Some of the criteria to choose, in terms of study-related issues, are the type and scope of the study (e.g., if the study is cross-sectional and different diseases will be compared, a generic measure is more appropriate), the study population (e.g., if is a pediatric or adult), how the study protocol will be administered (e.g., in person vs. distance), the type of outcomes needed (e.g., clinical, psychological, social, treatment, environmental, or

Table 11.2 HRQOL instruments for hemophilia available

Children (C/P version)	Age groups	Adults	Age focus
Cho-KLAT	4–7 (C/P), 8–12 (C/P), 13–17 (C/P)	A36 Hemofilia-QoL	> 17 years old
Haemo-QoL	4–7 (C/P), 8–12 (C/P), 13–17 (C/P)	Haemo-QoL-A	> 18 years old
QUAL HEMO	2–12 (C/P), 13–17	QUAL HEMO	> 18 years old
		Haem-A-QoL	> 18 years old
		HemoLatin-QoL	> 17 years old

C/P, Child/parents.

cost-related), and time for protocol completion (e.g., if is short, a brief measure will be recommended). On the other hand, in terms of instrument-related issues, the criteria to choose include who will fill out the questionnaire (e.g., if is the patient or other, proxy), the type of questionnaire needed (e.g., generic or disease-specific), psychometric characteristics available about the instrument (evidences of validity), feasibility of the PRO (acceptance, relevance, completion time) and the aspects covered by domains.

Health-related quality of life instruments for hemophilia

The instruments available to assess HRQoL across lifespan in hemophilia patients are described in Table 11.2. Three of the instruments are focused on the pediatric population (includes parents' view) and five are focus on adult assessment.

In this chapter we focus briefly on the A36Hemofilia-QoL and HemoLatin-QoL measures. The A36Hemofilia-QoL is an adult PRO which is used for patients over 17 years of age, includes 36 items, and takes 10 to 15 minutes to complete. It is a multidimensional instrument assessing nine relevant domains for hemophilia (i.e., physical health, daily activities, joint damage, pain, treatment satisfaction, treatment difficulties, emotional functioning, mental health, relationships and social activity). A global QoL index is possible to score as well [9,10]. The instrument was originally developed in Spain and several versions are currently available in different languages (Czech, Danish, English, Iranian, Norwegian, Polish, Sesotho, Spanish, Swedish, and Tagalog), and are being used by independent researchers. The manual for the questionnaire is available in Spanish and English, and a copy of the manual can be obtained from the authors. The evidence for the validity of the A36Hemofilia-QoL includes face and content validity, reliability and test–retest reliability, construct validity (concurrent with MOS-SF-36, EQ-5D and clinical markers, and discriminant over clinical markers), incremental validity (comparison with EQ-5D VAS) [9,10,14].

Another instrument, developed for use in adults and cross-culturally adapted for use in Latin America, is the HemoLatin-QoL. The questionnaire was developed for Latin-American countries and is available for two main languages, namely Latin-American Spanish and Brazilian Portuguese [5]. A psychometric field study is currently in progress. The preliminary version being tested consists of 47 items pertaining to 10 dimensions ("pain", "physical health", "emotional functioning", "social support", "activities and social functioning", "medical treatment", "mental health", "environment and resources satisfaction", "general wellbeing") and one single item for "general health". The psychometric study will help to refine the instrument and assist in the selection of best items to be maintained in the final version. Additional information about the questionnaire is available at the website www.hemolatin-qol.info.

Evidence of clinical indicators impacting HRQoL measured by PRO

There is evidence [10,15,16] that some clinical markers have a negative impact in the HRQoL of hemophilia patients, such as the number of hemarthroses in the prior year, the total number of bleeding episodes in the prior year, the number of damaged joints, the presence of human immunodeficiency virus (HIV) infection, the presence of hepatitis C virus (HCV) infection, presence of chronic pain (not related to bleeding), and the presence of inhibitors. The evidence of the negative impact of the presence of inhibitors on the HRQoL is true for children, adolescents and adults.

When inhibitors are present in adolescents and adults [15] the quality of life domains that are most affected, controlling for age effect, are poor mobility, low self-care, difficulty with daily activities, pain/discomfort, anxiety/depression (mood) in comparison to those without inhibitors.

For children and adolescents with inhibitors [10] the evidence includes low self-esteem, family attitude (over-protection), poor relationship with friends, difficulties with school activity, increase in the frequency of bleeding events, poor physical health, emotional distress related to the disease (mood), limited sports activity, and poor perceived health.

In terms of psychological process, the presence of inhibitors may exacerbate the sense of loss of control over the disease, and, as a consequence, lead to an increase in maladaptive behaviors (for example, not follow medical recommendations or engaging in high risk behaviors). In summary, poor relationship with friends (isolation), difficulties with daily activities, dealing with an over-protective family attitude, difficulties with school (sports) or work activities, contribute to experiencing feelings of being different from others, feelings of shame, leading to a perceived hemophilia-related stigma. Illness-related stigma has been related to decrease in wellbeing and perceived QoL in several health conditions.

Furthermore, hemophilia severity is related to treatment difficulties. Patients with mild and moderate levels of severity experience more treatment difficulties [14,17]. They probably have a general lack of knowledge and experience with the disease symptoms and poor self-care skills. Also, a negative affect (anxiety/depression) is a risk factor for treatment difficulties and dissatisfaction with treatment [14].

Conclusions

The modern management of hemophilia has greatly influenced not only survival of patients, their clinical symptoms and orthopedic outcome, but also their perceived QoL. Health outcome data, such as HRQoL, have become essential to optimize treatments and allocate resources in a cost-intensive chronic disease such as hemophilia where traditional outcome measures such as mortality are no longer significantly influenced by diverse treatment options. Capturing HRQoL is a unique way to assess the general wellbeing and perceived health of patients with hemophilia, their particular experiences related to the condition and satisfaction with treatment. And finally, there is evidence that HRQoL of men with hemophilia is affected by the disease severity and its complications. For that reason this outcome is an important key piece of data to take into account in clinical practice, and in any medical or pharmaceutical study.

References

1. Ravens-Sieberer U. Measuring and monitoring quality-of-life in population surveys: still a challenge for public health research. Soz.-Präventivmed 2001;46:201–4.
2. Revicki DA, Osoba D, Fairclough D, Barofsky I, Berzon I, Leidy NK, et al. Recommendations on health-related quality of life research to support labeling and promotional claims in the United States. Qual Life Res 2000;9:887–900.
3. Bullinger M. Quality of life-definition, conceptualization and implications – a methodologist's view. Thero Surg 1991;6:143–9.
4. Remor E., Young NI, von Mackensen S, Lopatina EG. Disease-specific quality of life measurement tools for haemophilia patients. Haemophilia 2004;10 (Suppl. 4): 30–34.

5. Remor E. Desarrollo de una medida específica para la evaluación de la calidad de vida en pacientes adultos viviendo con hemofilia en América-Latina: el Hemolatin-QoL. R Interam Psicol 2005;39:211–20.
6. Bullinger M, von Mackensen S, Fisher K, Khair K, Petersen C, Ravens-Sieberer U, et al. Pilot testing of the Haemo-QoL quality of life questionnaire for haemophiliac children in six European countries. Haemophilia 2002;8 (Suppl. 2): 47–54.
7. von Mackensen S, Bullinger M and the Haemo-QoL Group. Development and testing of an instrument to assess the quality of life of children with haemophilia in Europe (Haemo-QoL). Haemophilia 2004;10 (Suppl. 1): 17–25.
8. Young NL, Bradley CS, Blanchette V, Wakefield CD, Baranrd D, Wu JK, et al. Development of a health related quality of life measure for boys with haemophilia: the Canadian Hemophilia Outcomes – Kids Life Assessment Tool (CHO-KLAT). Haemophilia 2004;10 (Suppl. 1): 34–43.
9. Arranz P, Remor E, Quintana M, Villar A, Diaz JL, Moreno M, et al. Development of a new disease–specific quality-of-life questionnaire to adults living with haemophilia. Haemophilia 2004;10:376–82.
10. Remor E, Arranz P, Quintana M, Villar A, Jimenez-Yuste V, Diaz JL, et al. Psychometric field study of the new haemophilia quality of life questionnaire for adults: The 'Hemofilia-QoL'. Haemophilia 2005;11:603–610.
11. von Mackensen S, Scalone L, Ravera S, Mantovani L, Gringeri A. Assessment of health-related quality of life in patients with haemophilia with the newly developed haemophilia-specific instrument (Haem-A-QoL). Value Health 2005;8: A127 [abstract PHM5].
12. Guerois C, Lambert T, Peynet J, Fressinaud E, Chambost H, Trudeau E. Assessment of quality of life in hemophilia population: validation of the QUAL-HEMO, a French haemophilia age-group specific quality of life questionnaire. Haemophilia 2006;12 (Suppl. 2): PO804.
13. Rentz A, Flood E, Altisent C, Bullinger M, Klamroth R, Garrido RP, et al. Cross-cultural development and psychometric evaluation of a patient-reported health-related quality of life questionnaire for adults with haemophilia. Haemophilia 2008;14:1023–34.
14. Remor E. Predictors of treatment difficulties and satisfaction with hemophilia therapy in adult patients. J Coagul Disord 2010; The print version of the journal was concealed. The paper is available online at the follow URL. http://www.slm-hematology.com/uploads/media/JCD10022_-_Predictors_of_Treatment_Difficulties_and_Satisfaction_With_Hemophilia_Therapy_in_Adult_Patients.pdf.
15. Remor E, Arranz P, Miller R. Psychosocial impact of inhibitors on haemophilia patients' quality of life. In: Rodriguez-Merchan EC, Lee CA, eds. Inhibitors in Patients with Haemophilia. Oxford: Blackwell Science. 2002:187–92.
16. Morfini M, Haya S, Tagaraiello G, Pollman H, Quintana M, Siegmund B, et al. European study on orthopaedic status of haemophilia patients with inhibitors. Haemophilia 2007;13:606–612.
17. Lindvall K, Colstrup L, Loogna K, Wollter IM, Gronhaug S. Knowledge of disease and adherence in adult patients with hemophilia. Hemophilia 2010;16:592–6.

3 Inhibitors

12 Immunology of Inhibitor Development

Birgit M. Reipert, Christoph J. Hofbauer, Katharina N. Steinitz, Hans-Peter Schwarz and Frank M. Horling

Baxter Innovation GmbH, Vienna, Austria

Introduction

Circulating anticoagulants directed against antihemophilic factor were initially reported in the 1940s and 1950s [1]. Importantly, such anticoagulants were found not only in the blood of some patients with classic hemophilia, but also in women who developed a bleeding disorder within one or two years of childbirth, and in elderly women and men who did not have a prior history of bleeding disorders. Anticoagulants were described to impair blood clotting in all these clinical situations by inhibiting or inactivating antihemophilic factor [1].

Today we know that previously described anticoagulants against antihemophilic factor are neutralizing antibodies against the clotting factor VIII (FVIII), frequently referred to as FVIII inhibitors. The development of these antibodies in patients with congenital hemophilia A represents the most serious adverse event following replacement therapy with FVIII products. Their appearance in otherwise healthy individuals causes a severe autoimmune disease, known as acquired hemophilia A.

Why some patients with congenital hemophilia A develop antibodies against FVIII following replacement therapy while others do not is far from clear. The generation of antibodies is the result of a cascade of tightly regulated interactions between different cells of the innate and adaptive immune system in very distinct compartments. Any event that modulates the repertoire, the activation state or the migration pattern of immune cells will, therefore, have the potential to influence the risk of patients to develop antibodies against FVIII.

Immunology of antibody responses to proteins

The initial event in any antibody response against proteins is the recognition of proteins by specific naïve B cells which reside in and circulate through the follicles of peripheral lymphoid organs such as spleen, lymph nodes or mucosal lymphoid tissues. Proteins enter these lymphoid organs through the blood or lymph, often transported by dendritic cells that can recycle antigen to the cell surface in an intact form to make it available for binding by specific B cells [2]. Proteins bind to specific antigen receptors (B cell receptors) expressed on naïve B cells. Receptor binding causes the formation of antigen-receptor complexes that initiate the activation of intracellular signal-transduction pathways, which can eventually lead to B-cell activation and clonal expansion as well as differentiation into antibody-producing plasma cells. These plasma cells can be either short-lived or long-lived. The regulation of longevity has been the subject of intense research activities in recent years [3].

In principle, B-cell activation and differentiation may occur in a T-cell dependent or T-cell independent way (Figure 12.1). Multivalent antigens with repetitive epitopes can cross-link B cell receptors, thereby causing clustering of receptors which initiates B-cell activation. T-cell independent B-cell activation mainly involves B1 B cells and marginal zone B cells that express a restricted repertoire of germline-encoded antigen receptors with polyreactive specificities. Resulting plasma cells are short-lived and predominantly secrete antibodies of the IgM type with low affinity due to the lack of affinity maturation. B1 B cells are mainly located in the peritoneum and in mucosal sites. Marginal zone B cells, on the other hand, reside in the marginal zones surrounding lymphoid follicles in the spleen and are mainly involved in T-cell independent immune responses to blood-borne antigens [4].

Proteins such as FVIII are generally considered to be T-cell dependent antigens. B cells recognizing proteins require the help of specific CD4+ helper T cells to expand and differentiate into antibody-producing plasma cells. Interactions between B cells and CD4+ helper T cells not only initiate expansion and differentiation of B cells but also trigger isotype switching and affinity

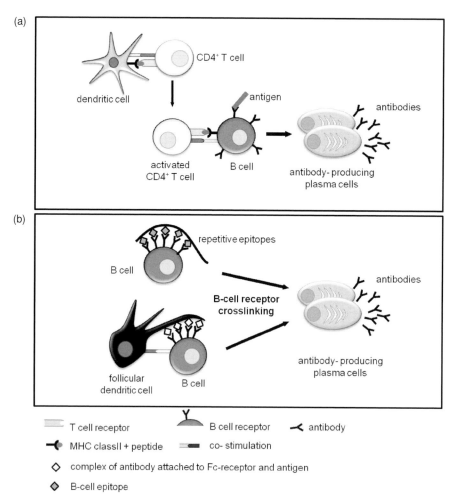

Figure 12.1 Schematic views of T-cell dependent (a) and T-cell independent (b) antibody responses .

maturation of antibodies, which results in the switch from IgM to IgG, IgA and IgE and, furthermore, in the generation of high-affinity antibodies. Isotype switching is caused by class-switch recombination, in which the gene segment coding for the constant region of the heavy chain of an immunoglobulin is changed and the gene segments coding for the variable region are maintained. Affinity maturation is induced by hypermutations of the immunoglobulin genes and subsequent survival of those B cells that produce the antibodies with the highest affinity [5].

A typical feature of T-cell dependent antibody responses against protein antigens is the differentiation of B cells into memory B cells that express high affinity B-cell receptors and respond very quickly and efficiently after re-encounter with the same protein. Different phases of T-cell dependent antibody responses occur in different anatomic sites within peripheral lymphoid organs. Early phases occur at the border between T-cell rich zones and primary follicles. Late phases require the specialized microenvironment of germinal centers [6].

Today, it is generally accepted that B cells require cognate interaction with CD4+ helper T cells to develop high affinity antibodies against protein antigens [7]. Initially, however, CD4+ helper

T cells need to interact with mature dendritic cells that present antigenic peptides in the context of the major histocompatibility complex (MHC) classII and express co-stimulatory molecules. CD4+ helper T cells recognize the peptide-MHC class II complex by their specific T-cell receptors. The nature of the initial interaction between CD4+ helper T cells and dendritic cells determines the outcome of the immune response against protein antigens. Only fully mature dendritic cells are considered to be able to trigger CD4+ helper T cells to facilitate differentiation of B cells into antibody-producing plasma cells that produce high-affinity antibodies. When CD4+ helper T cells interact with immature dendritic cells, they either undergo clonal deletion, anergy or develop into regulatory T cells that may induce tolerance rather than antibody responses. In this way, dendritic cells can be considered to be the key regulators of adaptive immunity against protein antigens [8]. Dendritic cells are derived from bone marrow and circulate as precursors in the blood before entering tissues where they become resident immature dendritic cells that are able to sense changes in their local environment [9]. Maturation of dendritic cells requires proinflammatory stimuli such as pathogen-associated molecular patterns (e.g. ligands for toll-like receptors) or inflammatory cytokines. Importantly, maturation signals for dendritic cells can also arise from damage-associated molecular patterns that are released during cell necrosis and tissue destruction [10].

The view on T-cell dependent and T-cell independent antibody responses has been slightly revised in recent years based on discoveries that have provided exceptions to the classic perception that isotype switch recombination of antibodies can only occur in the presence of T-cell help. Several new mechanisms for T-cell independent antibody responses have been described indicating the possibility of IgG and IgA production in the absence of classic T-cell help. Swanson et al. [11] described the enhancement of T-cell independent antibody responses by agonists for toll-like receptor 3 (TLR3). Triggering of TLR3 promoted the participation of follicular B cells in the immune response against a T-cell independent antigen resulting in the production of IgG antibodies. Similar to IgM antibodies, however, these IgG antibodies showed relatively low affinity, indicating a lack of affinity maturation. Another example for T-cell independent class-switch recombination is the induction of IgA production at mucosal sites where both T-cell dependent (Peyer's patches) and T-cell independent (lamina propria) mechanisms of class switch recombination to IgA have been described. Dendritic cells and epithelial cells in addition to classic T-cell help seem to be able to induce the class switch from IgM to IgA in B cells [12].

El Shikh et al. [13] recently reported that follicular dendritic cells (present in germinal centers) that periodically arrange immune complexes of T-dependent antigens bound to Fc receptors on their cell surface can also stimulate T-cell independent antibody responses against classic T-cell dependent antigens such as proteins by presenting them as repetitive epitopes to B cells. This mechanism would imply that once initial antibody responses against a protein have occurred, subsequent encounter with the same protein could result in both T-cell dependent and T-cell independent antibody responses.

What do we know about antibody responses against FVIII in patients?

For many years, most clinical studies have been restricted to the detection of antibodies that neutralize FVIII activity (FVIII inhibitors). The quantification of total binding antibodies directed against FVIII was almost neglected. Therefore, it was difficult to assess the overall immune response to FVIII associated with replacement therapy. FVIII inhibitors are quantified by measuring the Bethesda titer. The amount of antibody that neutralizes 50% of normal plasma FVIII activity is defined as one Bethesda unit (BU) [14]. More recently, a series of assay platforms for the detection of total binding antibodies against FVIII were presented based on the classic ELISA format, immunoblotting or bead-based formats [15,16]. These studies clearly indicated that neutralizing antibodies represent only part of the overall antibody spectrum directed against FVIII. As expected, there are binding antibod-

ies with specificity to FVIII that do not neutralize the protein's activity and, therefore, are not detectable using a Bethesda assay. Consequently, circulating antibodies against FVIII are found in a proportion of patients without FVIII inhibitors and even in some healthy individuals [16]. Most FVIII inhibitors bind to functionally important domains of FVIII and prevent its interaction with other coagulation factors such as factors IIa, IXa, X and von Willebrand factor or with phospholipids [17]. Other FVIII inhibitors seem to have catalytic activity and hydrolyze the protein [18]. Non-neutralizing anti-FVIII antibodies are directed against nonfunctional regions of FVIII and might influence the stability and/or the pharmacokinetic of FVIII [19].

Several findings indicated that CD4+ T cells are involved in the regulation of anti-FVIII antibody development in patients. Bray et al. reported that FVIII inhibitors decreased when CD4+ T cell levels dropped in patients with HIV infections [20]. Several authors have presented evidence that anti-FVIII antibodies isolated from patients with hemophilia A show signs of somatic hypermutations, a prerequisite for affinity maturation, which requires cognate interactions of B cells and CD4+ T cells. Another indication for the involvement of CD4+ T cells is the dominance of switched antibodies in the pool of FVIII inhibitors. Gilles et al. [19] and others reported that the antibody response to FVIII in patients is not isotypically restricted and involves all IgG subclasses with a preponderance of IgG1 and IgG4. IgE antibodies against FVIII have been reported in single cases which were associated with anaphylactic reactions observed after replacement therapy with FVIII [21]. More direct evidence for the involvement of CD4+ T cells comes from in vitro analyses of FVIII-specific T cells in peripheral blood cells obtained from patients. Results of these studies indicate that different subclasses of CD4+ T cells are involved in the regulation of anti-FVIII antibody responses [22,23]. However, more comprehensive longitudinal studies on the evolution of FVIII-specific CD4+ T cell responses are still missing. In particular, studies that focus on the very early events in the development of anti-FVIII antibodies are required to better understand how the immune system decides whether or not to develop antibodies against FVIII.

What have we learned from immune responses against FVIII in animal models?

In 1995, Bi et al. [24] introduced two murine models of hemophilia A that formed the basis for a series of experimental studies aimed at better understanding the regulation of antibody responses against FVIII. The two models express a typical phenotype of hemophilia A. One was generated by disrupting exon 16 and the other by disrupting exon 17 of the murine FVIII gene, in both cases causing a complete lack of FVIII protein in the circulation. Treatment with human FVIII elicits antibodies that are similar to those observed in patients with FVIII inhibitors [25]. The induction of these antibodies depends on cognate interactions between B cells and

CD4$^+$ T cells and can be prevented by inhibiting the activation of CD4$^+$ T cells or by blocking interactions of B cells and CD4$^+$ T cells [26]. Once induced, anti-FVIII antibodies persist in the circulation, corresponding to the long-term presence of anti-FVIII antibody-producing plasma cells in spleen and bone marrow [27].

Several groups have used hemophilic mice to test new concepts for modulating anti-FVIII immune responses. These concepts included blockade of co-stimulatory interactions between B cells and CD4$^+$ T cells, T-cell modulation by anti-CD3 antibodies, inhibition of anti-FVIII antibody responses by high doses of ligands for toll-like receptor 9, mutagenesis of key epitopes of FVIII, complex formation of FVIII with O-phospho-L-serine (OPLS), intrathymic FVIII injection, mucosal application of FVIII domains, use of peptide epitope surrogates, tolerogenic presentation of FVIII by immature dendritic cells, delivery of FVIII by transgenic apoptotic fibroblasts, inhibition of FVIII-specific memory B cells with high doses of FVIII and several gene therapy approaches. It remains to be seen if any of these experimental approaches can be translated into new therapeutic approaches for the prevention of FVIII inhibitor formation in patients.

Recently, Skupsky et al. [28] and Dimitrov et al. [29] presented evidence that the immunogenicity of FVIII in hemophilic mice is determined by the concomitant induction of proinflammatory signals that cause an induction of the innate immune system. These proinflammatory signals might be induced by proteins such as thrombin that are directly involved in the coagulation cascade. Based on Skupsky et al.'s findings the prevention of proinflammatory signals during application of FVIII could be expected to decrease the immunogenicity of FVIII. A recent paper by Kurnik et al. [30] indicated that this might indeed be the case. The authors presented clinical data showing that a new early prophylaxis regimen that avoids immunological "danger signals" might be able to reduce inhibitor formation in patients. However, larger clinical trials are required to prove this concept.

Conclusions

The generation of high affinity antibodies against protein antigens such as FVIII is believed to require cognate interactions between B cells and CD4$^+$ helper T cells to initiate somatic hypermutations of immunoglobulin genes for affinity maturation of antibodies and to facilitate class-switch recombination for generation of IgG, IgA or IgE antibodies. Subsequent encounter with the same protein might induce both T-cell dependent and T-cell independent antibody responses. Furthermore, based on current knowledge, it cannot be excluded that antibody responses against proteins such as FVIII could also occur in a T-cell independent way. Such antibodies should be of low affinity due to the lack of affinity maturation.

Several pieces of evidence suggest that the antibody response to FVIII in patients is regulated by CD4$^+$ T cells. The answer to the question why some patients develop antibodies while others do not requires more comprehensive longitudinal immunological studies that focus on early events in the development of anti-FVIII immune responses.

References

1. Margolius A, Jackson DP, Ratnoff O. Circulating anticoagulants: a study of 40 cases and a review of the literature. Medicine (Baltimore) 1961;40:145–202.
2. Wykes M, Pombo A, Jenkins C, MacPherson GG. Dendritic cells interact directly with naïve B lymphocytes to transfer antigen and initiate class switching in a primary T-dependent response. J Immunol 1998;161:1313–19.
3. Radbruch A, Muehlinghaus G, Luger EO, Inamine A, Smith KGC, Dörner T, Hiepe F. Competence and competition: the challenge of becoming a long-lived plasma cell. Nature Rev Immunol 2006;6:741–50.
4. Baumgarth N, Choi YS, Rothaeusler K, Yang Y, Herzenberg LA. B cell lineage contributions to antiviral host responses. Curr Top Microbiol Immunol 2008;319:41–61.
5. Wolniak KL, Shinall SM, Waldschmidt TJ. The germinal center response. Crit Rev Immunol 2004;24:39–65.
6. McHeyzer-Williams LJ, Malherbe LP, McHeyzer-Williams MG. Checkpoints in memory B-cell evolution. Immunol Rev 2006;211:255–68.
7. Rajewsky K. Clonal selection and learning in the antibody system. Nature 1996;381:751–8.
8. O'Shea JJ, Paul WE. Mechanisms underlying lineage commitment and plasticity of helper CD4$^+$ T cells. Science 2010;327:1098–102.
9. Steinman RM. Dendritic cells: understanding immunogenicity. Eur J Immunol 2007;37 (Suppl 1):S53–60.
10. Chen GY, Nunez G. Sterile inflammation: sensing and reacting to damage. Nature Rev Immunol 2010;10:826–37.
11. Swanson CL, Wilson TJ, Strauch P, Colonna M, Pelanda R, Torres RM. Type I IFN enhances follicular B cell contribution to the T cell-independent antibody response. J Exp Med 2010;207:1485–500.
12. Cerutti A. The regulation of IgA class switching. Nature Rev Immunol 2008;8:421–34.
13. El Shikh MEM, El Sayed RM, Szakal AK, Tew JG. T-independent antibody responses to T-dependent antigens: a novel follicular dendritic cell-dependent activity. J Immunol 2009;182;3482–91.
14. Verbruggen B, van Heerde WL, Laros-van Gorkom BAP. Improvements in Factor VIII Inhibitor Detection: From Bethesda to Nijmegen. Semin Thromb Hemost 2009;35:752–9.
15. van Helden PMW, van den Berg HM, Gouw SC, Kaijen PHP, Zuurveld MG, Mauser-Bunschoten EP, Aalberse RC, Vidarsson G, Voorberg J. IgG subclasses of anti-FVIII antibodies during immune tolerance induction in patients with hemophilia A. Br J Haematol 2008;142:644–52.
16. Krudysz-Amblo J, Parhami-Seren B, Butenas S, Brummel-Ziedins KE, Gomperts, ED, Rivard GE, Mann KG. Quantitation of anti-factor VIII antibodies in human plasma. Blood 2009;113:2587–94.
17. Ananyeva NM, Lacroix-Desmazes S, Hauser CAE, Shima M, Ovanesov MV, Khrenov AV, Saenko EL. Inhibitors in hemophilia A: mechanisms of inhibition, management and perspectives. Blood Coagulation Fibrinolysis 2004;15:109–24.
18. Lacroix-Desmazes S, Moreau A, Sooryanarayana, Bonnemain C, Stieltjes N, Pashov A, Sultan Y, Hoebeke J, Kazatchkine MD, Kaveri

SV. Catalytic activity of antibodies against factor VIII in patients with hemophilia A. Nature Med 1999;5:1044–7.

19. Gilles JG, Arnout J, Vermylen J, Saint-Remy JM. Anti-factor VIII antibodies of hemophiliac patients are less frequently directed towards nonfunctional determinants and do not exhibit isotypic restriction. Blood 1993;892:2452–61.

20. Bray GL, Kroner BL, Arkin S, Aledort LW, Hilgartner MW, Eyster ME, Ragni MV, Goedert JJ. Loss of high-responder inhibitors in patients with severe hemophilia A and human immunodeficiency Virus Type 1 Infection. Am J Hematol 1993;42:375–9.

21. Kadar JG, Schuster J, Hunzelmann N. IgE-mediated anaphylactic reaction to purified and recombinant factor VIII in a patient with severe haemophilia A. Haemophilia 2007;13:104–5.

22. Jacquemin M, Vantomme V, Buhot C, Lavend'homme R, Burny W, Demotte N, Chaux P, Peerlinck K, Vermylen J, Maillere B, van der Bruggen P, Saint-Remy JM. CD4 +T-cell clones specific for wild-type factor VIII: a molecular mechanism responsible for a higher incidence of inhibitor formation in mild/moderate hemophilia A. Blood. 2003;101:1351–8.

23. Ettinger RA, James EA, Kwok WW, Thompson AR, Pratt KP. Lineages of human T-cell clones, including T helper 17/T helper 1 cells, isolated at different stages of anti-factor VIII immune responses. Blood. 2009;114:1423–8.

24. Bi L, Lawler AM, Antonarakis SE, High KA, Gearhart JD, Kazazian HH. Targeted disruption of the mouse factor VIII gene produces a model of haemophilia A. Nature Genet 1995;10:119–21.

25. Reipert BM, Ahmad RU, Turecek PL, Schwarz HP. Characterization of antibodies induced by human factor VIII in a murine knockout model of hemophilia A. Thromb Haemost 2000;84:826–32.

26. Qian J, Collins M, Sharpe AH, Hoyer LW. Prevention and treatment of factor VIII inhibitors in murine hemophilia A. Blood 2000;95:1324–29.

27. Hausl C, Maier E, Schwarz HP, Ahmad RU, Turecek PL, Dorner F, Reipert BM. Long-term persistence of anti-factor VIII antibody-secreting cells in hemophilic mice after treatment with human factor VIII. Thromb Haemost 2002;87:840–45.

28. Skupsky J, Zhang AH, Su Y, Scott DW. A role for thrombin in the initiation of the immune response to therapeutic factor VIII. Blood 2009;114:4741–8.

29. Dimitrov JD, Dasgupta S, Navarrete AM, et al. Induction of heme oxygenase-1 in factor VIII-deficient mice reduces the immune response to therapeutic factor VIII. Blood 2009;115:2682–5.

30. Kurnik K, Bidlingmaier C, Engl W, Chehadeh H, Reipert B, Auerswald G. New early prophylaxis regimen that avoids immunological danger signals can reduce FVIII inhibitor development. Haemophilia 2010;16:256–62.

13 Epidemiology of Inhibitors

Johanna G. van der Bom

Leiden University Medical Center, Leiden, The Netherlands

Introduction

During the first decade of the 21st century, knowledge about the etiology of inhibitors has advanced rapidly with the discovery of several factors that contribute to the incidence of inhibitors, particularly the role of treatment related factors [1]. The most intriguing observations are those that suggest that avoiding the presence of endogenous danger signals early during the replacement treatment of patients with hemophilia A reduces their risk to develop inhibitors by inducing tolerance to exogenous factor VIII. If true, it might be possible to prevent inhibitors in a significant number of patients. Figure 1 illustrates inhibitor occurrence in eight patients who developed inhibitors before the age of one year.

Hemophilia B versus hemophilia A

We have learned about inhibitor etiology from observing differences between patients with hemophilia A and B. Hemophilia A and B are traditionally thought of as one bleeding disorder caused by the deficiency of two different clotting factors. Yet, there are many more differences between patients who have a deficiency of factor VIII and patients who have a deficiency of factor IX [2]. One difference is their risk of inhibitor development which is only about 2% among patients with hemophilia B, whereas it is about 25 percent among patients with severe hemophilia A [3]. This difference may among other things be explained by a difference in molecular size of factor IX and factor VIII. Infusion of a larger "non-self" molecule will present more "non-self" epitopes and may therefore carry a higher risk to induce the development of inhibitory antibodies [4].

Severe, moderate, mild hemophilia

Similarly, observed differences in incidence of inhibitors between patients with different severities of hemophilia have provided insight into the role of the types of mutations in the clotting factor gene and their resulting hemophilia phenotype on inhibitor occurrence. It is now generally agreed that the mutation in the gene for factor VIII or IX that bring about the clotting factor deficiency has a great impact on inhibitor incidences. Mutations that totally prevent endogenous synthesis of factor VIII protein, such as large deletions, non-sense mutations and the prevalent intron 22 inversions are associated with a much higher incidence of inhibitors as compared to missense and splice-site mutations [5]. In mild to moderate hemophilia, missense mutations represent the main mutation type, with a relatively low inhibitor incidence of 5%. These patients synthesize some endogenous protein that appears to be sufficient to induce immune tolerance. However, in patients with missense mutations clustered in the A2 and C2 domains (C1/C2 junction), the risk of inhibitor formation is fourfold greater than in patients with mutations outside this region, indicating that inhibitor incidence in missense mutations is also dependent on localization of the mutation [6,7].

Incidences of inhibitors vary between and within families

In addition to the hemophilia causing mutation in the gene for factor VIII and IX, variants of other genes are related to a patient's risk to develop inhibitors. A positive family history of inhibitors is related to the incidence of inhibitors even among

Current and Future Issues in Hemophilia Care, First Edition. Edited by Emérito-Carlos Rodríguez-Merchán and Leonard A. Valentino.
© 2011 John Wiley & Sons, Ltd. Published 2011 by Blackwell Publishing Ltd.

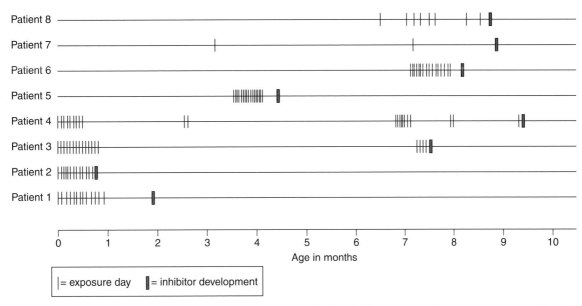

Figure 13.1 Factor VIII exposure patterns in eight patients with severe hemophilia A who developed inhibitors. For example patient 1 was exposed 12 days during his first month, and an inhibitor was found when he was two months old. (Reproduced from Van Der Bom JG, ter AP, van den Berg HM, Psaty BM, Weiss NS: Assessment of incidence of inhibitors in patients with haemophilia. Haemophilia 2009;15:707–711.)

patients with the same factor 8 gene defect, suggesting that other genetic variants, besides the factor 8 gene mutation, contribute to a patient's individual risk of inhibitor development [8]. These are likely to be located at many positions in many different genes [9]. Genetic variants that have so far been associated with inhibitor development include variants in the genes for the major histocompatibility complex (MHC) class II molecules [10,11], genes coding for interleukin 10, tumor necrosis factor alpha, and cytotoxic T-lymphocyte antigen 4 [12–16].

Genetic and non-genetic risk factors

Inhibitor development is a multifactorial disease; it is for a large part explained by genetics, but environmental factors also contribute to its occurrence. The associations between genetic variants and inhibitor incidence are relatively easily studied and interpreted. Observed differences in incidence of inhibitors between patients with different genotypes can be seen as experiments with a Mendelian randomization. They are therefore not confounded by behavioral or environmental exposures [17]. Yet, one needs to make sure that the number of exposure days is comparable between groups. If not, an observed difference in incidence may be explained by difference in cumulative number of exposure days.

Studies examining potential effects of non-genetic risk factors, however, are much more challenging. If a randomized controlled trial is possible it will provide the most reliable evidence. Unfortunately, for almost all questions about non-genetic risk factors randomized controlled trials are neither feasible nor ethical. Therefore, all our current knowledge about risk factors, including

the effects of different treatment regimens comes from observational studies. The design and analysis of observational studies on risk factors for inhibitors are severely hampered by the pattern of occurrence of inhibitors, with a relatively high risk early during the treatment and a much lower risk later during treatment. Also typical and frequently ignored is the total absence of risk of inhibitors in the absence of factor infusions. For example, the observed relative risk of inhibitors after intensive factor treatment will be extremely high if it is compared to the risk of inhibitors in the absence of treatment [6,18].

Early and late inhibitors

For the most part, inhibitors develop early in a patient's treatment life. Figure 13.2 illustrates the occurrence of inhibitors according to the cumulative number of days with factor VIII infusions (exposure days) among patients with severe hemophilia A. About 50 percent of all inhibitors occur before a patient's 13th exposure day. After approximately 50 days of exposure to the deficient clotting

---

Box 13.1 Facts that need to be considered in the design, analyses and interpretation of studies on risk factors of inhibitors in hemophilia.

- In the absence of factor, the risk to develop inhibitors is zero.
- Early during replacement therapy the risk to develop inhibitors is high —25% for severe hemophilia A.
- After about 75 exposure days, the risk to develop inhibitors is very low – less than 0.5 percent per year for severe hemophilia A.

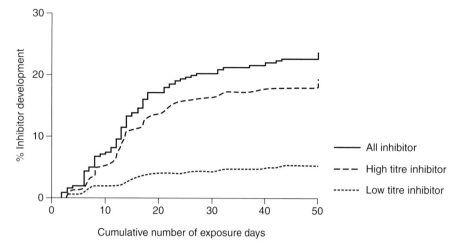

Figure 13.2 Incidence of inhibitors according to cumulative number of exposure days among patients with severe hemophilia A. (Reproduced from Gouw SC, Van Der Bom JG, Marijke van den BH. Treatmentrelated risk factors of inhibitor development in previously untreated patients with hemophilia A: the CANAL cohort study. Blood 1-6-2007;109:4648–54.)

factor, hemophilia patients become relatively tolerant [19,20], and the incidence of inhibitor development is reduced to a figure that is probably less than four per 1000 patients per year [21,22]. Because of this phenomenon of emergent tolerance after about 50 infusions, incidence figures are preferably reported separately for "early inhibitors" which occur during the first 50 to 100 exposure days and "late inhibitors" which occur after 100 exposure days [23]. Similarly, it is reasonable to assume that knowledge about risk factors for inhibitors occurring early cannot readily be generalized to inhibitors that occur later during treatment.

Assessment and comparison of incidences of early inhibitors

To assess the incidence of inhibitors in previously untreated patients (PUPs), ideally a group of newly treated patients with hemophilia, unselected with regard to characteristics associated with inhibitors, is identified and completely followed for 150 exposure days for the development of inhibitors. For example, it might be possible to include all consecutive patients who are, or have been, for the first time in their life treated in a certain region, or at one or several hemophilia treatment centers.

Minimally-treated patients
Patients who have previously been treated briefly elsewhere (outside the study region or the study treatment centers), sometimes called minimally-treated patients, confound the estimate of incidence, because they did not develop inhibitors during their first few exposure days. Including such patients will lead to a lower observed incidence of inhibitors in the study population and therefore underestimation of the risk of developing inhibitors.

However, under the assumption that inhibitor risk depends only on the cumulative number and not on the frequency and circumstances of dosing of previous exposures, it is possible to

adjust for such underestimation during the analysis of the data. To do that the data need to be separated according to each cumulative exposure day. There would be 150 separate strata; one for each consecutive exposure day. Minimally-treated patients would contribute information to the period of time during which they were being monitored for the development of inhibitors and not before this time. This technique is called left censoring.

Referred patients
Sometimes patients with hemophilia are referred to a specific hemophilia treatment center, because one or several of their family members with hemophilia have developed inhibitors. Given the role of genetic factors in the development of inhibitors, these patients inherently have an increased risk of developing inhibitors themselves. Including such patients in the study population will lead to a higher observed cumulative incidence and therefore a relative overestimation of the risk of developing inhibitors. In general, it will not be possible to adjust for this bias.

Atypical patient population
The risk of developing inhibitors has been associated with treatment intensity and several other clinical factors [24]. It is therefore important to assess the incidence of inhibitors in a clearly described homogeneous patient population. If a center at which the study is performed is a referral center for patients with a more severe bleeding pattern, these patients will be treated more intensively and this may lead to a higher observed cumulative incidence. Consequently, from this study population the estimated risk of developing inhibitors will be higher than the risk obtained from other populations. A score to measure a patient's risk of developing inhibitors may be used to separate patients with different a priori risks [25]. This allows for reporting incidences of inhibitors according to more homogeneous risk profiles.

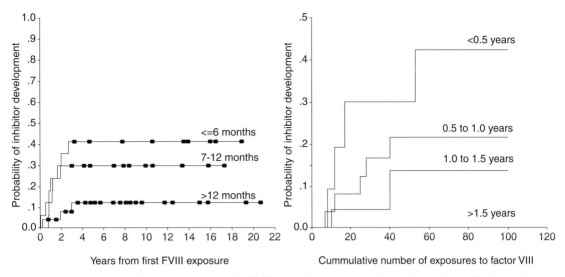

Figure 13.3 Association between age at first factor VIII exposure and risk of inhibitor development among patients with severe hemophilia A in two independent cohort studies. This was later explained by confounding by other risk factors (Reproduced from van der Bom JG, Mauser-Bunschoten EP, Fischer K, van den Berg HM: Age at first treatment and immune tolerance to factor VIII in severe hemophilia. Thromb Haemost 2003;89:475–9. Lorenzo JI, Lopez A, Altisent C, Aznar JA: Incidence of factor VIII inhibitors in severe haemophilia: the importance of patient age. Br J Haematol 2001;113:600–603.)

Follow-up

Preferably, all patients would be followed until their 100th exposure day following initiation of treatment with the clotting factor. Patients who are not followed until the 100th exposure day may affect the observed incidence in a study in either direction. If their loss to follow-up is due to end of study, and therefore independent of the patients' risk of developing inhibitors, then a Kaplan–Meier life table will validly estimate the risk of developing inhibitors before the 150th exposure day [10].

If, however, the patients' loss to follow-up is not the results of end of study, but for other reasons, then it is always possible that these "lost" patients had either a higher or a lower risk of developing inhibitors.

Confounding

If the incidence of inhibitors differs between groups with a different risk factor status, this difference may be a consequence of the risk factor, but it may also be explained by other differences between the patients in the groups. This is called confounding. Confounding explained the observed association between age at the start of treatment with factor VIII and increased inhibitor incidence [8].

A higher incidence of inhibitors in patients starting factor VIII replacement therapy before the age of six months had been found in several independent cohort studies [26,27] (Figure 13.3). However, subsequent studies showed that the observed association between age at first treatment and the risk of inhibitors may have been confounded by other determinants of inhibitor development, such as treatment intensity. After adjustment for these confounders, age

at first treatment was no longer associated with inhibitor risk [3,8]. Thus, patients who were treated at a younger age tended to have a more severe phenotype of hemophilia, which leads to more intensive treatment periods. At present, age at start of first treatment is no longer considered an independent risk factor of inhibitor development.

Assessment and comparison of incidences of inhibitors occurring in multitransfused patients

New inhibitor formation in heavily treated patients with hemophilia A is rare. It occurs with an incidence between 1.5 to 3.8 per 1000 patient years [28]. The causes of such failure of tolerance are currently unknown. Some have suggested that the risk increases with age and continuous infusion of factor VIII [28,29]. The evidence to support this, however, is still scarce.

Methodological considerations

Ideally, a large group of patients with hemophilia who share a similar treatment history of at least 150 exposure days, unselected with regard to characteristics associated with inhibitors, would be identified and all of them followed for an equal number of exposure days for the development of inhibitors. This would provide the proportion of PTPs developing inhibitors in the chosen number of exposure days, i.e. the cumulative incidence of inhibitors in for example 1000 exposure days in PTPs. The closest estimates for this figure come from pivotal trial programs for recombinant factor products.

Cumulative incidence (%) of inhibitors in PTPs

Recently, a comprehensive review of the incidence of inhibitors in pivotal trials of recombinant factor VIII products presented cumulative incidences of inhibitors after starting the use of a new factor VIII product, in the range between 0.9 to 2.9% [30]. Yet, these reported figures refer to notably different cumulative numbers of exposure days, and are therefore difficult to interpret. The reported number of exposure days to recombinant factor VIII in the patients treated in these studies ranged between 14 and 1632. The patient with 14 exposure days has had much less opportunity to develop inhibitors than the one with 1632 days. Therefore, incidence estimates need to be corrected for these varying numbers of exposure days. A Kaplan–Meier life table in relation to the number of exposure days can provide a corrected estimate of cumulative incidence. A Kaplan–Meier life table takes into account "censored" data, in specific losses from the study population before the final outcome is observed.

In addition, the cumulative incidence is only meaningful if it is reported together with the number of exposure days for which the incidence applies.

Incidence rate (per patient-year or per exposure-day) of inhibitors in PTPs

Due to the low prevalence of hemophilia and the very infrequent occurrence of inhibitors in PTPs it is almost unfeasible to directly estimate the cumulative incidence of inhibitors in PTPs. A potential valid alternative is the incidence rate. Under the assumption that the incidence of inhibitors does no longer depend on previous exposures to the deficient clotting factor, incidence rate may provide a perfectly valid estimate of inhibitor incidence. An example is the nationwide study in the UK that described an incidence rate of inhibitors 3.8 per 1000 patient-years in PTPs with severe hemophilia A [31]. Patients enter the study population, i.e. contribute to the denominator of the incidence rate, if they fulfill the inclusion criteria, for example reach a given age, live in a certain region, or use a specific product. And, they leave the study population, i.e. no longer contribute to the denominator, when they no longer fulfill these criteria. All the individual periods of follow-up are summed and jointly make the denominator of the incidence rate. The numerator is, like in the cumulative incidence, the number of patients who have developed an inhibitor while they were contributing follow-up time (person-years or exposure-days) to the denominator. The advantage of exposure days in the denominator is that days without exposure do not disturb the estimate of inhibitor incidence, because the denominator of incidence is only composed of days at which clotting factor was used.

An alternative to incidence rates according to patient-years or exposure-days can be the incidence rate according to units of clotting factor. One report presented an incidence of inhibitors of 89 per 6.48×10^9 IU factor VIII among recipients of a certain brand of recombinant factor VIII as observed between 1993 and 2002 [32]. If separated according to PUPs and PTPs this figure

provides a valuable estimate for the comparison of the incidence of inhibitors among patients receiving different factor VIII products.

Factor VIII product

The most important necessary cause of inhibitor development in all patients with hemophilia is of course the repeated intravenous administration of exogenous factor VIII. Exogenous factor VIII can either be purified from plasma of healthy blood donors or produced by recombinant techniques. The production process of factor VIII may influence its molecular structure and possibly also its immunogenicity. So far there was one production step that was clearly associated with more inhibitors. Virus inactivation of factor VIII from healthy donors by pasteurization yielded a factor VIII product that caused inhibitors in a considerable number of patients in the early 1990s in Belgium and the Netherlands [33,34]. This experience lead to the recommendation of the International Society of Thrombosis and Hemostasis Scientific Subcommittee that immunogenicity of new factor VIII product should always be studied in patients who have been treated with factor VIII on at least 150 exposure days [35]. Neo-antigenicity of a new product can be noticed relatively easy because the baseline risk in these patients is very low.

New bioengineered factor VIII products may be produced with the intention to induce fewer inhibitors than established products. Such lower risk can of course only be demonstrated in patients who still have a measurable risk to develop inhibitors, thus patients early during their treatment. Therefore, if a new factor VIII product is claimed to induce fewer inhibitors, this would have to be shown in a cohort of previously untreated patients with severe hemophilia with a known risk of inhibitors. The risk for inhibitor development can be estimated with an inhibitor risk score [27]. Table 13.1 shows how the inhibitor risk of a previously untreated patient with severe hemophilia A can be calculated.

Ever since the introduction of recombinant factor concentrates on the market in 1990, there have been worries about a higher risk of inhibitor development of recombinant as compared to plasma derived concentrates. Observational studies that directly compare the incidence of early inhibitors in patients with hemophilia A treated with different products are scarce. The conclusion of the most recent meta-analysis of studies reporting incidences of inhibitors in previously untreated patients exposed to plasma-derived and recombinant products is that the observed difference in incidence may either be true or be due to other factors, including differences in risk profiles of the patients in the studies and differences in the frequency and accuracy of inhibitor testing [36]. The ongoing SIPPET study will be the first randomized study comparing incidences of inhibitors in plasma-derived products with that of recombinant products [37].

Future research challenges

Standardized electronic documentation of treatment of patients with hemophilia will help to assess associations between potential

Table 13.1 Risk score to be used to predict inhibitor risk at the first factor VIII treatment of a patient with severe hemophilia A. The last column in the first table indicates the score given for each risk factor. These need to be summed for one patient. The sum of the scores can be translated to the probability of inhibitors in the lower panel. Presented are all combinations of predictors and their corresponding predicted probability of inhibitor development. (Reproduced from Ter Avest PC, Fischer K, Elisa MM, Santagostino E, Jimenez Y, V, van den Berg HM, Van Der Bom JG. J Thromb Haemost 7-10-2008.)

	Regression coefficient*	Odds ratio	P-value	Score
Positive family history of inhibitors	1.131	3.1	<0.001	2
High risk gene mutation type	1.086	3.0	0.005	2
Intensive treatment at 1ˢᵗ treatment.	1.769	5.9	<0.001	3

Total points in score	Probability	Family history of Inhibitors	Gene mutation type	Intensive treatment at 1ˢᵗ factor VIII exposure
0	0.09	Absent	Low risk	Absent
2	0.22	Absent	High risk	Absent
3	0.36	Absent	Low risk	Present
4	0.47	Present	High risk	Absent
5	0.63	Absent	High risk	Present
7	0.84	Present	High risk	Present

risk factors and the incidence of inhibitors in hemophilia. Improved collection of treatment and outcome data from unselected cohorts of patients, in addition to the use and development of statistical models that take the specific inhibitor risk pattern into account will lead to further understanding of the etiology of inhibitors. Together with knowledge from basic science studies it may be possible to prevent inhibitors in a significant number of patients.

Conclusions

Knowledge about the etiology of inhibitors comes both from basic science studies and from epidemiological studies. Epidemiological studies examine associations between inhibitor occurrence and potential risk factors. The typical pattern of occurrence of inhibitors, with a relatively high risk early during the treatment and a much lower risk later during treatment, together with a total absence of risk in the absence of factor infusions, are unique to the problem of inhibitors in hemophilia and need to be considered carefully in research addressing inhibitor risk factors.

References

1. Astermark J, Altisent C, Batorova A, Diniz MJ, Gringeri A, Holme PA, Karafoulidou A, Lopez-Fernandez MF, Reipert BM, Rocino A, Schiavoni M, von DM, Windyga J, Fijnvandraat K: Non-genetic risk factors and the development of inhibitors in haemophilia: a comprehensive review and consensus report. Haemophilia 2010;16:747–766.

2. Tagariello G, Iorio A, Santagostino E, Morfini M, Bisson R, Innocenti M, Mancuso ME, Mazzucconi MG, Pasta GL, Radossi P, Rodorigo G, Santoro C, Sartori R, Scaraggi A, Solimeno LP, Mannucci PM: Comparison of the rates of joint arthroplasty in patients with severe factor VIII and IX deficiency: an index of different clinical severity of the 2 coagulation disorders. Blood 2009;114:779–784.

3. Gouw SC, van den Berg HM, le Cessie S, van der Bom JG: Treatment characteristics and the risk of inhibitor development: a multicenter cohort study among previously untreated patients with severe hemophilia A. J Thromb Haemost 2007;5:1383–1390.

4. Reipert BM, van Helden PM, Schwarz HP, Hausl C: Mechanisms of action of immune tolerance induction against factor VIII in patients with congenital haemophilia A and factor VIII inhibitors. Br J Haematol 2007;136:12–25.

5. Oldenburg J, Ananyeva NM, Saenko EL: Molecular basis of haemophilia A. Haemophilia 2004;10 Suppl 4:133–139.

6. Eckhardt CL, Menke LA, van Ommen CH, van der Lee JH, Geskus RB, Kamphuisen PW, Peters M, Fijnvandraat K: Intensive peri-operative use of factor VIII and the Arg593→Cys mutation are risk factors for inhibitor development in mild/moderate hemophilia A. J Thromb Haemost 2009;7:930–937.

7. Oldenburg J, Pavlova A: Genetic risk factors for inhibitors to factors VIII and IX. Haemophilia 2006;12 Suppl 6:15–22.

8. Gouw SC, van der Bom JG, Marijke van den BH: Treatment-related risk factors of inhibitor development in previously untreated patients with hemophilia A: the CANAL cohort study. Blood 2007;109:4648–4654.

9. Yang J, Benyamin B, McEvoy BP, Gordon S, Henders AK, Nyholt DR, Madden PA, Heath AC, Martin NG, Montgomery GW, Goddard ME, Visscher PM: Common SNPs explain a large proportion of the heritability for human height. Nat Genet 2010;42:565–569.

10. Frommel D, Allain JP, Saint-Paul E, Bosser C, Noel B, Mannucci PM, Pannicucci F, Blomback M, Prou-Wartelle O, Muller JY: HLA antigens

and factor VIII antibody in classic hemophilia. European study group of factor VIII antibody. Thromb Haemost 1981;46:687–689.

11. Oldenburg J, Picard JK, Schwaab R, Brackmann HH, Tuddenham EG, Simpson E: HLA genotype of patients with severe haemophilia A due to intron 22 inversion with and without inhibitors of factor VIII. Thromb Haemost 1997;77:238–242.

12. Pavlova A, Delev D, Lacroix-Desmazes S, Schwaab R, Mende M, Fimmers R, Astermark J, Oldenburg J: Impact of polymorphisms of the major histocompatibility complex class II, interleukin-10, tumor necrosis factor-alpha and cytotoxic T-lymphocyte antigen-4 genes on inhibitor development in severe hemophilia A. J Thromb Haemost 2009;7:2006–2015.

13. Aly AM, Aledort LM, Lee TD, Hoyer LW: Histocompatibility antigen patterns in haemophilic patients with factor VIII antibodies. Br J Haematol 1990;76:238–241.

14. Frommel D, Allain JP, Saint-Paul E, Bosser C, Noel B, Mannucci PM, Pannicucci F, Blomback M, Prou-Wartelle O, Muller JY: HLA antigens and factor VIII antibody in classic hemophilia. European study group of factor VIII antibody. Thromb Haemost 1981;46:687–689.

15. Lippert LE, Fisher LM, Schook LB: Relationship of major histocompatibility complex class II genes to inhibitor antibody formation in hemophilia A. Thromb Haemost 1990;64:564–568.

16. Wieland I, Wermes C, Eifrig B, Holstein K, Pollmann H, Siegmund B, Bidlingmaier C, Kurnik K, Nimtz-Talaska A, Niekrens C, Eisert R, Tiede A, Ebenebe C, Lakomek M, Hoy L, Welte K, Sykora KW: Inhibitor-Immunology-Study. Different HLA-types seem to be involved in the inhibitor development in haemophilia A. Hamostaseologie 2008;28 Suppl 1:S26–S28.

17. Davey SG, Ebrahim S: What can Mendelian randomisation tell us about modifiable behavioural and environmental exposures? BMJ 2005;330:1076–1079.

18. Kempton CL, Soucie JM, Miller CH, Hooper C, Escobar MA, Cohen AJ, Key NS, Thompson AR, Abshire TC: In non-severe hemophilia A the risk of inhibitor following intensive factor treatment is greater in older patients: a case-control study. J Thromb Haemost 2010;8:2224–31.

19. White GC, DiMichele D, Mertens K, Negrier C, Peake IR, Prowse C, Schwaab R, Yoshioka A, Ingerslev J: Utilization of previously treated patients (PTPs), noninfected patients (NIPs), and previously untreated patients (PUPs) in the evaluation of new factor VIII and factor IX concentrates. Recommendation of the Scientific Subcommittee on Factor VIII and Factor IX of the Scientific and Standardization Committee of the International Society on Thrombosis and Haemostasis. Thromb Haemost 1999;81:462.

20. Briet E, Rosendaal FR, Kreuz W, Rasi V, Peerlinck K, Vermylen J, Ljung R, Rocino A, Addiego J, Lorenzo JI: High titer inhibitors in severe haemophilia A. A meta-analysis based on eight long-term follow-up studies concerning inhibitors associated with crude or intermediate purity factor VIII products. Thromb Haemost 1994;72:162–164.

21. Darby SC, Keeling DM, Spooner RJ, Wan KS, Giangrande PL, Collins PW, Hill FG, Hay CR: The incidence of factor VIII and factor IX inhibitors in the hemophilia population of the UK and their effect on subsequent mortality, 1977–99. J Thromb Haemost 2004;2:1047–1054.

22. McMillan CW, Shapiro SS, Whitehurst D, Hoyer LW, Rao AV, Lazerson J: The natural history of factor VIII:C inhibitors in patients with hemophilia A: a national cooperative study. II. Observa-

tions on the initial development of factor VIII:C inhibitors. Blood 1988;71:344–348.

23. van der Bom JG, ter AP, van den Berg HM, Psaty BM, Weiss NS: Assessment of incidence of inhibitors in patients with haemophilia. Haemophilia 2009;15:707–711.

24. Astermark J, Altisent C, Batorova A, Diniz MJ, Gringeri A, Holme PA, Karafoulidou A, Lopez-Fernandez MF, Reipert BM, Rocino A, Schiavoni M, von DM, Windyga J, Fijnvandraat K: Non-genetic risk factors and the development of inhibitors in haemophilia: a comprehensive review and consensus report. Haemophilia 2010;16:747–766.

25. Ter Avest PC, Fischer K, Elisa MM, Santagostino E, Jimenez Y, V, van den Berg HM, van der Bom JG: Risk stratification for inhibitor development at first treatment for severe haemophilia A: a tool for clinical practice. J Thromb Haemost 2008;6:2048–54.

26. Lorenzo JI, Lopez A, Altisent C, Aznar JA: Incidence of factor VIII inhibitors in severe haemophilia: the importance of patient age. Br J Haematol 2001;113:600–603.

27. van der Bom JG, Mauser-Bunschoten EP, Fischer K, van den Berg HM: Age at first treatment and immune tolerance to factor VIII in severe hemophilia. Thromb Haemost 2003;89:475–479.

28. Kempton CL, Soucie JM, Abshire TC: Incidence of inhibitors in a cohort of 838 males with hemophilia A previously treated with factor VIII concentrates. J Thromb Haemost 2006;4:2576–2581.

29. von Auer AC, Oldenburg J, von DM, Escuriola-Ettinghausen C, Kurnik K, Lenk H, Scharrer I: Inhibitor development in patients with hemophilia A after continuous infusion of FVIII concentrates. Ann NY Acad Sci 2005;1051:498–505.

30. Peerlinck K, Hermans C: Epidemiology of inhibitor formation with recombinant factor VIII replacement therapy. Haemophilia 2006;12:579–590.

31. Darby SC, Keeling DM, Spooner RJ, Wan KS, Giangrande PL, Collins PW, Hill FG, Hay CR: The incidence of factor VIII and factor IX inhibitors in the hemophilia population of the UK and their effect on subsequent mortality, 1977–99. J Thromb Haemost 2004;2:1047–1054.

32. Ewenstein BM, Gomperts ED, Pearson S, O'Banion ME: Inhibitor development in patients receiving recombinant factor VIII (Recombinate rAHF/Bioclate): a prospective pharmacovigilance study. Haemophilia 2004;10:491–498.

33. Peerlinck K, Arnout J, Gilles JG, Saint-Remy JM, Vermylen J: A higher than expected incidence of factor VIII inhibitors in multitransfused haemophilia A patients treated with an intermediate purity pasteurized factor VIII concentrate. Thromb Haemost 1993;69:115–118.

34. Rosendaal FR, Nieuwenhuis HK, van den Berg HM, Heijboer H, Mauser-Bunschoten EP, van der MJ, Smit C, Strengers PF, Briet E: A sudden increase in factor VIII inhibitor development in multitransfused hemophilia A patients in The Netherlands. Dutch Hemophilia Study Group. Blood 1993;81:2180–2186.

35. White GC, DiMichele D, Mertens K, Negrier C, Peake IR, Prowse C, Schwaab R, Yoshioka A, Ingerslev J: Utilization of previously treated patients (PTPs), noninfected patients (NIPs), and previously untreated patients (PUPs) in the evaluation of new factor VIII and factor IX concentrates. Recommendation of the Scientific Subcommittee on Factor VIII and Factor IX of the Scientific and Standardization Committee of the International Society on Thrombosis and Haemostasis. Thromb Haemost 1999;81:462.

36. Iorio A, Halimeh S, Holzhauer S, Goldenberg N, Marchesini E, Marcucci M, Young G, Bidlingmaier C, Brandao LR, Ettingshausen CE, Gringeri A, Kenet G, Knofler R, Kreuz W, Kurnik K, Manner D, Santagostino E, Mannucci PM, Nowak-Gottl U: Rate of inhibitor development in previously untreated hemophilia A patients treated with plasma-derived or recombinant factor VIII concentrates: a systematic review. J Thromb Haemost 2010;8:1256–65.

37. Mannucci PM, Gringeri A, Peyvandi F, Santagostino E: Factor VIII products and inhibitor development: the SIPPET study (survey of inhibitors in plasma-product exposed toddlers). Haemophilia 2007;13 Suppl 5:65–68.

14 Early Tolerization to Minimize Inhibitors in PUPs with Hemophilia A

Günter Auerswald and Karin Kurnik

Klinikum Bremen-Mitte, Ambulanz für Thrombose und Hämostasestörungen, Prof.-Hess Kinderklinik, Bremen, Germany

Introduction

The aim of hemophilia A treatment is to prevent or to treat bleeding episodes, mainly by substitution of the missing coagulation factor. Major milestones have been the development of safe and effective factor (F) VIII concentrates, either plasma-derived or recombinant, the introduction of prophylaxis and home-self-infusion for patients with severe hemophilia A, and the development of therapies for immune tolerance induction.

The most problematic and costly complication of the treatment of hemophilia A that remains to be overcome is the development of inhibitory antibodies (FVIII inhibitors) to FVIII replacement therapy, particularly in previously untreated patients (PUPs). It is now becoming clear that inhibitor development is a complex, multi-factorial immune response involving both patient-specific and treatment-related factors [1–3]. It has been shown that patients with severe defects in the F8 gene, such as large deletions, inversions (most commonly intron 22 inversion) and stop mutations are significantly more likely to develop inhibitors than are those with more minor defects such as missense mutations, small deletions or insertions and splice site mutations [1].

However, the F8 gene defect alone is not the sole determinant of inhibitor risk. In a large scale family study, the Malmö International Brother Study (MIBS) [4], siblings with severe hemophilia A and intron 22 inversion showed an inhibitor concordance rate of only 40%, suggesting some other factor was involved [4,5].

MIBS study group and development of inhibitors

The MIBS study group found a strong association between polymorphisms in the promoter regions of the IL10 and the TNF-alpha genes and the development of FVIII inhibitors [6,7]. Both IL10 and TNF-alpha are known to be involved in the regulation of antibody responses and could, therefore, be of major importance in the regulation of the development of FVIII inhibitors. Furthermore, the study group reported an association of a decreased risk of developing FVIII inhibitors with a polymorphism in the CTLA-4 gene [8]. The same polymorphism was previously shown to be associated with the development of antibody-dependent autoimmune diseases [9].

Severe mutations in the F8 gene are predicted to cause a complete deficit of any endogenous FVIII production. In these circumstances, FVIII cannot be presented to the immune system during negative selection of high-affinity autoreactive T cells in the thymus [10,11] and central immune tolerance against FVIII cannot establish itself. The MIBS study group found a strong association between polymorphisms in the promoter regions of the IL10 and the TNF-alpha genes and the development of FVIII inhibitors [6,7]. Both IL10 and TNF-alpha are known to be involved in the regulation of antibody responses and could, therefore, be of major importance in the regulation of the development of FVIII inhibitors. Furthermore, the study group reported an association of a decreased risk of developing FVIII inhibitors with a polymorphism in the CTLA-4 gene [8]. The same polymorphism was previously shown to be associated with the development of antibody-dependent autoimmune diseases [9].

Severe mutations in the F8 gene are predicted to cause a complete deficit of any endogenous FVIII production. In these circumstances, FVIII cannot be presented to the immune system during negative selection of high-affinity autoreactive T cells in the thymus [10,11] and central immune tolerance against FVIII cannot establish itself. FVIII in FVIII products that are given for replacement therapy to patients who carry such mutations would therefore be seen as a foreign protein by their immune system. Why

Current and Future Issues in Hemophilia Care, First Edition. Edited by Emérito-Carlos Rodríguez-Merchán and Leonard A. Valentino.
© 2011 John Wiley & Sons, Ltd. Published 2011 by Blackwell Publishing Ltd.

some of these patients develop FVIII inhibitors while others do not is far from clear. For many years immunologists believed that the immune system's primary goal was to discriminate between self and non-self [12,13].

Matzinger (1994) introduced the concept that the primary driving force of the immune system is the need to detect and protect against danger [14]. If a foreign or a self-antigen is not dangerous, immune tolerance is the expected outcome [14]. In recent years, it has been suggested that the ability of the immune system to sense danger is part of a more generalized protection against danger [14]. If a foreign or a self-antigen is not dangerous, immune tolerance is the expected outcome [14]. In recent years, it has been suggested that the ability of the immune system to sense danger is part of a more general surveillance, defense and repair system that enables multicellular organisms to control whether their cells are alive or dead and to recognize when microorganisms intrude [15–18]. Danger is transmitted by various signals that are associated either with pathogens or with tissue and cell damage [15–18]. Pathogens express pathogen-associated molecular patterns (PAMPS) that are recognized by pattern recognition receptors such as toll-like receptors (TLR), Nod1-like receptors (NLRs) or Rig-I like receptors (RLRs) that are expressed on a range of cells of the innate and the adaptive immune system.

Once these receptors are triggered, several signaling pathways are activated that can induce inflammatory responses and the activation of specific anti-pathogen immune responses. Evidence is accumulating that trauma, ischemia and tissue damage can cause inflammatory responses that are very similar to responses induced by pathogens [15–18]. Damaged cells release so called damage-associated molecular patterns (DAMPs) that recruit and activate receptor-expressing cells of the innate immune system, including dendritic cells, granulocytes, monocytes or eosinophils, and thus directly or indirectly promote adaptive immune responses [15–18].

Based on the increasing evidence that both pathogen-associated as well as cell-damage associated molecules present danger signals that can stimulate inflammatory responses of the innate immune system and thereby up-regulate antibody responses, the prevention of such danger signals during treatment with FVIII products could decrease the risk for the development of FVIII inhibitors in previously untreated patients with severe hemophilia A. The aim should be to expose the patient to FVIII in the absence of immunological danger signals by avoiding the first treatments with FVIII in the context of a severe bleeding episode or during infection, by avoiding surgery during the first 20 exposure days (ED) and by avoiding vaccinations on the same day as FVIII treatments. Furthermore, any hemorrhage that occur should be treated early by giving higher doses immediately, thereby avoiding long and intensive treatment and shortening the time of tissue damage.

The overall risk of developing inhibitors to FVIII during the first 150 exposure days is 20–30% for PUPs [19]. Of those developing inhibitors, 50% will do so within the first 20 and 95% during the first 50 days [19]. If the patient can be brought through this high

risk period without inhibitor development, the subsequent risk is low [20].

We therefore decided to test the efficacy of a novel strategy to overcome the high risk of inhibitor development during the first 50 exposure days of a prophylaxis using a regimen specifically designed to induce tolerance to the administered FVIII and to minimize inhibitor development.

Munich and Bremen experience

In two centers in Germany (Munich and Bremen) twenty-six previously untreated patients with severe hemophilia A (all <1% FVIII baseline activity) with a variety of F8 gene mutations, were treated with a prophylaxis regimen designed to induce immune tolerance by avoiding immunological danger signals [21].

The incidence of inhibitor development in this group was compared with that in a historical control group of 30 children, matched for severity of disease and presence of high-risk F8 gene mutations, treated with a standard joint protection prophylaxis regimen. Both study and control group consists of consecutive PUPs treated in the respective hemophilia center during a given time period. Full patient details for both groups are given in Table 14.1.

According to the German hemophilia treatment guidelines, prophylaxis in children with hemophilia is standard of care [22]. Patients in the study group were treated with low dose prophylaxis, starting with 250 IU once weekly (corresponds to approximately 25 IU/kg/week) as soon as a bleeding tendency manifested, either through soft tissue and muscle hemorrhage or a significant tendency for hematomas (Figure 14.1).

Treatment was also introduced for "safety" reasons as bleeding prophylaxis after trauma (i.e. head trauma without signs of bleeding). In patients with joint bleeding, prophylaxis was introduced at the higher dose of 25 IU/kg twice weekly, and in those with severe joint or life threatening hemorrhage, at 25–50 IU/kg three times weekly. When required due to the severity of bleeding, the dose was increased from once to twice to three times per week. For tolerization, as has been demonstrated with immune tolerance induction programs used for inhibitor patients, it seems to be important to always give the FVIII doses on the same day and to avoid interrupting the prophylaxis regimen even when additional on demand FVIII doses are necessary to manage an acute hemorrhage. This treatment regimen beginning with once weekly infusions is very practical, since it provides early protection (to some extent) against hemorrhage, allows the child and his family to adapt to the demands of prophylaxis, and usually does not require placement of a central venous access device.

Patients in the control group were treated with a standard joint-protection prophylaxis regimen consisting of 40–50 IU/kg FVIII given three times weekly, starting at or after the first joint or other severe hemorrhage.

Fifty-six of the 58 subjects studied had 20 or more exposure days to FVIII therapy. Data from these subjects were analyzed for

	Control group (standard prophylaxis regimen) N = 30	Study group (new prophylaxis regimen) N = 26	Statistical significance
Demographics – Bremen			
Born between	03/1995–12/2000	01/2001–07/2007	
Ethnicity	All Caucasian	All Caucasian	Not significant
Demographics – Munich			
Born between	01/2002–09/2004	01/2005–10/2007	
Ethnicity	All Caucasian	All Caucasian	Not significant
Genetic factors			
Severity of hemophilia A	All <1% FVIII activity	All <1% FVIII activity	Not significant
FVIII mutation type:			
High risk (%)	24 (80)	18 (69)	Not significant
Low risk (%)	5 (17)	8 (31)	Not significant
Unknown (%)	1 (3)		

Table 14.1 Patient-related risk factors for inhibitor development in the study group compared with the control group

inhibitor development and both patient-related and treatment-related factors which might have affected inhibitor development.

Fourteen of the 30 subjects given standard prophylaxis and one of the 26 subjects given the new prophylaxis regimen developed an inhibitor. By Fisher's exact test, the difference between the groups was highly significant (P = 0.0003, odds ratio 0.048, 95% CI: 0.001 to 0.372) (Table 14.2).

Eight subjects given standard prophylaxis but none of those given the new regimen were high responders. By Fisher's exact test, the difference between groups was again significant (P = 0.005, odds ratio for high response 0.00, 95% CI: 0.00 to 0.57) (Table 14.2). Inhibitors in the control group developed after a median of 11 exposure days (range: 3–170 EDs) which is in agreement with a recent international study [23].

There were no significant differences between the study and control groups in any patient related factors (Table 14.1), nor in the majority of treatment-related factors (Table 14.3). In a logistic regression model for inhibitor development with factors for study group (standard vs. new regimen prophylaxis), genetic risk for inhibitor development (low vs. high), and type of factor concentrate (recombinant vs. plasma-derived), only study group (type of prophylaxis regimen) had a significant effect (P = 0.005). Logistic regression analysis was not performed for the risk of high responder inhibitors due to lack of events in patients given the new regimen.

There were however highly significant differences between groups for the prophylaxis-related factors: age at the start of prophylaxis and the number of exposure days before the introduction of prophylaxis (Table 14.4).

Age at start of prophylaxis was available for 23 of the 30 subjects in the standard prophylaxis group and all 26 subjects given the new regimen. The median age at start of prophylaxis was 19 months (range 0.8 to 87) for those given standard prophylaxis and 10.7 months (range 0.5 to 24.5) for those given the new regimen. By the Wilcoxon test, this difference is highly significant (P < 0.0006).

Standard prophylaxis had been introduced after a median of 30 exposure days (range 1 to infinity) whereas the new regimen was introduced after a median of one exposure day (range 0 to 14). By the Wilcoxon test, this difference too is highly significant (P < 0.0001). As a post-hoc analysis, these results should be interpreted as hypothesis generating. Confirmation in a prospectively planned, historically-controlled study would be warranted.

Discussion

It may be considered that the overall risk of developing an inhibitor reflects the level of danger signals perceived by the patient's immune system. It is not, therefore, surprising that on-demand

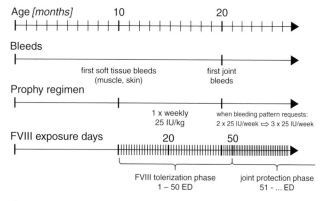

Figure 14.1 Treatment scheme for previously untreated patients receiving the new prophylaxis regimen.

Table 14.2 Inhibitor development in the study group compared with the control group

	Control group (standard prophylaxis regimen) N = 30	Study group (new prophylaxis regimen) N = 26	Statistical significance
Inhibitors (%)	14 (47)	1 (3.8)	Highly significant: $P = 0.0003$ Odds ratio = 0.048 (95% CI: 0.001 to 0.372)
High responders (%)	8 (27)	0	Highly significant:
Low responders (%)	6 (20)	1 (3.8)	$P = 0.005$ Odds ratio of high response = 0.00 (95% CI: 0.00 to 0.57)

treatment which is, by definition, given in the presence of bleeding should cause inhibitor development more frequently than prophylaxis.

The value of prophylactic factor replacement therapy in the prevention of severe joint bleeding and arthropathy is now well established [24], and is increasingly being adopted as the standard approach to treatment of hemophilia A. However, even in those countries, such as Sweden, where prophylaxis is virtually universal there has been no reduction in the overall incidence of inhibitors in PUPs [25]. The prophylaxis regimens employed have

Table 14.3 Treatment-related risk factors for inhibitor development in the study group compared with the control group

	Control group (standard prophylaxis regimen) N = 30	Study group (new prophylaxis regimen) N = 26	Statistical significance
Product type:			
rFVIII (%)	16 (53)	15 (58)	Not significant
pdFVIII (%)	14 (47)	11 (42)	
Age at 1st exposure:			
Median (months)	9.8	8.1	Not significant
Range (months)	0.1–22	0–21	
Reason for 1st exposure:			
Bleed (%)	21 (70)	12 (46)	Not significant:
Safety (%)	9 (30)	14 (54)	$P = 0.103$
Total EDs:			
Median	500	100	Not significant
range	(1 with 26 EDs)	(only 4 <100 EDs)	
Surgery:			
within the first 20 EDs	3	2	Not significant
Vaccination:			
Given I.M.	1	All no	Not significant
Given on a FVIII day	All no	All no	

Table 14.4 Prophylaxis related factors for inhibitor development in the study group compared with the control group

	Control group (standard prophylaxis regimen) N = 30	Study group (new prophylaxis regimen) N = 26	Statistical significance
Age at start of prophylaxis:			
Median (months)	(n = 23)	(n = 26)	Highly significant:
Range (months)	19	10.7	$P < 0.0006$
	0.8–87	0.5–24.5	
EDs before prophylaxis:			
Median	30	1	Highly significant:
range	1–infinity	0–14	$P < 0.0001$

been designed for joint protection, with relatively high doses of concentrate such as 50 IU/kg three times per week. Because they are usually introduced at or just after the first significant joint hemorrhage, the FVIII is being introduced at a time when there are strong immunological danger signals present, to an immune system which has already been "primed" by previous on-demand therapy. Therefore, prophylaxis might start too late to prevent inhibitor formation.

An effective prophylactic regimen for the treatment of PUPs without the development of inhibitors must take into account and avoid known danger signals, such as bleeding associated with tissue damage, immunological challenges such as vaccination, or infection. This would permit the immune system to develop tolerance to the foreign protein in a "non-threatening" situation. The results utilizing this approach demonstrate that with an early start of low dose prophylaxis administered once weekly the incidence of inhibitors, even in high-risk patients might be dramatically reduced from the normally expected level, which in PUPs has historically been around 30% [1,19].

However, we are aware of the fact that our results can only be considered as hypothesis generating and need to be confirmed in a larger prospective clinical study. Our results also suggest that early introduction of FVIII is a more satisfactory way of avoiding inhibitors than is attempting to delay the use of FVIII, for example by treating bleeding with rFVIIa [26]. Starting with prophylaxis early in life, in our study at a median age of 8.1 months, was not associated with an increased inhibitor risk, a finding that is well in line with other recent studies [27,28].

A low-dose, escalating regimen may also provide a better long-term outcome for patients, with less frequent hemarthroses and better joint outcomes, due to the earlier start of prophylaxis. The beneficial effect on joint outcomes is hard to explain, since a weekly prophylaxis regimen cannot maintain FVIII levels above 1%. Nevertheless, the benefits of a similar regimen has been demonstrated in a 10-year study of tailored primary prophylaxis in Canada [29]. This regimen differs from our proposed regimen in that higher doses are used, prophylaxis is only introduced after the first joint hemorrhage has occurred and dose escalation is done only after the occurrence of several episodes of hemorrhage or the development of a target joint.

As well as its key role in preventing inhibitor development, the new prophylaxis regimen offers a number of other advantages. With once weekly administration, it is not necessary to insert a central venous access device (CVAD) such as a Port-A-Cath®, (Smiths Medical), thereby avoiding surgery. If the initial dosage proves inadequate, it may still be possible to avoid the need for a CVAD by increasing the individual dose rather than increasing the frequency of dosing. Avoiding the need for a CVAD is probably a major advantage for the induction of immune tolerance to FVIIII because any surgical procedure is likely to be associated with some form of tissue damage together with the generation of danger signals. Once weekly administration of FVIII concentrate is also simpler for parents, requiring only one infusion each week,

so that adherence is improved with a consequent improvement in outcome. There is also a pharmacoeconomic benefit in that lower doses and less frequent infusions provide a considerable cost savings compared with standard prophylactic regimens.

Conclusions

The results from our recent study suggest that an early start of prophylaxis is associated with a decreased rate of inhibitor development in patients with severe hemophilia A and this is possibly due to minimizing exposure to immunological danger signals during the first 20 exposure days. Once the patients have developed tolerance to FVIII, usually after about 20 to 50 EDs on the low dose regimen, and venous access permitting, prophylaxis may be changed to the more typical three times weekly regimen which has proven optimal joint protection (Figure 14.1).

References

1. Oldenburg J, Pavlova A. Genetic risk factors for inhibitors to factors VIII and IX. Haemophilia 2006;12 (Suppl 6):15–22.
2. Astermark J, Lacroix-Desmazes S, Reding MT. Inhibitor development. Haemophilia 2008;14 (Suppl 3):36–42.
3. Lee CA, Lillicrap D, Astermark J. Inhibitor development in hemophiliacs: the roles of genetic versus environmental factors. Semin Thromb Hemost 2006;32 (Suppl 2):10–14.
4. Astermark J, Oldenburg J, Escobar M, White GC, Berntorp E. The Malmo International Brother Study (MIBS). Genetic defects and inhibitor development in siblings with severe hemophilia A. Haematologica 2005;90:924–931.
5. Santagostino E. Can the genetic profile predict inhibitor development in hemophilia A? J Thromb Haemost 2007;5:261–262.
6. Astermark J, Oldenburg J, Pavlova A, Berntorp E, Lefvert AK. Polymorphisms in the IL10 but not in the IL1beta and IL4 genes are associated with inhibitor development in patients with hemophilia A. Blood 2006;107:3167–3172.
7. Astermark J, Oldenburg J, Carlson J et al. Polymorphisms in the TNFA gene and the risk of inhibitor development in patients with hemophilia A. Blood 2006;108:3739–3745.
8. Astermark J, Wang X, Oldenburg J, Berntorp E, Lefvert AK. Polymorphisms in the CTLA-4 gene and inhibitor development in patients with severe hemophilia A. J Thromb Haemost 2007;5:263–265.
9. Gough SC, Walker LS, Sansom DM. CTLA4 gene polymorphism and autoimmunity. Immunol Rev 2005;204:102–115.
10. Palmer E. Negative selection – clearing out the bad apples from the T-cell repertoire. Nat Rev Immunol 2003;3:383–391.
11. Siggs OM, Makaroff LE, Liston A. The why and how of thymocyte negative selection. Curr Opin Immunol 2006;18:175–183.
12. Bretscher P, Cohn M. A theory of self-nonself discrimination. Science 1970;169:1042–1049.
13. Burnet FM. A modification of Jerne's theory of antibody production using the concept of clonal selection. CA Cancer J Clin 1976;26:119–121.

14. Matzinger P. Tolerance, danger, and the extended family. Annu Rev Immunol 1994;12:991–1045.

15. Bianchi ME. DAMPs, PAMPs and alarmins: all we need to know about danger. J Leukoc Biol 2007;81:1–5.

16. Lotze MT, Zeh HJ, Rubartelli A et al. The grateful dead: damage-associated molecular pattern molecules and reduction/oxidation regulate immunity. Immunol Rev 2007;220:60–81.

17. Kaczorowski DJ, Mollen KP, Edmonds R, Billiar TR. Early events in the recognition of danger signals after tissue injury. J Leukoc Biol 2008;83:546–552.

18. Kono H, Rock KL. How dying cells alert the immune system to danger. Nat Rev Immunol 2008;8:279–289.

19. EMEA. Report on expert meeting on FVIII products and inhibitor development, Feb 28–Mar 2, 2006. EMEA/CHMP/BPWP/123835/2006, http://www.emea.europa.eu/pdfs/human/bpwg/12383506en.pdf, Accessed April 27, 2009.

20. Hay CR. The epidemiology of factor VIII inhibitors. Haemophilia 2006;12 (Suppl 6):23–28.

21. New early prophylaxis regimen that avoids immunological danger signals can reduce FVIII inhibitor development; Haemophilia 2009;16 (2):256–262.

22. Executive Committee of the German Medical Association on the recommendation of the Scientific Advisory Board. Cross-sectional Guidelines for Therapy with Blood Components and Plasma Derivatives; 4th revised edition, 2008; http://www.bundesaerztekammer.de/page.asp?his=0.6.3288.6716, accessed at: June 4, 2009.

23. Gouw SC. van den Berg HM, Le Cessie S and van der Bom JG. Treatment characteristics and the risk of inhibitor development: a multicenter cohort study among previously untreated patients with severe hemophilia A. Journal of Thrombosis and Haemostasis 2007;5:1383–1390.

24. Coppola A, Di CM, De SC. Primary prophylaxis in children with haemophilia. Blood Transfus 2008;6 (Suppl 2):4–11.

25. Knobe KE, Sjorin E, Tengborn LI, Petrini P, Ljung RC. Inhibitors in the Swedish population with severe haemophilia A and B: a 20-year survey. Acta Paediatr 2002;91:910–914.

26. Rivard GE, Lillicrap D, Poon MC et al. Can activated recombinant factor VII be used to postpone the exposure of infants to factor VIII until after 2 years of age? Haemophilia 2005;11:335–339.

27. Gouw SC, van der Bom JG, and van den Berg HM for the CANAL Study group. Treatment-related risk factors of inhibitor development in previously untreated patients with severe hemophilia A: the CANAL cohort study. Blood 2007;109:4648–4654.

28. Chalmers EA, Brown SA, Keeling D, Liesner R, Richards M, Stirling D, Thomas A, Vidler V, Williams MD, Young D on behalf of the paediatric working party of UKHCDO. Early factor VIII exposure and subsequent inhibitor development in children with severe haemophilia A. Haemophilia 2007;13 (Suppl 2):149–155.

29. Blanchette VS, Rivard GE, Pai MK, Israels SJ, McLimont M, Feldman BM. 10 Year Musculoskeletal Outcomes with Tailored Primary Prophylaxis: The Canadian Hemophilia Prophylaxis Study [abstract]. Blood 2007;110:Abstract 84.

15 Prediction of Inhibitors in Severe Hemophilia

H. Marijke van den Berg[1,2] and Kathelijn Fischer[2]

[1]Meander Hospital, Amersfoort, The Netherlands
[2]University Medical Center Utrecht, The Netherlands

Introduction

The most important side effect of hemophilia A treatment is the development of alloantibodies to factor VIII. These antibodies interfere with infused factor VIII and can completely block the haemostatic potential of the clotting product. Although in those cases alternative treatment options are available, they are less effective in treating bleeding. Especially in severe hemophilia inhibitors develop in the early phase of treatment. Clinically important inhibitors occur in about 25% of all previously untreated patients (PUPs) with severe hemophilia A [1]. The mean number of exposure days before inhibitors develop is 10–15 days. As a consequence, inhibitors often appear at a very early age, which makes it difficult to start immune tolerance treatment. Difficult venous access in combination with the high bleeding tendency in toddlers makes the diagnosis of an inhibitor a nightmare both for families and clinicians.

Increased awareness of inhibitor formation arose in the 1980s, when clotting factors became available in sufficient quantities. Moreover, when it was established that some clotting factor products were associated with an increased incidence of inhibitor development, frequent testing for inhibitors became standard practice. This occurred around the time of the introduction of recombinant factor VIII products. In the registration studies in naïve patients (PUPs) that were to follow, high inhibitor incidences were detected, even up to over 30% for some recombinant products. Because the study designs of the PUP studies varied widely and were suffering from (1) small patient numbers; (2) different frequencies of testing; (3) missing of genetic factors, etc., it was impossible to recognize whether the nature of the clotting product as such could explain the different incidences [2–4].

During the last decades a serious search for risk factors of inhibitor development was started. This chapter reviews the development and uptake of a prediction rule for inhibitor development in severe hemophilia A.

Endogenous (genetic) risk factors

It has been established that the molecular factor VIII gene defect is a strong individual predictor of inhibitors. Patients with a single nucleotide missense mutation have a lower risk for inhibitor formation, while the risk is high in patients with major gene deletions [5,6]. In several small studies Afro-Americans were shown to have a higher likelihood to develop inhibitors [7]. This finding, which might be related to different HLA patterns, still awaits confirmation [8]. Independent of mutation type, a positive family history for inhibitor development appears to be associated with increased inhibitor risk as well [9,10].

Recently, polymorphisms in the immune-regulating genes coding for interleukin 10 (IL-10), tumor necrosis factor alpha (TNF-α), and cytotoxic T-lymphocyte associated protein-4 (CTLA-4) were found to be associated with inhibitor development [11–14].

Non-genetic factors

A very interesting observation was that several non-genetic factors are independent risk factors for inhibitor development. These include age at first exposure to factor VIII, vaccination, infection, and intensive treatment [15–18]. Very important was the observation that early regular prophylaxis may protect patients with severe hemophilia against the development of inhibitors [19,20]. Since genetic factors cannot be changed in an individual patient, the observation that treatment-related factors also have independent influences on inhibitor development, enables the identification

Current and Future Issues in Hemophilia Care, First Edition. Edited by Emérito-Carlos Rodríguez-Merchán and Leonard A. Valentino.
© 2011 John Wiley & Sons, Ltd. Published 2011 by Blackwell Publishing Ltd.

Table 15.1 Positive and negative predictive values and calibration of the risk score in the CANAL cohort and validation cohort. (Reproduced from Ter Avest PC, Fischer K, Mancuso ME, Santagostino E, Yuste VJ, van den Berg HM, et al. Risk stratification for inhibitor development at first treatment for severe hemophilia A: a tool for clinical practice. J Thromb Haemost 2008 Dec;6(12):2048–54.)

Risk categories CANAL cohort	Total number of patients	Predicted inhibitors	Observed inhibitors	Positive predictive value	Negative predictive value
Low 0 points	95	8	6	0.06	0.68
Medium 2 points	170	38	39	0.23	0.73
High >2 points	67	36	38	0.57	0.83
Risk categories Validation cohort	**Total number of patients**	**Predicted inhibitors**	**Observed inhibitors**	**Positive predictive value**	**Negative predictive value**
Low 0 points	20	2	1	0.05	0.64
Medium 2 points	28	6	8	0.29	0.75
High >2 points	16	8	8	0.50	0.81

of patients with higher risks of inhibitor development and the adaptation of the treatment regimen accordingly.

How to predict inhibitors

In severe hemophilia, inhibitors occur at a median of 10 to 15 exposure days. When we want to influence the risk profile, we should be able to predict it at the start of factor VIII treatment. For the development of a prediction score Ter Avest et al. used data from the CANAL study [18]. The CANAL study is a multicenter retrospective cohort study of 332 patients with severe hemophilia A (factor VIII levels <0.01 IU/ml), born between 1990 and 2000, in 14 hemophilia treatment centers. Data were available on patient characteristics and on all first 50 exposure days. The outcome of interest was "clinically relevant inhibitor", which was defined as at least two positive inhibitor titers and decreased recovery.

The majority of the CANAL patients were Caucasian (89%), and family history of hemophilia was positive in 152 (46%) patients. Inhibitors developed in 83 out of 332 patients (25%). These patients received their first factor VIII at a median age of 11 months (interquartile range (IQR) 6–15 months), while the median number of exposure days (ED) at the time of inhibitor development was 14 (IQR 8–23).

The prediction model was meant to detect patients at the start of treatment. Therefore the following risk factors were included: family history of inhibitors, factor VIII gene mutation type, intensive treatment at first treatment episode, age at first exposure to factor VIII, and reason for first treatment with factor VIII [10]. Intensive treatment was defined as factor VIII treatment for at least five consecutive days at first exposure. Using the coefficients from the regression analysis, a prediction score was established. It included positive family history (2 points), high risk factor VIII gene mutations (2 points), and intensive treatment at first exposure (3 points). With an overall risk of 25% inhibitor development, the score was able to differentiate between patients at

low risk (0 points, i.e. no risk factors), predicted to have 6% inhibitor development, and those with intensive treatment who were at high risk (>2 points), with a predicted 57% risk of inhibitor development (Table 15.1).

In fact, the incidence of inhibitors in patients with intensive treatment was 60.8% (31/51) compared to 18.5% (52/281) in those without intensive treatment at first exposure. This results in an attributable risk of 42.3%, suggesting a very strong effect of intensive treatment at first exposure.

External validation

To validate the risk score, data from a different cohort was used. With generosity of Baxter, Bayer and Wyeth (now Pfizer), we had obtained the original data of patients who had participated in the original four multicenter recombinant factor VIII product registration studies (Kogenate®, Kogenate Bayer®, Refacto®, Recombinate®) assessing safety, efficacy, and inhibitor risk in PUPs with hemophilia A [15].

The same inclusion criteria were applied as were used in CANAL, but patients who already contributed to the CANAL cohort and patients without information on the gene defect were excluded. Eventually, the validation cohort consisted of 64 patients with severe hemophilia A. Patient characteristics and treatment variables in the validation cohort were comparable to those of the CANAL cohort. Seventeen out of 64 patients (27%) developed a clinically relevant inhibitor at a median of 11 exposure days (IQR 8–18 days), age at first treatment and the distribution of ethnicity being similar to those of the CANAL cohort. The prediction rule performed well in the validation cohort. Comparison between the validation and the CANAL cohort (Table 15.2) revealed similar positive predictive value of a score of more than 2 points; 50% and 57%, respectively. The negative predictive values were similar as well: for a score below 2, negative predictive value was 81% in the validation cohort versus 83% in the CANAL cohort.

Table 15.2 Results of the survey from 42 centers

Factors possibly increasing risk of inhibitor development

	1	2	3	4	5	Missing	Mean (SD)
Major FVIII defect	0	0	0	15	27		4.64 (0.49)
Family history of inhibitors	0	0	1	19	22		4.50 (0.55)
Non-Caucasian ethnicity	0	4	6	22	9	1	3.88 (0.87)
Early exposure to FVIII product	3	9	19	9	0	3	2.85 (0.86)
Early intensive FVIII treatment	1	1	6	19	14	1	4.07 (0.91)
Concomitant infection	0	1	23	16	2		3.45 (0.63)
Use of recombinant FVIII	2	10	24	5	1		2.83 (0.79)
Factors possibly reducing risk of inhibitor development							
Delayed start of FVIII treatment	2	12	11	14	2	1	3.05 (1.02)
Initial use of vWF containing product	2	9	21	9	0	1	2.90 (0.80)
Early start of FVIII prophylaxis	1	3	12	16	8	2	3.68 (0.97)
Avoidance of elective surgery	0	0	10	17	12	3	4.05 (0.76)
Would factors reducing risk influence management?							
Delayed start of FVIII treatment	15	5	1	3	12	8	2.78 (1.81)
Initial use of vWF containing product	21	6	4	2	5	4	2.05 (1.45)
Early start of FVIII prophylaxis	10	2	1	6	18	5	3.54 (1.74)
Avoidance of elective surgery	4	0	2	6	26	4	4.32 (1.28)

Score: 1 = very unlikely; 2 = likely; 3 = uncertain; 4 = likely; 5 = very likely; mean = mean score; SD = standard deviation, indicating level of diversion of the answers.

Acceptance of prediction score

A separate part of the development of a prediction score is its acceptance in clinical practice. A survey was constructed which contained the following risk factors: major gene defects, family history for inhibitors, non-Caucasian ethnic origin, early exposure to factor VIII (age <6 months), early intensive replacement therapy, concomitant infection during factor VIII replacement therapy, and whether recombinant factor VIII products were considered to have a higher likelihood to develop inhibitors. The following factors were considered as potentially able to reduce inhibitor development: delayed onset of factor VIII treatment (1st exposure >6 months of age), initial exposure with a vWF-containing factor VIII product, early onset of prophylaxis, and avoidance of early elective therapy. For the likelihood rating a 5-point Likert scale was used, ranging from 1–5 with 1 for very unlikely and 5 for very likely.

The survey was administrated in March 2009 [21], 5.5 months after the publication of the original prediction score by Ter Avest et al. [10]. The responses of 42 centers were available for analysis. These centers were responsible for 2642 patients with severe hemophilia A <18 years of age. In addition to genetic factors, respondents considered early intensive treatment the most important factor for inhibitor development, with a score of 4.07 out of 5. Factors likely to reduce inhibitor development were early onset of prophylaxis (score 3.68) and avoidance of early surgery (4.05). Likewise, most would agree that a high-risk patient in

need of intensive therapy should continue with early prophylaxis in order to prevent inhibitor development (score 3.54).

Compared to US and Canadian hematologists, a trend towards earlier introduction of early prophylaxis was observed amongst European hematologists, as a strategy to prevent inhibitor development. Out of 23 European centers, 15 (65%) would start early prophylaxis in high-risk patients, whereas only 7/13 (54%) US and Canadian centers were inclined to start early prophylaxis in order to prevent inhibitor development.

Discussion

The introduction of a composite risk score enables risk prediction for inhibitor development in an individual patient at the time of first treatment. The score makes it possible to select patient populations with virtually no risk of inhibitor development. More importantly, it selects patients at a risk of over 50%. The prediction score also enables hematologists to select individual patients in whom peak treatment moments should be delayed by the avoidance of early elective surgery. If delay of the intensive treatment period is impossible, continuation of prophylaxis seems to be an effective approach to prevent inhibitor development or else to modify the clinical course from the development of a high into low titer inhibitor.

Although growing numbers of factors with impact on inhibitor development have been identified, in our analysis most did not influence risk in individual patients. The recognition that intensive treatment is a stronger risk factor than large gene defects has thrown a new light on both genetic and non-genetic factors. Intensive treatment is used with large hemorrhage and for the hemostatic coverage for surgical events. It is hypothesized that the intensive treatment period acts as a danger signal, triggering the activation of the immunologic system [22,23]. Since it is possible to prevent bleeding with early prophylactic therapy, it seems a logical approach to start treatment with factor VIII very early in young children with one or more genetic risk factors. Thus not only are large hemorrhages are prevented, but it also exposes the immunologic system to the foreign factor VIII in the absence of a danger signal. The latter seems to explain the lower incidence of inhibitor development in patients on prophylaxis [24–26]. For full prophylaxis, it is necessary to infuse factor VIII three times weekly or every other day, which often requires the implantation of a central venous catheter. Over the last decade, however, prophylaxis is often started with once weekly infusions [27]. The CANAL study shows that a protective effect of prophylaxis is also present with once weekly dosing. This was recently corroborated by a very interesting study by two German centers, who reported a substantial decrease in inhibitor development when using a low-dose (25 IU/kg once weekly) factor VIII regimen for the first 20 exposure days [28]. For the patients with large hemorrhages at first exposure to factor VIII and in need of intensive treatment, prophylaxis should be initiated and continued until at least 50 exposure days have been reached.

Conclusions

The introduction of new clinical guidelines takes time and it can only be successful when there is high acceptance among clinicians. The prediction score has been developed using data from the CANAL study, which has run mainly in Europe. Not surprisingly therefore it was shown that the hematologists in the USA and Canada were less inclined to start early prophylaxis than their European colleagues [21].

The presented inhibitor risk score did not include several established risk factors, such as ethnicity and surgery, because the variation we observed in these variables was insufficient in the CANAL cohort. It is possible that future studies will reveal that these factors, and other risk factors yet to be discovered, can improve the prediction of inhibitor risk in patients with severe hemophilia A. In addition, the effect of peak treatment after a low number of exposures to FVIII needs to be assessed.

Since the prediction score has been developed, many physicians have adopted the strategy of early prophylaxis in patients with severe hemophilia and a high-risk mutation or in need of intensive treatment. Further clinical data on this important subject is expected from the Rodin study (www.rodinstudy.eu). This is a large collaborative study, which aims to collect data of 800 children with severe hemophilia A born between 1 January 2000 and 1 January 2010. The aims of the Rodin study are to add addi-

tional factors to the prediction score and to demonstrate whether modified management enables the reduction of total inhibitor incidence.

References

1. Wight J, Paisley S. The epidemiology of inhibitors in haemophilia A: a systematic review. Haemophilia 2003 Jul;9(4):418–35.
2. Lusher JM, Arkin S, Abildgaard CF, Schwartz RS. Recombinant factor VIII for the treatment of previously untreated patients with hemophilia A. Safety, efficacy, and development of inhibitors. Kogenate Previously Untreated Patient Study Group. N Engl J Med 1993 Feb 18;328(7):453–9.
3. Bray GL, Gomperts ED, Courter S, Gruppo R, Gordon EM, Manco-Johnson M, et al. A multicenter study of recombinant factor VIII (recombinate): safety, efficacy, and inhibitor risk in previously untreated patients with hemophilia A. The Recombinate Study Group. Blood 1994 May 1;83(9):2428–35.
4. Courter SG, Bedrosian CL. Clinical evaluation of B-domain deleted recombinant factor VIII in previously untreated patients. Semin Hematol 2001 Apr;38(2 Suppl 4):52–9.
5. Schwaab R, Brackmann HH, Meyer C, Seehafer J, Kirchgesser M, Haack A, et al. Haemophilia A: mutation type determines risk of inhibitor formation. Thromb Haemost 1995 Dec;74(6): 1402–6.
6. Schroder J, El-Maarri O, Schwaab R, Muller CR, Oldenburg J. Factor VIII intron-1 inversion: frequency and inhibitor prevalence. J Thromb Haemost 2006 May;4(5):1141–3.
7. Aledort LM, Dimichele DM. Inhibitors occur more frequently in African-American and Latino haemophiliacs. Haemophilia 1998 Jan;4(1):68.
8. Viel KR, Ameri A, Abshire TC, Iyer RV, Watts RG, Lutcher C, et al. Inhibitors of factor VIII in black patients with hemophilia. N Engl J Med 2009 Apr 16;360(16):1618–27.
9. Aledort LM, Dimichele DM. Inhibitors occur more frequently in African–American and Latino haemophiliacs. Haemophilia 1998 Jan;4(1):68.
10. Ter Avest PC, Fischer K, Mancuso ME, Santagostino E, Yuste VJ, van den Berg HM, et al. Risk stratification for inhibitor development at first treatment for severe hemophilia A: a tool for clinical practice. J Thromb Haemost 2008 Dec;6(12):2048–54.
11. Astermark J, Wang X, Oldenburg J, Berntorp E, Lefvert AK. Polymorphisms in the CTLA-4 gene and inhibitor development in patients with severe hemophilia A. J Thromb Haemost 2007 Feb;5(2): 263–5.
12. Astermark J, Oldenburg J, Carlson J, Pavlova A, Kavakli K, Berntorp E, et al. Polymorphisms in the TNFA gene and the risk of inhibitor development in patients with hemophilia A. Blood 2006 Dec 1;108(12):3739–45.
13. Astermark J, Oldenburg J, Pavlova A, Berntorp E, Lefvert AK. Polymorphisms in the IL10 but not in the IL1beta and IL4 genes are associated with inhibitor development in patients with hemophilia A. Blood 2006 Apr 15;107(8):3167–72.
14. Astermark J, Oldenburg J, Escobar M, White GC, Berntorp E. The Malmo International Brother Study (MIBS). Genetic defects and inhibitor development in siblings with severe hemophilia A. Haematologica 2005 Jul;90(7):924–31.

15. Gouw SC, van den Berg HM, le CS, van der Bom JG. Treatment characteristics and the risk of inhibitor development: a multicenter cohort study among previously untreated patients with severe hemophilia A. J Thromb Haemost 2007 Jul;5(7):1383–90.

16. Lorenzo JI, Lopez A, Altisent C, Aznar JA. Incidence of factor VIII inhibitors in severe haemophilia: the importance of patient age. Br J Haematol 2001 Jun;113(3):600–3.

17. Sharathkumar A, Lillicrap D, Blanchette VS, Kern M, Leggo J, Stain AM, et al. Intensive exposure to factor VIII is a risk factor for inhibitor development in mild hemophilia A. J Thromb Haemost 2003 Jun;1(6):1228–36.

18. Gouw SC, van der Bom JG, Marijke van den BH. Treatment-related risk factors of inhibitor development in previously untreated patients with hemophilia A: the CANAL cohort study. Blood 2007 Jun 1;109(11):4648–54.

19. Morado M, Villar A, Jimenez YV, Quintana M, Hernandez NF. Prophylactic treatment effects on inhibitor risk: experience in one centre. Haemophilia 2005 Mar;11(2):79–83.

20. Santagostino E, Mancuso ME, Rocino A, Mancuso G, Mazzucconi MG, Tagliaferri A, et al. Environmental risk factors for inhibitor development in children with haemophilia A: a case–control study. Br J Haematol 2005 Aug;130(3):422–7.

21. van den Berg HM, Chalmers EA. Clinical prediction models for inhibitor development in severe hemophilia. J Thromb Haemost 2009 Jul;7 Suppl 1:98–102.

22. Matzinger P. The danger model: a renewed sense of self. Science 2002 Apr 12;296(5566):301–5.

23. Reipert BM, van Helden PM, Schwarz HP, Hausl C. Mechanisms of action of immune tolerance induction against factor VIII in patients with congenital haemophilia A and factor VIII inhibitors. Br J Haematol 2007 Jan;136(1):12–25.

24. Sharathkumar A, Lillicrap D, Blanchette VS, Kern M, Leggo J, Stain AM, et al. Intensive exposure to factor VIII is a risk factor for inhibitor development in mild hemophilia A. J Thromb Haemost 2003 Jun;1(6):1228–36.

25. Morado M, Villar A, Jimenez Y, V, Quintana M, Hernandez NF. Prophylactic treatment effects on inhibitor risk: experience in one centre. Haemophilia 2005 Mar;11(2):79–83.

26. Santagostino E, Mancuso ME, Rocino A, Mancuso G, Mazzucconi MG, Tagliaferri A, et al. Environmental risk factors for inhibitor development in children with haemophilia A: a case–control study. Br J Haematol 2005 Aug;130(3):422–7.

27. Astermark J, Petrini P, Tengborn L, Schulman S, Ljung R, Berntorp E. Primary prophylaxis in severe haemophilia should be started at an early age but can be individualized. Br J Haematol 1999 Jun;105(4):1109–13.

28. Kurnik K, Bidlingmaier C, Engl W, Chehadeh H, Reipert B, Auerswald G. New early prophylaxis regimen that avoids immunological danger signals can reduce FVIII inhibitor development. Haemophilia 2010 Mar;16(2):256–62.

16 Genetic Basis for Inhibitor Development

Johannes Oldenburg and Anna Pavlova

University Clinic Bonn, Bonn, Germany

Introduction

Inhibitors, i.e. antibodies that inhibit or inactivate replacement therapy with factor VIII (FVIII) or factor IX (FIX), develop in 20–30% of patients with hemophilia A and up to approximately 3% of patients with hemophilia B [1] as a result of a T cell-dependent activation of immune response [2,3]. Patient-specific, non-modifiable genetic factors comprise a large group of variables which have an impact on the risk of inhibitor development. Genetic markers predisposing patients to inhibitor production include mutations in the *F8* or *F9* genes, variety in MHC alleles and polymorphisms in immune-response genes (*IL-10, TNF, CTLA-4*). Family history and ethnic origin additionally modify inhibitor development risk.

Inhibitors in patients with hemophilia A

Family history, race and ethnicity

It has long been recognized that some families with HA are more predisposed to develop inhibitors than others, suggesting that this risk is partly determined by inheritance. The risk of inhibitor formation increases significantly in families with a history of inhibitors. Observations by Astermark et al. [4] of 388 families showed that 48% of patients develop inhibitors in families with a positive inhibitor history, compared to 15% in families with no history of inhibitors. In the Malmö International Brother Study (MIBS), a relative risk (RR) of 3.2 for formation of an inhibitor was observed for patients whose older brother had an inhibitor [5]. Cox Gill reported a higher incidence of inhibitor formation in hemophilia siblings (50%), compared to that observed in more extended hemophilic relatives (9%) [6]. Data published by

Santagosino et al. (20% vs. 2%) and Gouw et al. (46% vs. 26%) confirmed the association of inhibitor-positive family history with an increased risk of antibody development [7,8].

Ethnicity represents another influential factor of inhibitor development. In African Americans, the susceptibility to inhibitor development is reported to be twice as high as in Caucasian patients (51.9% vs. 25.8%), although the common hemophilia genotypes are similarly distributed among all racial groups [4,9,10,11]. The reason for this discrepancy has not been determined, but may reflect inherited racial differences in HLA antigens, in other immune response genes and in *F8* polymorphisms. In this respect, the exclusive presence of H3 or H4 *F8* haplotype in black hemophiliacs, distinct from the H1 and H2 in all racial groups, has been recently proposed as an inhibitor risk factor for this ethnic group [12].

Factor 8 genotype

The strongest predictor of inhibitor development is the type of *F8* gene defect, which determines the disease severity. Two major groups of *F8* gene alteration in the context of inhibitor development are recognized: (i) high-risk mutations (null mutations such as large deletions, intron 22 and intron 1 inversions, nonsense mutations, non-A-run small deletions, splice site mutations at conserved positions) which are associated with no circulating antigen and phenotypically always related to severe HA phenotype; and (ii) low-risk mutations (missense mutations, duplications and small deletions/insertions within the A-run, splice-site mutations at non-conserved positions) causing the expressed FVIII protein to be non-functional and resulting in either a severe or, in most cases, a mild/moderate HA phenotype.

Combined data from the HAMSTeRS mutation register and Bonn Centre show that patients with large deletions are at the highest risk (∼51%) for developing inhibitors. This risk increases around 2-fold when the deletion affects more than one domain

Current and Future Issues in Hemophilia Care, First Edition. Edited by Emérito-Carlos Rodríguez-Merchán and Leonard A. Valentino.

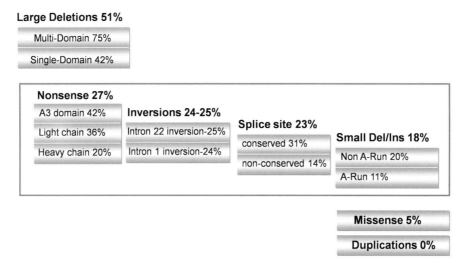

Figure 16.1 Inhibitor prevalence (as percentage) for patients with hemophilia A with various mutations types.

(75%) compared to single domain deletions (42%) (Figure 16.1). In contrast, patients with missense mutations and duplications exhibit the smallest risk (<5%). The remaining *F8* mutation types predispose patients to inhibitor formation risks in the moderate range of 18–27% [13]. Interestingly, within the group of high-risk null mutations and corresponding lack of circulating FVIII protein, the incidence of inhibitors show high diversity ranging from 72% for large multi-domain deletions to 20–25% for intron-1 and intron-22 inversions (Figure 16.1). Variety in inhibitor occurrence is even found among patients exhibiting the same mutation type. Patients with nonsense mutations in the light chain and especially in the A3 domain are more predisposed to develop inhibitors than those carrying nonsense mutations localised to the heavy chain (42% vs. 20%). The reasons for these differences in inhibitor risk within the group of null mutations are not yet understood.

Missense mutations represent only a proportionally small group of *F8* gene defects with respect to inhibitor development. They are associated with the presence of endogenous, but functionally altered, protein that is sufficient to induce immune tolerance. Missense mutations account for 15% of mutations in severe HA and almost all mutations in mild and moderate HA. Generally, they are associated with a low inhibitor risk. However, in patients with missense mutations clustered in the C1/C2 and A2 domains, the risk of inhibitor development is increased up to four-fold [14–16]. Moreover, some specific mutations seem to be associated with a particular high risk for inhibitor development. An Arg593 to Cys mutation in the A2 domain of FVIII is associated with a cumulative inhibitor incidence of 16.2% (6/37) of reported patients in the HAMSTeRS database. Similarly, Tyr2105Cys, Arg2150His, Pro2300Leu and Trp2229Cys mutations in the C1/C2 domain are linked to increased inhibitor formation risk. The prevalence of inhibitors in these mutations can be as high as 40%, similar to that observed for patients with severe *F8* gene defects [17].

The *Factor 8* missense mutations associated with inhibitors are not randomly distributed within the *F8* gene. Inhibitors are reported more commonly in patients with mutations clustered within the light chain than with mutations within the heavy chain (A1 and A2), suggesting that the A3, C1 and C2 domains of FVIII are critical for the immunogenicity of the protein. The reasons for this phenomenon are still not well-understood, but as C1/C2 domains mediate the binding of FVIII to vWF and phospholipid membranes, it is reasonable to hypothesize that any changes in the three-dimensional structure of FVIII in this region may directly affect the immunogenicity.

A correlation between the mutation type and type of inhibitors (low/high titer) has been observed by Oldenburg et al. (unpublished data). Nearly 80% of inhibitor patients with large deletions develop high titer antibodies, while only in 30% of patients bearing missense mutations high responders are detected.

To what extent the causative *F8* gene mutation influences inhibitor risk could be determined by the rate of concordance between siblings. Recently, the MIBS showed a high level of concordance (69.9%) among brothers for the presence or absence of inhibitors [5,18]. However, concordance for the presence of inhibitors among inhibitor families was only 42.4%. Moreover, Cox Gill showed that concordance for inhibitor status amongst second and third-degree hemophilic relatives was very much lower [6].

All these data strongly imply that other factors beside the *F8* gene mutations additionally contribute to determining the individual risk of inhibitor development and provide further support for a potential role of polymorphisms in immune response genes.

The major histocompatibility complex and immune response genes

Varieties in the major histocompatibility complex (MHC), an important component in the immune response pathway, have been suggested to influence the inhibitor development. Despite its key role in the recognition and presentation of FVIII for initiating either tolerance or the immune response, conflicting results have been reported regarding the predisposition or the protective role of various HLA alleles [19]. Two studies of HLA class II complex among homogeneous patients characterized for the presence of the intron 22 inversion indicate that certain HLA haplotypes may confer either increased or decreased inhibitor risk [20,21]. These authors showed correlations between inhibitor formation and HLA class I/II genotypes where A3, B7, C7, DQB0602 and DR15 were associated with inhibitor development with odds ratios of 1.9–4.0, whereas DR13 and DQB0603 appeared to be associated with a decreased risk with an odds ratio of 0.1–0.7. A recent study in a case–control, mutation matched cohort of 260 patients with and without inhibitors confirms the higher prevalence of DR1501 (0.20 vs. 0.11) and DQB0602 (0.16 vs. 0.09) in patients with inhibitors [22]. Interestingly, no correlation of any HLA allele with inhibitor formation was found in the MIBS cohort [23]. It can be hypothesized that in the MIBS brother pairs, who have 50% of their alleles in common, other factors may mask the involvement of HLA.

The search for other determinants of genetic susceptibility for inhibitor formation has been extended to genes involved in the immune response. Functional polymorphisms of pro- and anti-inflammatory cytokines are important modulators of the immune response. An imbalance in cytokine secretion may affect the clinical outcome following initial exposure to supplemented FVIII protein. Expression and production of cytokines are, in part, genetically determined and are influenced by certain polymorphisms in these genes. These polymorphisms putatively modulate the cytokine synthesis/release upon antigenic stimulation, thus promoting or inhibiting the expansion of inhibitor-producing B-cell clones. Current knowledge of the influence of polymorphisms on the *IL-10, TNF-α* and *CTLA-4* genes with respect to inhibitor formation is highlighted in the analysis of individuals from the MIBS and in a case controlled study on 260 severe hemophilia A patients with and without inhibitors [22–24]. An association between a 134 bp allele in the promoter region of the *IL-10* gene and *IL10-1082G* allele and the risk of developing an inhibitor have been demonstrated [22,24]. A clear predominance of the IL-10 high-producer GCC haplotype was observed in patients with inhibitors (0.55 vs. 0.32; P = 0.0065) [24]. Inhibitors were identified in 72.7% of the patients with the *TNFα-308A/A* genotype, compared with only 39.7% for the *TNFα-308G/G* [23]. The *CTLA-4* genotype has the potential to exert a minor effect on the immune response to FVIII by modulating the level of this co-stimulatory molecule at the cell surface.

Inhibitors in patients with hemophilia B

The incidence of FIX inhibitors is about 3% of all HB patients. The mutation profile for HB demonstrates heterogeneity with respect to molecular defects with a high prevalence of missense mutations.

Overall, 75% of genetic alterations in *F9* mutation databases are missense mutations (75% vs. 14.5% in HA), while 25% represent all other gene defects (25% vs. 85.5% for HA) [13,25]. Similar data are reported by Belvini et al. where missense mutations have a prevalence of 69.5%, followed by nonsense mutations (14.4%), small deletions (6.4%), splice site mutations (5.9%), large deletions (2.5%) and promoter mutations (1.3%) [26].

For both HA and HB, inhibitor formation is associated with same mutation types. Large gene deletions or rearrangements are indicative of high risk for inhibitor development and account for approximately 50% of inhibitors in HB, compared to other null-mutations with inhibitor formation rates of approximately 20%. The different proportions of high risk, null-mutation genotypes for hemophilia B and A patients may explain, to some extent, the lower incidence of inhibitor development in FIX-deficient patients. However, within specific mutation type, such as nonsense mutation, the inhibitor prevalence is also much lower in HB than HA (6% vs. 30%). In both, HA and B missense mutations represent a very low risk of inhibitor development. Only 1% of case with severe HB and missense mutation are present with inhibitors in F9 mutation database [25].

Several arguments could be speculated for the lower inhibitor prevalence in HB than HA [27]. (1) The relatively smaller size of the FIX protein, compared to the FVIII protein, suggests fewer immunogenic epitopes to be recognized against which antibodies can be formed. (2) An overall lower proportion of null-mutations in HB (25%) compared with that in HA (85.5%) and specific mutation profile, with predominant presence of missense mutations in HB [13,25]. Since fewer CRM+ than CRM− individuals with HB develop inhibitors, it is further postulated that CRM+ patients develop tolerance to the endogenously encoded protein that extends to the exogenous FIX used in replacement therapy [28]. (3) Furthermore, the structural homology and considerable conservation of amino acid sequence between FIX and other Vitamin K-dependent clotting factors (factors II, VII, IX, X, protein C and S) may confer some tolerance to FIX and could be a reason for the lower FIX immunogenicity [27,29].

Several clinical features are specific for FIX inhibitors. The occurrence of an allergic, anaphylactic reaction to FIX-containing products is a peculiar phenominon concomitant with FIX inhibitor development [27,30,31]. Fifty-one (58%) of the 88 FIX inhibitor patients reported in ISTH registry of FIX inhibitors were associated with an allergic manifestation. Seventy-five percent of them presented with total gene deletion [27]. Although the experience with immune tolerance induction (ITI) in HB patients with inhibitors is limited, the poor outcome of ITI is another characteristic that distinguishes HB from HA inhibitors. Furthermore, approximately 38% of FIX inhibitor patients develop nephrotic syndrome as a complication of ITI [27]. Thus, in patients with hemophilia B, a genetic analysis of the *F9* gene directly after diagnosis of bleeding disorder is recommended because the result may point to patient risk for developing an allergic reaction. Those patients should be closely supervised by a physician during the first 20 FIX concentrate administrations.

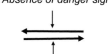

Low Risk Genetic Factors	Environmental Factors	High Risk Genetic Factors
- Negative family history	*- Early prophylaxis*	- Positive family history
- Non-severe haemophilia	*- Absence of danger signals*	- Severe haemophilia
- Caucasian origin		- African origin
- Missense mutation		- Null mutation
- IL10 134 allele negative	*- Early event-based treatment*	- IL10 134 allele positive
-TNFα A2 allele negative	*- Intensive treatment*	-TNFα A2 allele positive
-CTLA4 -318 allele positive	*- Continuous infusion*	-CTLA4 -318 allele negative
	- Danger signals	

Figure 16.2 Genetic and environmental risk factors associated with inhibitor development in hemophilia A.

Conclusions

In conclusion, inhibitor development in HA and HB is considered to be a multifactorial event including both genetic and environmental risk factors. While the inherited genetic risk factors cannot be changed, it is thought that on a given genetic background, defined by the type of *F8/F9* genes mutations and polymorphisms of immune response genes, the environmental factors may allow to move a "high risk" patient to a "low risk" patient (Figure 16.2) by choosing treatment regimes less prone to inhibitor development, such as initiation of early prophylaxis in the absence of hemorrhage [32].

References

1. Berntorp E, Shapiro A, Astermark J, et al. Inhibitor treatment in haemophilias A and B: summary statement for the 2006 international consensus conference. Haemophilia 2006;12(Suppl 6):1–7.
2. Saint-Remy JM, Lacroix-Desmazes S, Oldenburg J. Inhibitors in haemophilia: pathophysiology. Haemophilia 2004;10(Suppl 4): 146–51.
3. Astermark J. Why do inhibitors develop? Principles of and factors influencing the risk for inhibitor development in haemophilia. Haemophilia 2006;12(Suppl 3):52–60.
4. Astermark J, Berntorp E, White GC, et al. MIBS Study Group. The Malmo international brother study (MIBS): further support for genetic predisposition to inhibitor development in hemophilia patients. Haemophilia 2001;7:267–72.
5. Astermark J, Oldenburg J, Escobar M, et al. Malmo International Brother Study Group. The Malmo international brother study (MIBS). Genetic defects and inhibitor development in siblings with severe hemophilia. A. Haematologica 2005;90:924–31.
6. Cox Gill J. The role of Genetics in Inhibitor Formation. Thromb Haemost 1999; 82:500–4.
7. Santagostino E, Mancuso ME, Rocino A, et al. Environmental risk factors for inhibitor development in children with haemophilia A: a case-control study. Br J Haematol 2005;130(3):422–7.
8. Gouw SC, van den Berg HM, le Cessie S, et al. Treatment characteristics and the risk of inhibitor development: a multicenter cohort study among previously untreated patients with severe hemophilia A. J Thromb Haemost 2007;5(7):1383–90.
9. Lusher JM. First and second generation recombinant factor VIII concentrates in previously untreated patients: recovery, safety, efficacy, and inhibitor development. Semin Thromb Hemost 2002;28(3):273–6 [Review].
10. Addiego JE, Kasper C, Abildgaard T *et al*. Increased frequency of inhibitors in African American hemophilic patients. Blood 1994;1:293a.
11. Scharrer I, Bray GL, Neutzling O. Incidence of inhibitors in haemophilia A patients – a review of recent studies of recombinant and plasma-derived factor VIII concentrates. Haemophilia 1999;5:145–54.
12. Viel KR, Ameri A, Abshire TC,et al. Inhibitors of factor VIII in black patients with hemophilia. N Engl J Med 2009;16;360(16):1618–27.
13. Oldenburg, J. Pavlova, A. Genetic risk factors for inhibitors to factors VIII and IX. Haemophilia 2006;12(Suppl. 6):15–23.
14. Suzuki H, Shima M, Arai M, et al. Factor VIII Ise (R2159 C) in a patient with mild haemophilia A, an abnormal factor VIII with retention of function but modification of C2 epitopes. Thromb Haemost 1997;77:862–7.
15. Jacquemin M, Lavend'homme R, Benhida A, et al. A novel cause of mild/moderate haemophilia A: mutations scattered in the factor VIII C1 domain reduce factor VIII binding to von Willebrand factor. Blood 2000;96:958–65.
16. Liu ML, Shen BW, Nakaya S, et al. Haemophilic factor VIII C1- and C2-domain missense mutations and their modeling to the 1.5-angstrom human C2-domain crystal structure. Blood 2000;96: 979–87.
17. Hay CR. Factor VIII inhibitors in mild and moderate severity haemophilia A. Haemophilia 1998;4:558–63.
18. Berntorp E, Astermark J, Doonfield SM, et al. Haemophilia Inhibitor Genetics Study – evaluation of a model for studies of complex diseases using linkage and associated methods. Haemophilia 2005;11:427–9.
19. White GC II, Kempton CL, Grimsley A, et al. Cellular immune responses in haemophilia: why do inhibitors develop in some, but not all haemophiliacs? J Thromb Haemost 2005;3:1676–81.
20. Oldenburg J, Picard J, Schwaab R, et al. HLA genotype of patients with severe haemophilia A due to intron 22 inversion with and without inhibitors to factor VIII. Thromb Haemost 1997;77:238–42.
21. Hay CR, Ollier W, Pepper L, et al. HLA class II profile: a weak determinant of factor VIII inhibitor development in severe haemophilia A. UKHCDO inhibitor working party. Thromb Haemost 1997;77:234–7.
22. Pavlova A, Delev D, Lacroix-Desmazes S, et al. Impact of polymorphisms of the major histocompatibility complex class II,

interleukin-10, tumor necrosis factor-alpha and cytotoxic T-lymphocyte antigen-4 genes on inhibitor development in severe hemophilia A. J Thromb Haemost 2009;7(12):2006–15.

23. Astermark J, Oldenburg J, Carlson J, et al. Polymorphisms in the TNFA gene and the risk of inhibitor development in patients with hemophilia A. Blood 2006;108:3739–45.

24. Astermark J, Oldenburg J, Pavlova A, et al. MIBS Study Group. Polymorphisms in the IL10 but not in the IL1beta and IL4 genes are associated with inhibitor development in patients with hemophilia A. Blood 2006;107:3167–72.

25. Green P. A Database of Point Mutations and Short Additions and Deletions in the Factor IX Gene. Haemophilia B Mutation Database, King's College London, University of London, London, Version 13, 2004. http://www.kcl.ac.uk/ip/petergreen/haemBdatabase.html (accessed April 2, 2007).

26. Belvini D, Salviato R, Radossi P, et al. AICE HB Study Group. Molecular genotyping of the Italian cohort of patients with hemophilia B. Haematologica 2005;90:635–42.

27. Warrier I. Inhibitors in haemophilia B. In: Lee C, Berntorp E, Hoot KW (eds). Textbook of Hemophilia, 2005. Oxford: Blackwell Publishers, 2005:97–100.

28. Ljung, R.C. Gene mutations and inhibitor formation in patients with hemophilia B. Acta Haematologica 1995;94:49–52.

29. Oldenburg J, Schröder J, Brackmann HH, et al. Environmental and genetic factors influencing inhibitor development. Semin Hematol. 2004;41(1 Suppl 1):82-8 [Review].

30. Warrier I, Ewenstein B, Koerper M, et al. FIX inhibitors and anaphylaxis in hemophilia B. J Pediatr Haematol Oncol 1997;19:23–27.

31. Thorland EC, Dost JB, Lusher J, et al. Anaphylactic response to FIX replacement therapy in haemophilia B patients: complete gene deletions confer the highest risk. Haemophilia 1999;5:101–105.

32. Kurnik K, Bidlingmaier C, Engl W, et al. New early prophylaxis regimen that avoids immunological danger signals can reduce FVIII inhibitor development. Haemophilia 2010;16(2):256–62.

17 Non-Genetic Risk Factors for Inhibitor Development

Lisa N. Boggio and Mindy L. Simpson

Rush University Medical Center, Chicago, IL, USA

Introduction

The most serious complication of hemophilia is the development of inhibitors. Patients with inhibitors have more clinically serious or life-threatening bleeding episodes. Bleeding is more difficult to control as patients do not respond to factor VIII or IX infusions and often must be treated with bypassing agents such as recombinant factor VIIa or activated prothrombin complex concentrates. The cost of this therapy is greatly increased over that of patients without an inhibitor [1]. Inhibitors develop in 20–30% of patients with severe hemophilia A and up to 5% in those with severe Hemophilia B. Both patient-related (genetic) and treatment-related risk factors have been postulated to increase the risk of inhibitor formation. The genetic risks for inhibitor formation are discussed in Chapter 16. Here we will discuss non-genetic risk factors for inhibitor formation.

First treatment exposure

The effect of initial treatment on inhibitor development is complex. The age at which patients start infusions of replacement factor is variable. Some patients may start therapy prior to any major bleeding events, as in primary prophylaxis, and others may start out of the need to treat an acute bleeding episode. Therefore it is difficult to assess the risk associated with inhibitor development as it relates to the age at first exposure to replacement factor [2]. Several studies have attempted to look at age as a risk factor, but there is no consensus. Early studies which evaluated age as an independent variable for risk found that the younger a patient starts factor treatment, the higher the risk of inhibitor development with the highest rate of inhibitor formation in patients exposed to fac-

tor VIII products at earlier than 6 months of age [3]. However, later studies were not able to confirm these results when they took other confounding variables into account such as mutation type, factor product, and treatment intensity [4,5].

In addition to age, conditions at the first exposure time have been evaluated including the factor product (recombinant vs. plasma-derived), the reason or situation (surgery, bleeding, or prophylaxis), and the intensity of treatment. The CANAL Study (Concerted Action on Neutralizing Antibodies in severe hemophilia A) looked at 366 patients with severe hemophilia A in an attempt to identify risk factors for inhibitor development [5]. In the CANAL Study, patients were more likely (65% risk) to develop inhibitors if their initial exposure to factor replacement was related to a surgical procedure versus 23% risk when treatment was initiated for bleeding and 22% risk for prophylaxis initiation. The CANAL Study also reported that patients treated for the first time in response to bleeding or surgery had a 3.3-fold increased risk of inhibitor development if they required at least 5 consecutive days of factor VIII infusion (so-called peak treatment moments) compared to patients requiring 1-2 days of treatment.

Treatment regimens

Prophylaxis vs. on-demand

Treatment regimens consisting of prophylaxis versus episode-based or on-demand therapy have been evaluated for the risk of subsequent inhibitor development. Several studies suggest that prophylaxis treatment may offer a protective effect against the development of inhibitors [4–6]. There was a 60% decreased risk of inhibitor development for patients on regular prophylaxis in the CANAL Study compared to on-demand treatment [5]. Additionally, there is a suggestion that starting prophylaxis early (within the first 20 exposure days) and with a low dose regimen may

---

Current and Future Issues in Hemophilia Care, First Edition. Edited by Emérito-Carlos Rodríguez-Merchán and Leonard A. Valentino.
© 2011 John Wiley & Sons, Ltd. Published 2011 by Blackwell Publishing Ltd.

reduce inhibitor formation [7]. However, there is a higher risk of inhibitor development within the first 50 exposure days of either regimen, and this risk decreases after 200 exposure days.

Continuous vs. bolus infusions

Factor dosing is typically given as bolus infusions, but this allows the patient's factor levels to swing high and low as the body utilizes the concentrate. In situations where it would be preferable to maintain a more constant factor concentration mimicking the natural situation, such as with surgery and major bleeding, continuous infusion of factor has been tried with success. With the continuous infusion, it is possible to avoid the deep troughs that might be associated with bleeding risk and it has been shown to decrease the overall total factor consumption, so is more cost-effective [8]. In a pediatric study of bolus versus continuous infusions, the continuous infusion regimen saved 30% factor VIII concentrate usage over the bolus treatment regimen and both treatments were equally safe and effective [9]. However, there is a concern that continuous infusions may be associated with inhibitor formation. It is difficult to study the association of continuous infusions and inhibitors as most patients who receive continuous infusion for surgery or major bleeding will subsequently move on to a bolus infusion treatment regimen for days to weeks following the event. In a retrospective German study, they found that out of 250 continuous infusions, 10 inhibitors were reported including five severe, one moderate, and four mild hemophilia patients of which two were previously untreated patients and 8 were previously treated patients [10]. Typically the mild patients and previously treated patients would be thought to represent a lower risk group for developing inhibitors. Therefore the German study suggested that perhaps the continuous infusion treatment regimen increased the risk of inhibitor development in these otherwise lower risk patient groups. Further study is needed to assess this relationship.

Intensity of treatment

In the setting of more intensive treatment, there is generally an increased inhibitor development risk. This situation is more complex in that it relates to the dose, duration, and reason for treatment. The CANAL Study defined a "major peak treatment moment" as one where a patient receives factor for a minimum of five consecutive days related to bleeding or surgery. In the CANAL Study, an increased risk of inhibitor development was shown during major peak treatment moments compared to those with a 1–2 day factor exposure [5]. If the major peak treatment moment happened to be the first factor treatment exposure for a patient, there was a 3.3-fold increased risk of inhibitor development compared to a relative risk of 2.0 for a major peak treatment moment at any exposure day according to the CANAL Study results. The mean dose of factor VIII exposure during 5 consecutive days was related to inhibitor risk. Compared to doses <35 IU/kg, patients receiving a dose of 35–50 IU/kg showed a 1.4 times higher risk and at a dose of >50 IU/kg the risk of inhibitor formation was 3.3 times greater [5]. Therefore, it is recommended to minimize intensive treatment when possible, especially for previously untreated patients.

Factor concentrates

Choices exist in factor concentrates available to patients including recombinant and plasma-derived factor products. In the 1990s, there were two pasteurized plasma-derived factor VIII concentrates that were related to increased inhibitor development in previously treated patients, where the inhibitors disappeared after cessation of the specific product. This showed a direct relationship between a product type and inhibitor development [11]. Other products have not had such clear evidence for inhibitor formation but it is suggested that very high purity factor concentrates (such as monoclonal or recombinant products) may be more antigenic than older, less pure products.

Multiple theories exist as to why plasma-derived products may have a lower risk of inhibitor development. Von Willebrand factor (vWF) present in many plasma-derived products has been hypothesized to reduce immunogenicity of factor VIII by masking B- and T- cell epitopes or by altering the tertiary structure of factor VIII. Alternatively, transforming growth factor-β is a contaminant in some plasma-derived factor concentrates, and this may affect cytokine production and the interactions between antigen-presenting cells and T cells [11].

A study by Chalmers evaluated children treated by either recombinant factor VIII product or plasma derived factor VIII product. The overall incidence of inhibitor development was 27% with a recombinant product compared to 14% in patients treated with plasma-derived product [12]. In contrast, the CANAL Study did not show a clearly lower risk of inhibitors with plasma-derived products; but it did conclude that some but not all plasma-derived products might confer a diminished risk of inhibitor development [13]. With unresolved risk association between product and inhibitors, further study is needed.

Switching between factor concentrates has also been suggested as an inhibitor risk. Studies of previously treated patients indicate that the immunogenicity of products and product switching carry a small risk for inhibitor development. Further information is needed to assess the risk in previously untreated patients [2].

Immune system challenges

Immune challenges also play a role in inhibitor development. Healthy blood donors have been shown to have anti-factor VIII antibodies without clinical sequellae [14]; however pathologic immune responses may develop only after "dangerous" insults [15] such as inflammation, autoimmune disease, infection, vaccinations, surgery, or infiltration of factors VIII/IX into tissues during a major bleed.

How are inhibitors formed? Factor VIII is taken up by antigen presenting cells (APC) and is degraded into protein fragments. Certain fragments are expressed on the surface of the APC with a major histocompatibility complex (MHC) class-II molecule. This is recognized by CD4+ cells which in turn stimulate B cells to

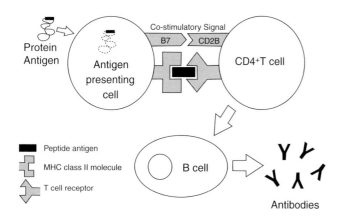

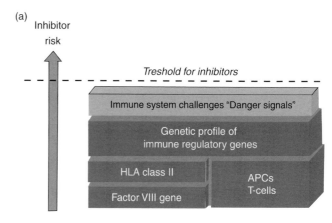

Figure 17.1 Protein is expressed on the surface of the antigen presenting cell with a MHC class II molecule. This is recognized by T cells which then stimulate B cells to make antibodies. (Reproduced from Reding, M.T. Immunological aspects of inhibitor development. Haemophilia, 2006; 12(Suppl 6): p. 30–5; discussion 35–6.)

produce antibodies (Figure 17.1). This process occurs in congenital and acquired hemophilia patients and in healthy controls [16] although the response is less intense in those without a clinical inhibitor [17], suggesting that the intensity of the response has a critical role in inhibitor formation. CD4 expressing cells can differentiate into different T-cell subsets which in turn can produce IL-4 and IL-10. These increase antibody production of B-cells. Polymorphisms in IL-10 gene, tumor necrosis factor alpha (TNFα) and cytotoxic T-lymphocyte antigen-4 (CTLA-4) have been associated with inhibitor development [18,19]. Patients with these polymorphisms may be more sensitive to inflammatory stimuli in the production of inhibitors [17].

Due to the small numbers of subjects in most studies, it is difficult to separate the role of genetic influences versus environmental influences, however a higher genetic "platform" as proposed by Astermark requires less environmental influences to achieve inhibitor formation (Figure 17.2).

Bleeding and surgery

Surgery and hemorrhage expose potentially immunogenic factors and other inflammatory cytokines in the extravascular space [20,21]. Many studies have looked at the role of major bleeding in inhibitor formation. In a study of 77 patients, reported by Ragni et al., hemophilia A patients with inhibitors were more likely to have had central nervous system bleeding (35% compared to 1.7% of controls). Of those 77 patients, African-American patients with inhibitors were more likely to have the central nervous system hemorrhage as their first bleeding event, typically within the first 6 months of life and preceding their inhibitor formation [22]. With major bleeding events, it may be difficult to determine whether the hemorrhage or the need for more intense treatment could potentiate inhibitor formation. Similarly, some studies have implicated surgery as a risk factor for inhibitor formation. In the CANAL

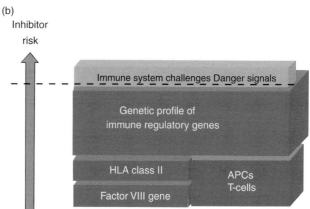

Figure 17.2 Schematic model of patients with a "safe" (a) or "unsafe" (b) platform for inhibitors to be developed, and the potential impact of immune system challenges (danger signals) in association with factor VIII replacement therapy to reach the detrimental "threshold". (Reproduced from Astermark, J., Inhibitor development: patient-determined risk factors. Haemophilia, 2010; 16(102): 66–70.)

study, the risk of inhibitor formation was 3.3-fold increased when surgery was performed in the context of the first factor exposure versus a 1.4-fold increase in risk when surgery occurred after first factor exposure [5]. However, in an alternative study by Santagostino including previously treated and first-exposure patients, there was no statistically significant increase in inhibitor patients having had surgery versus non-inhibitor patients [6]. In general, it is recommended to minimize intensive treatment as possible, especially during immune system challenges.

Vaccination and infection

Controversy surrounds the optimal way to vaccinate persons with bleeding disorders. All agree that the vaccines are beneficial and prevent infections, especially in persons likely to be exposed to blood products. There is an increased risk of bleeding after intramuscular injections. It has been suggested that intramuscular vaccination is more efficient, however giving factor replacement prior to vaccination may further activate the immune system and lead to inhibitor formation [23]. Few studies have prospectively evaluated this issue. Only one study by Santagostino et al. evaluated 60 cases and 48 controls for the development of inhibitors. Subjects had severe or moderately severe hemophilia A and received factor VIII with vaccination and during infection. There was no difference in the development of inhibitors in this group (20 cases, 23 controls) [6]. Acute hepatitis infection or seroconversion to hepatitis B surface antigen positivity was reported with a higher frequency in inhibitor patients (31.6% vs. 7.7% in controls), but most patients in this study were exposed prior to vaccine availability [22]. There have been no reports of increased inhibitor formation with the wide-spread use of recombinant hepatitis A and B vaccination.

Antenatal issues and breast feeding

Exposure to factor VIII in utero or via breast milk may be protective against inhibitor formation [24]. Breast feeding, in addition to passive protection against infections, may also stimulate the immune system of the baby through oral tolerance [25]. Human milk fat globule (HMFG) has sequence homology with human factors VIII and V and ingestion may induce tolerance to factor VIII [24]. A few studies have looked at this issue and have not noted a protective effect of breast feeding [5,6,22,26]. Other perinatal issues, such as amniocentesis, villocentesis, premature birth, and mode of delivery, were not found to affect inhibitor formation in these studies.

Conclusions

Inhibitor development is caused by a complex interaction between genetic and environmental factors. Identification of these factors may help in reducing the incidence of inhibitor development and therefore improve the quality of life for patients with hemophilia. This chapter emphasizes the fact that there is little evidence supporting our clinical practice. Several environmental factors have been identified, but analysis of these factors is limited by the small amount of studies as well as by the small numbers of patients included in these studies.

The European Haemophilia Treatment Standardisation Board (ETHSB) recently completed a review of this topic and surveyed their members regarding these issues. The board recommends that caution be taken in patients with intensive treatment especially previously untreated patients during surgical procedures. Elective surgical procedures requiring intensive factor replacement should be avoided. Vaccinations should be given subcutaneously without concomitant factor infusions [2].

It is our practice to screen all patients for risk of inhibitors via a thorough family history. Ideally genetic testing should be performed in all patients; however this is limited by payment and insurance constraints. Vaccinations are given without concomitant factor products and not more than one vaccination may be

given into a single muscle group on each occasion. Factor infusion is limited until the first hemarthrosis or serious bleeding occurs. All patients are encouraged to participate in prospective trials to quantify the risk of inhibitor formation.

References

1. Gringeri, A., et al. Cost of care and quality of life for patients with hemophilia complicated by inhibitors: the COCIS Study Group. Blood, 2003;102(7):2358–63.
2. Astermark, J., et al. Non-genetic risk factors and the development of inhibitors in haemophilia: a comprehensive review and consensus report. Haemophilia, 2010;16(5):747–66.
3. Lorenzo, J.I., et al. Incidence of factor VIII inhibitors in severe haemophilia: the importance of patient age. Br J Haematol, 2001;113: 600–603.
4. Morado, M., et al. Prophylactic treatment effects on inhibitor risk: experience in one centre. Haemophilia, 2005;11:79–83.
5. Gouw, S.C., van der Bom, J.G., van den Berg, H.M. Treatment-related risk factors of inhibitor development in previously untreated patients with hemophilia A: the CANAL cohort study. Blood, 2007;109(11):4648–54.
6. Santagostino, E., et al. Environmental risk factors for inhibitor development in children with haemophilia A: a case-control study. Br J Haematol, 2005;130(3):422–7.
7. Kurnik, K., et al. New early prophylaxis regimen that avoids immunological danger signals can reduce FVIII inhibitor development. Haemophilia, 2010;16:256–62.
8. Hathaway, W.E., et al. Comparison of continuous and intermittent factor VIII concentrate therapy in hemophilia A. Am J Hematol, 1984;17:85–8.
9. Bidlingmaier, C., Deml, M.M., Kurnik, K. Continuous infusion of factor concentrates in children with haemophilia A in comparison with bolus injections. Haemophilia, 2006;12:212–17.
10. Von Auer, C.H., et al. Inhibitor Development in Patients with Hemophilia A after Continuous Infusion of FVIII Concentrates. Ann NY Acad Sci, 2005;1051:498–505.
11. Gouw, S.C., van den Berg, H.M. The multifactorial etiology of inhibitor development in hemophilia: genetics and environment. Semin Thromb Hemost, 2009;35:723–34.
12. Chalmers, E.A., et al. Early factor VIII exposure and subsequent inhibitor development in children with severe haemophilia A. Haemophilia, 2007;13:149–55.
13. Gouw, S.C., et al. Recombinant versus plasma-derived factor VIII products and the development of inhibitors in previously untreated patients with severe haemophilia A: the CANAL cohort study. Blood, 2007;109:4693–7.
14. Gilles, J.G., Saint-Remy, J.M. Healthy subjects produce both anti-factor VIII and specific anti-idiotypic antibodies. J Clin Invest, 1994. 94(4): p. 1496–505.
15. Matzinger, P. Tolerance, danger, and the extended family. Annu Rev Immunol, 1994;12:991–1045.
16. Reding, M.T., et al. Sensitization of CD4+ T cells to coagulation factor VIII: response in congenital and acquired hemophilia patients and in healthy subjects. Thromb Haemost, 2000;84(4):643–52.
17. Reding, M.T. Immunological aspects of inhibitor development. Haemophilia, 2006;12(Suppl 6): p. 30–5; discussion 35–6.

18. Astermark, J., et al. Polymorphisms in the IL10 but not in the IL1beta and IL4 genes are associated with inhibitor development in patients with hemophilia A. Blood, 2006;107(8):3167–72.

19. Astermark, J. Inhibitor development: patient-determined risk factors. Haemophilia, 2010;16(102):66–70.

20. Astermark, J. Why do inhibitors develop? Principles of and factors influencing the risk for inhibitor development in haemophilia. Haemophilia, 2006;12(Suppl 3):52–60.

21. Oldenburg, J., et al. Environmental and genetic factors influencing inhibitor development. Semin Hematol, 2004;41(1 Suppl 1): 82–8.

22. Ragni, M.V., et al. Risk factors for inhibitor formation in haemophilia: a prevalent case-control study. Haemophilia, 2009;15(5):1074–82.

23. Makris, M., Conlon C.P., Watson H.G. Immunization of patients with bleeding disorders. Haemophilia, 2003;9(5):541–6.

24. Yee, T.T., Lee C.A.. Oral immune tolerance induction to factor VIII via breast milk, a possibility? Haemophilia, 2000.6(5): p. 591.

25. Hanson, L.A. Breastfeeding provides passive and likely long-lasting active immunity. Ann Allergy Asthma Immunol, 1998;81(6): p. 523–33; quiz 533–4, 537.

26. Knobe, K.E., et al. Breastfeeding does not influence the development of inhibitors in haemophilia. Haemophilia, 2002;8(5):657–9.

4 Inhibitor Treatment

18 Immune Tolerance Induction Programs

Jan Blatny[1] and Prasad Mathew[2]

[1]Children's University Hospital Brno, Brno, Czech Republic
[2]University of New Mexico, Albuquerque, NM, USA

Introduction

Development of inhibitors is one of the most serious complications of hemophilia treatment today. They occur in up to 25–30% of patients with severe hemophilia A, up to 7% of patients with moderate to mild hemophilia A and in about 3–5% of patients with hemophilia B [1]. Despite the significant improvement in our understanding of the mechanisms of inhibitor development, which helps us to avoid or diminish known triggers and risk factors for inhibitor development, there are still and probably always will be persons with hemophilia who will have to face all the problems and difficulties related to inhibitors.

It is unlikely for the vast majority of persons with hemophilia to develop inhibitors after 150 exposure days (ED). The highest risk is during the first 50 ED. Thus, inhibitors often appear during early childhood, especially in children with severe hemophilia (median age of development 1.7–3.3 years of age). Inhibitors associated with mild FVIII deficiency tend to appear later in life, reflecting the infrequency of bleeding episodes in these patients and thus decreased need for treatment. They are often associated with a familial predisposition and the presence of high-risk mutations that induce change in the FVIII molecule resulting in a functional FVIII defect [2]. For more than 30 years, the treatment of choice for inhibitor eradication in hemophilia patients has been immune tolerance induction (ITI).

Historical perspectives in ITI

The ultimate goal for the treatment of hemophilia patients with inhibitors is to achieve immune tolerance, in order to make substitution therapy with FVIII or FIX effective again. Different methods were designed to achieve immune tolerance in patients. One of the first regimens that was used was the Bonn protocol [3], which used a high-dose FVIII regimen over relatively long period of time (in months, up to 2–3 years), followed by the Malmö treatment model (Swedish) which uses extracorporeal immunoadsorption with protein A columns and administration of cyclophosphamide, high doses of FVIII and intravenous gammaglobulin (IVIG) [4]. This protocol is no longer used in Sweden for ITI as the responses were not always durable. The low-dose van Creveld (Dutch) protocol relies on FVIII administration every other day at a dose of 25 IU/kg. The dose is decreased each time the absolute FVIII recovery exceeds 30% [5]. Other models using both high and low-dose regimens have been developed in many centers.

The aim of the recent International Immune Tolerance Study (I-ITI) was to find out which dosing regimen gave a better chance for inhibitor eradication. This study compared two dosing arms – a high-dose arm (100 IU/kg twice a day) and a low-dose arm (50 IU/kg three times a week). It was stopped early due to excessive bleeding in the low-dose arm, though the primary end-point of success in ITI appeared to be similar for both arms [6]. Regimens for ITI for factor IX inhibitors are lacking in the published literature.

It is not the intention of this chapter to describe the immune tolerance protocols in detail, as they are easily available in the published literature. Rather, the chapter will focus on the factors which may influence the decision-making process when dealing with the patients who are or who may be candidates for immune tolerance induction.

Which ITI regimen to use?

This question does not have an easy or an unambiguous answer! Of the protocols available for use, there are differences in the

---

Current and Future Issues in Hemophilia Care, First Edition. Edited by Emérito-Carlos Rodríguez-Merchán and Leonard A. Valentino.
© 2011 John Wiley & Sons, Ltd. Published 2011 by Blackwell Publishing Ltd.

principles of the respective regimens. All of the regimens target FVIII deficiency with inhibitors. Some of them (e.g. the Malmö protocol) use immune suppression to speed up and enforce immune tolerance to the factor administered during the treatment. Such regimens are often of shorter duration and are less expensive. Other regimens rely on induction of immune tolerance through repeated long-term exposure to factor concentrates and may have different dosing schemes (e.g. the high-dose Bonn protocol or the low-dose regimens such as the van Creveld protocol). If the aim is to avoid exposure of the patient to immune suppression medications – then one tends to use the latter regimens. When choosing the regimen for ITI, the decision may also be influenced by the resources available. Although this is not a medical limitation, it may play an important role in a significant number of patients treated worldwide. On average, the overall success rate of ITI regimens is very similar, being over 70% in general [7].

Author comment: To answer the question "Which regimen to use?": Based on current knowledge, we recommend the use of high-dose protocols (FVIII of about 200 IU/kg/day) in "poor risk patients" (vide infra – pre-ITI inhibitor titer higher than 10 Bethesda units (BU) and/or high historical peak inhibitors titer over 200 BU and/or time since inhibitor diagnosis exceeding 5 years). In good risk patients the dose of FVIII used during ITI is probably not that crucial. This recommendation may be revised in the future once the final report of the international ITI (I-ITI) study becomes available.

When to start ITI?

It is recommended that ITI ideally be initiated within the first year after inhibitor development [8]. While the maximal peak historical inhibitor titer might influence the decision whether to start immune tolerance at all, the pre-ITI inhibitor titer seems to be important regarding the decision of when to start immune tolerance. It appears that pre-ITI titer below 10 BU positively affects both the success and time required to achieve tolerance. Some authors suggest that waiting until the inhibitor titer falls below 5 BU might further improve the results of ITI [7]. The average time from the appearance of the inhibitor until the fall of the titer below 10 BU is about 6 months [9]. It is, however, assumed that during this interval, there is no further exposure to FVIII. This means that all exposure to FVIII is discontinued (both prophylaxis and on demand therapy) and bleeding episodes are treated with a bypassing agent. This is the reason, why rFVIIa is the preferred therapy for acute bleeding management in these settings [10].

Another critical factor, the time from inhibitor development till the start of immune tolerance, may also play an important role in deciding when to start ITI. Thus if the waiting period for the inhibitor to decline below 10 BU is longer than 1–2 years, the advantage of low pre-ITI inhibitor titer might become doubtful and one would consider initiating ITI despite the inhibitor

still being over 10 BU. Another reason when it may be necessary to start ITI regardless of the inhibitor titer, is the clinical situation, when there is a severe life and/or limb threatening acute bleeding or there is a risk of significant increase of morbidity during the "waiting period" (e.g. risk of target joint development etc.).

Author comment: To answer the question, "When to start ITI": We recommend using the scheme suggested at a consensus panel of opinion leaders in 2007 – see Figure 18.1.

Which product to use?

Data suggest that ITI using either monoclonal or recombinant FVIII concentrates gives success rates of about 70%. On the other hand, studies mainly from German centers, suggest that using plasma-derived concentrates rich in VWF (von Willebrand factor) increases the likelihood of successful tolerization [11]. Results from the Italian prospective surveillance study showed that six of 13 patients at high risk for poor response to ITI, including three patients who previously had failed ITI, were successfully tolerized when using high-purity FVIII concentrate containing VWF [12].

Meta-analysis of data from the IITR and the NAITR however found no association between outcome of ITI and the product used. In both studies, the overall success rates were equivalent of about 70%. So far, there are no prospective, randomized trial results available comparing FVIII/VWF with monoclonal or recombinant concentrates. The ongoing RESIST (Rescue Immune Tolerance) study may, however, provide this data.

Author comment: To answer the question "Which product to use?": Currently most patients can be tolerized using the product which led to inhibitor development. Switching to other product for the first attempt of ITI is not recommended at this time.

Who is the ideal patient for a successful ITI?

Based on meta-analysis of the data from the International Immune Tolerance registry (IITR) and The North American Immune Tolerance Registry (NAITR), two significant ITI outcome predictors were identified: historical peak inhibitor titer and the titer at initiation of immune tolerance induction [13]. Inverse correlation between historical peak titer and success of ITI was also observed in the German ITI registry [14]. Furthermore, separate evaluations of possible outcome predictors based solely on IITR confirmed these findings showing that the group with a good outcome was characterized by the favorable success predictors (pre-titer <10 BU, time from inhibitor detection to treatment <5 years, treatment dose >100 IU/kg) and the group with a poorer outcome was defined by the opposite features associated with a poorer prognosis. The two cohorts were evaluated with reference to the probabilities of success and treatment duration as end-points. This analysis demonstrated that treatment duration was significantly shorter in

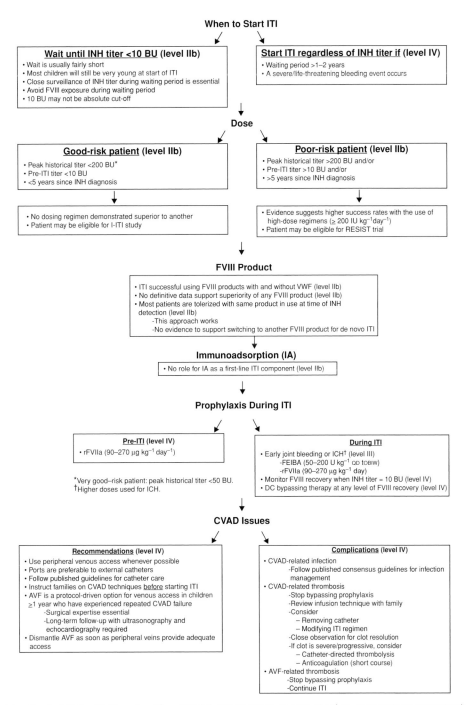

When to Start ITI

Wait until INH titer <10 BU (level IIb)
• Wait is usually fairly short
• Most children will still be very young at start of ITI
• Close surveillance of INH titer during waiting period is essential
• Avoid FVIII exposure during waiting period
• 10 BU may not be absolute cut-off

Start ITI regardless of INH titer if (level IV)
• Waiting period >1–2 years
• A severe/life-threatening bleeding event occurs

Dose

Good-risk patient (level IIb)
• Peak historical titer <200 BU*
• Pre-ITI titer <10 BU
• <5 years since INH diagnosis

Poor-risk patient (level IIb)
• Peak historical titer >200 BU and/or
• Pre-ITI titer >10 BU and/or
• >5 years since INH diagnosis

• No dosing regimen demonstrated superior to another
• Patient may be eligible for I-ITI study

• Evidence suggests higher success rates with the use of high-dose regimens (≥ 200 IU kg⁻¹day⁻¹)
• Patient may be eligible for RESIST trial

FVIII Product
• ITI successful using FVIII products with and without VWF (level IIb)
• No definitive data support superiority of any FVIII product (level IIb)
• Most patients are tolerized with same product in use at time of INH detection (level IIb)
    -This approach works
    -No evidence to support switching to another FVIII product for de novo ITI

Immunoadsorption (IA)
• No role for IA as a first-line ITI component (level IIb)

Prophylaxis During ITI

Pre-ITI (level IV)
• rFVIIa (90–270 μg kg⁻¹ day⁻¹)

*Very good-risk patient: peak historical titer <50 BU.
†Higher doses used for ICH.

During ITI
• Early joint bleeding or ICH† (level III)
    -FEIBA (50–200 U kg⁻¹ OD toBIW)
    -rFVIIa (90–270 μg kg⁻¹ day)
• Monitor FVIII recovery when INH titer = 10 BU (level IV)
• DC bypassing therapy at any level of FVIII recovery (level IV)

CVAD Issues

Recommendations (level IV)
• Use peripheral venous access whenever possible
• Ports are preferable to external catheters
• Follow published guidelines for catheter care
• Instruct families on CVAD techniques before starting ITI
• AVF is a protocol-driven option for venous access in children ≥1 year who have experienced repeated CVAD failure
    -Surgical expertise essential
    -Long-term follow-up with ultrasonography and echocardiography required
• Dismantle AVF as soon as peripheral veins provide adequate access

Complications (level IV)
• CVAD-related infection
    -Follow published consensus guidelines for infection management
• CVAD-related thrombosis
    -Stop bypassing prophylaxis
    -Review infusion technique with family
    -Consider
        – Removing catheter
        – Modifying ITI regimen
    -Close observation for clot resolution
    -If clot is severe/progressive, consider
        – Catheter-directed thrombolysis
        – Anticoagulation (short course)
• AVF-related thrombosis
    -Stop bypassing prophylaxis
    -Continue ITI

Figure 18.1 Suggested algorithm for initiating ITI. (Reproduced from DiMichele DM, Hoots WK, Pipe SW, Rivard GE, Santagostino E. International workshop on immune tolerance induction: consensus recommendations. Haemophilia. 2007 Jul;1(Suppl 1):1–22.)

patients with favorable predictors. In fact, most of the patients (65%) with good prognostic indicators achieved tolerance within one year, compared to the poor prognostic group in which a 65% success rate was not achieved for at least 31 months. This finding has also significant economic impact!

Author comment: Based on published literature, patients with positive prognostic factors (pre-ITI inhibitor titer below 10 BU, low historical peak inhibitor titer less than 200 BU and time since inhibitor diagnosis

to ITI start less than 5 years), have the greatest chance of achieving a successful ITI.

When to use bleeding prophylaxis during ITI and which bypassing agent to choose?

It has been known for many years, that prophylaxis with FVIII can prevent joint damage in persons with hemophilia without inhibitors. The efficacy of this approach has been confirmed by the randomized controlled US joint Outcome Study reported by Manco-Johnson in 2007 [15]. Increasingly, prophylaxis of bleeding is also being used in patients with inhibitors, either prior to or during ITI, if they suffer significant and/or frequent bleeds.

aPCC (activated prothrombin complex concentrate) has been used for prophylaxis during ITI for over 30 years. It has been a part of the Bonn protocol and is still used in patients at high risk of bleeding. Different authors have used different dosing schemes for aPCC for bleeding prophylaxis during ITI, but in general, depending on the bleeding severity and/or pattern, the dose has ranged from 50–100 IU/kg/day. In all reported cases use of aPCC have led to significant decrease of both frequency and severity of bleedings during ITI.

At the time of introduction of the first immune tolerance regimens, aPCC was the only available bypassing agent. Thus, historically rFVIIa (recombinant activated FVII) was less likely to be used for prophylaxis during ITI. In addition, due to its shorter half-life (around 3 hours) and even more rapid clearance in children, it was deemed by many to be ineffective for the prophylaxis when administered only once per day. In 2001 Saxon et al. first reported that rFVIIa at a dose of 90 μg/kg once daily significantly reduced the number of target joint bleedings in a boy with hemophilia and inhibitors undergoing ITI. This finding suggests that rFVIIa may have a much longer biological effect, than indicated just by its half-life. Similar findings were then confirmed by others [16,17]. It has been shown that treatment with bypassing agents outside the setting of ITI is not associated with increased risk of thrombosis in patients with hemophilia and inhibitors. Whether it would be so within the setting of ITI is not known at this time, though reports attest to its safety when used during ITI.

Author comment: To answer the question : "When to use bleeding prophylaxis during ITI and which bypassing agent to choose?": We recommend the use rFVIIa for bleeding prophylaxis prior to initiation of ITI at a dose of 90–270 μg/kg daily, when necessary to prevent significant bleeding episodes until the inhibitor titer declines. For further prophylaxis during ITI both aPCC or rFVIIa can be used. When using aPCC the dosing regimens may vary from 50–200 IU/kg daily to twice a week (not to exceed 200 IU/kg/day). Once there is evidence of any level of FVIII recovery present, bypassing prophylactic therapy may be discontinued.

Central venous access devices

Central venous access devices (CVAD) are often used in patients during treatment with ITI regimens. In certain settings (low-dose, low-frequency ITI regimens, especially in older children and/or adults) it may not be necessary to place CVAD to start ITI. Using peripheral venous access is the most safe and preferred way of factor administration outside or within ITI. However in small children and especially in protocols, where high doses of factor concentrates are administered daily, placement of CVAD is often

necessary. There are two major types of CVAD suitable for this purpose: either tunnelled external catheters or fully implantable catheters (known as ports). Ports are mostly used in hemophilia patients mainly because of lower risk of infection. Published guidelines and local/institutional standards and recommendations for implantation and maintenance of CVAD should always be used. All available measures should be taken to prevent infection and thrombosis of CVAD.

When to stop ITI?

The definition of successful immune tolerance based on the consensus recommendation established during the Second International Conference on Immune Tolerance, in Bonn, Germany, in 1997, are as follows: undetectable inhibitor level (<0.6 BU), FVIII plasma recovery >66% of predicted, FVIII half-life ≥6 h after a 72 h FVIII washout period, and the absence of anamnesis upon further FVIII exposure. A similar definition was also adopted by the I-ITI study group which also defined the criteria for partial success as a reduction of the inhibitor titer to <5 BU; FVIII recovery of less than 66% of predicted; and FVIII half-life of <6 h after a 72 h FVIII washout period associated with a clinical response to FVIII therapy and no increase in the inhibitor titer exceeding 5 BU over a 6-month period of on-demand treatment or 12 months of prophylaxis.

The panel also defined failure of ITI as follows: Failure to fulfil criteria for full or partial success within 33 months and/or less than a 20% reduction in the inhibitor titer for any 6-month period during ITI after the first 3 months of treatment. This implies that 9 months is the minimum period for ITI and 33 months is the maximum duration of ITI, although the decision to continue immune tolerance would be at the discretion of the individual physician and patient characteristics.

Incomplete response or ITI failure

The time to response to an ITI regimen may vary ranging from weeks to several years. Results from the NAITR showed that patients who were using FVIII doses over 50 U/kg/day achieved tolerance more quickly, compared to those who were using lower dose/frequency regimens. Thus one strategy for slow responding patients might be to increase the dose or to give more time for the current regimen to induce tolerance.

Another option for patients, whose response to ITI using monoclonal or recombinant factor concentrates is slow or suboptimal, is to switch them to a plasma-derived VWF rich factor concentrate. This recommendation is based on results derived mainly from experience of some European centers and is also supported by certain results of IITR analysis [18,19].

Rituximab (a monoclonal antiCD20 antibody) may improve the results in some patients who are difficult to tolerize [20].

Immune tolerance in hemophilia B patients

Inhibitors are much less frequent in hemophilia B patients. Their incidence is around 3%, but the vast majority are high responding alloantibodies. The development of inhibitors in hemophilia B patients is associated with large or complete deletions in FIX gene. These mutations are also often associated with severe allergic and/or anaphylactic reactions to FIX appearing concurrently with, or after development of FIX inhibitors. The inhibitors and allergic reactions may be associated with the development of nephrotic syndrome during ITI therapy. The success rate of ITI in these patients is low and adverse events are often reported during ITI (10 times higher than in persons with FVIII inhibitors [7]). The ISTH (International Society of Thrombosis and Hemostasis) registry on FIX inhibitors reported a success rate of only 15% success (five out of 34 patients) Two of the successfully tolerized patients had low-responding inhibitors and 38% of FIX inhibitors patients undergoing ITI developed nephrotic syndrome [21,22]. Based on current knowledge, no recommendations for immune tolerance in patients with hemophilia B and inhibitors are available, and parameters used for outcome prediction in hemophilia A patients should not be used for patients with hemophilia B. If ITI is initiated, it should be done with extreme caution and screening tests for nephrotic syndrome should be done routinely and repeatedly during the course of ITI in these patients.

Conclusions

Immune tolerance induction is the treatment of choice for patients with hemophilia A and inhibitors, preferably during childhood. ITI should be commenced after inhibitor titer declines below 10 BU, ideally within 1–2 years after inhibitor development, but not later than 5 years. During this "waiting period", bypassing agents like rFVIIa should be used to treat bleeding episodes as it does not induce an immune response (anamnesis). In emergency situations (significant risk of increased morbidity) ITI might be initiated regardles of inhibitor titer.

High-dose regimens should be used preferably for patients with poor outcome predictors. Low-dose regimens may take a longer time for successful tolerization and might be associated with more frequent bleeding periods during ITI. ITI should be terminated when success parametres are met or often after 33 months. Currently there are no firm recommendations for ITI in patients with hemophilia B with inhibitors.

References

1. DiMichele DM, Hoots WK, Pipe SW, Rivard GE, Santagostino E. International workshop on immune tolerance induction: consensus recommendations. Haemophilia. 2007 Jul;13 Suppl 1:1–22.

2. Hay CR. Factor VIII inhibitors in mild and moderate severity haemophilia A. Haemophilia. 1998 Jul; 4(4):558–63.

3. Brackmann HH, Gormsen J. Massive factor-VIII infusion in haemophiliac with factor-VIII inhibitor, high responder. Lancet. 1977 Oct 29;2(8044):933.

4. Nilsson IM, Berntorp E, Freiburghaus C. Treatment of patients with factor VIII and IX inhibitors. Thromb Haemost. 1993 Jul 1;70(1): 56–9.

5. Mauser-Bunschoten EP, Roosendaal G, van den Berg HM. Low-dose immune tolerance therapy: the van Creveld model. Vox Sang. 1996; 70 Suppl 1:66–7.

6. Corrected Minutes of International ITI Investigators Meeting ASH 2009 - New Orleans December 6, 2009 [cited 2010 Nov 22]. Available from: http://www.itistudy.com/

7. DiMichele DM, Kroner BL; North American Immune Study Group. The North American Immune Tolerance Registry: practices, outcomes, outcome predictors. Thromb Haemost. 2002 Jan;87(1): 52–7.

8. Auerswald G, von Depka Prondzinski M, Ehlken B, Kreuz W, Kurnik K, Lenk H, et al. Treatment patterns and cost-of-illness of severe haemophilia in patients with inhibitors in Germany. Haemophilia. 2004 Sept;10(5):499–508.

9. DiMichele DM, Hay CR. The international immune tolerance study: a multicenter prospective randomized trial in progress. J Thromb Haemost. 2006 Oct;4(10):2271–3.

10. Brackmann HH, Effenberger E, Hess L, Schwaab R, Oldenburg J. NovoSeven in immune tolerance therapy. Blood Coagul Fibrinolysis. 2000 Apr;11 Suppl 1:S39–44.

11. Kreuz W, Escuriola-Ettinghausen C, Auerswald G. Immune-tolerance induction in haemophilia A patients with inhibitors: the choice of concentrate affecting success. Haematologica. 2001;86 Suppl 4: 16–20.

12. Gringeri A. Immunotolerance induction (ITI) with high purity FVIII/VWF concentrates in inhibitor patients with a high risk of a poor response to ITI: a prospective surveillance. J Thromb Haemost. 2005;3 Suppl 1:A207.

13. Kroner BL. Comparison of the International immune tolerance registry and The North American immune tolerance registry. Vox Sang. 1999; 77 Suppl 1:33–7.

14. Lenk H; ITT Study Group. The German registry of immune tolerance treatment in haemophilia – 1999 update. Haematologica. 2000 Oct;85(10 Suppl): 45–7.

15. Manco-Johnson MJ, Abshire TC, Shapiro AD, Riske B, Hacker MR, Kilcoyne R, et al. Prophylaxis versus episodic treatment to prevent joint disease in boys with severe hemophilia. N Engl J Med. 2007 Aug 9;357(6):535–44.

16. Morfini M, Auerswald G, Kobelt RA, Rivolta GF, Rodriguez-Martorell J, Scaraggi FA, et al. Prophylactic treatment of haemophilia patients with inhibitors: clinical experience with recombinant factor VIIa in European Haemophilia Centers. Haemophilia. 2007 Sep;13(5): 502–7.

17. Blatny J, Kohlerova S, Zapletal O, Fiamoli V, Penka M, Smith O. Prophylaxis with recombinant factor VIIa for the management of bleeding episodes during immune tolerance treatment in a boy with severe haemophilia A and high-response inhibitors. Haemophilia. 2008 Sep;14(5):1140–2.

18. Auerswald G, Spranger T, Brackmann HH. The role of plasma-derived factor VIII/von Willebrand factor concentrates in the

treatment of hemophilia A patients. Haematologica. 2003 Jun;88(6): EREP05.

19. DiMichele DM, Hay CR. The international immune tolerance study: a multicenter prospective randomized trial in progress. J Thromb Haemost. 2006 Oct;4(10):2271–3.

20. Carcao M, St Louis J, Poon MC, Grunebaum E, Lacroix S, Stain AM, et al. Rituximab for congenital haemophiliacs with in-hibitors: a Canadian experience. Haemophilia. 2006 Jan;12(1):7–18.

21. Key NS. Inhibitors in congenital coagulation disorders. Br J Haematol. 2004 Nov;127(4):379–91.

22. Chitlur M, Warrier I, Rajpurkar M, Lusher JM. Inhibitors in factor IX deficiency a report of the ISTH-SSC international FIX inhibitor registry (1997–2006). Haemophilia. 2009 Sep;15(5):1027–31.

19 Prophylaxis in Hemophilia A Patients with Inhibitors

Leonard A. Valentino[1] and Guy Young[2]

[1]Rush University Medical Center, Chicago, IL, USA
[2]UCLA Health System, Los Angeles, CA, USA

Introduction

Prophylaxis, the routine scheduled replacement of coagulation factor VIII (FVIII), is considered optimal care for patients with severe hemophilia A (FVIII activity <1%) and is recommended by the National Hemophilia Foundation, the World Health Organization, and the World Federation of Hemophilia. Observational studies [1–4] and the prospective randomized controlled US Joint Outcome Study [5] have established the efficacy of prophylaxis in preventing hemarthrosis and the subsequent development of arthropathy, target joints, and disability. In addition, prophylaxis has been shown to protect against life-threatening hemorrhage, including recurrent central nervous system bleeding following intracranial hemorrhage (ICH), and to indirectly improve academic performance [6] and quality of life (QOL) [7]. Prophylaxis also has the potential to achieve cost benefit by reducing absenteeism from school and work, increasing productivity, and decreasing the need for emergency department visits, hospitalization, and orthopedic interventions and other surgeries [3,7].

Increasingly, bypassing agent prophylaxis (BAP) is being used in hemophilia A patients with inhibitors, reflecting both the favorable experience with FVIII prophylaxis documented over the last four decades and the compelling need for bleed prevention in the inhibitor population. Up to 30% of patients with severe hemophilia A develop alloantibodies that neutralize the hemostatic effect of therapeutically administered FVIII [8]. Approximately 70% of these inhibitory antibodies are high-responding and anamnestic, exhibiting a substantial rise in titer (≥5 Bethesda units [BU]) following exposure to clotting factor replacement [9]. Compared with bleeding in hemophilia patients without inhibitors, bleeding associated with high-titer, high-responding inhibitors is more difficult to control because the hemostatic effect of bypassing therapy is unpredictable and does not reach the overall success rates ob-

tained with FVIII replacement. Furthermore, no laboratory assays are clinically available that correlate with bypassing agent dosing or efficacy. Consequently, individuals with inhibitors are at increased risk for severe joint disease that may develop after only a few bleeding episodes.

Plasma-derived activated prothrombin complex concentrate (aPCC; FEIBA® VH and FEIBA® NF, Baxter Healthcare Corporation, Westlake Village, CA) and recombinant activated factor VII (rFVIIa; NovoSeven®, Novo Nordisk, Bagsvaerd, Denmark) are the only current factor treatment options used to treat acute bleeding in patients with high-titer anti-FVIII antibodies. Both agents are also used for BAP, and outcome data are accumulating.

Clinical experience with bypassing agent prophylaxis

The first reports of prophylaxis in inhibitor patients appeared in the literature in the mid 1970s. Every-other-day infusion of prothrombin complex concentrate at doses of 30 to 50 U/kg was found to decrease joint bleeding and improve mobility in a small number of patients [10,11]. Concurrent with these investigations, Brackmann and Gormsen described the successful use of the aPCC FEIBA in preventing breakthrough bleeding in patients undergoing immune tolerance induction (ITI) with high-dose FVIII, a protocol that has become known as the Bonn regimen [12].

By the mid-1990s, the use of BAP had become more widespread, and between 2000 and 2010, 15 reports of >5 patients receiving prophylaxis with aPCC or rFVIIa prophylaxis were published, some as meeting abstracts (Table 19.1) [13–26]. These reports are primarily retrospective in nature and included small numbers of patients who had a variety of bleeding patterns and hemophilia treatment histories and were treated with a wide range of prophylactic regimens. To date, one long-term prospective study [24]

Table 19.1 Experience with BAP

Investigator	No. of patients	Prophylaxis dose	Duration of prophylaxis, median (range)	Outcome	Adverse events (AEs)*
Brackmann [13]	22 (all undergoing ITI)	aPCC: 50 U/kg BID	7 months (0.7–15)	Orthopedic outcome unchanged in 7/22 patients; clinical improvement in 6/22 patients	No TEs
Kreuz [14]	22	aPCC: 50 U/kg QD 100 U/kg BID	N/S	Median annual incidence of joint hemorrhage = 1	No life-threatening bleeding or TEs
Hilgartner [15]	7	aPCC: 50–100 U/kg QOD-TIW	3 years (3.6–5)	Decrease in annual target joint bleeds in 4/6 cases	No AEs or TEs
Schino [16]	7	aPCC: 50–100 U/kg QOD	12 months	50–90% reduction in bleed frequency	No AEs or TEs
DiMichele & Négrier [17]	14	aPCC: 69 U/kg (15–100) QD-QW	19.5 months (0.25–26)	53% mean decrease in bleed frequency	No AEs or TEs
Cheng [18]	5	aPCC: 50 or 75 U/kg BIW or QW	11.3 months (1.4–12)	80% mean total reduction in bleeding	No AEs
Ewing [19]	7	aPCC: 75 U/kg QOD or TIW	4.5 years (2.5–6.0)	64% reduction in annual hemarthroses	No AEs or TEs
Konkle [25]	22	rFVIIa: 90 or 270 μg/kg QOD	3 months	45–59% reduction in bleed frequency	No AEs or TEs
Morfini [26]	13	90–330 μg/kg BID-QW	4 months to 4 years	Decrease in mean number of bleeds from 2.5 per month to 0.6 per month	No AEs
Leissinger [20]	5	aPCC: 50, 75, or 100 U/kg QD or TIW	15 months (6–24)	73–83% mean total reduction in bleeding (per 6 months)	No AEs or TEs
Lambert [21]	13	aPCC: 77.4 ± 8.6 U/kg QD-QOD	11.9 months (1.7–54.6)	58% mean decrease in annual bleed rate	No AEs or TEs
Valentino [22]	6	aPCC:100 U/kg QD	818 days (41–1552)	Pronounced reduction in bleeding	No AEs
Jiménez-Yuste [23]	5	aPCC: 50 U/kg QOD or TIW	13 months (11-24)	Reduction in bleeding in 4/5 patients	No life-threatening bleeding or TEs
	5	rFVIIa: 90 or 100 μg/kg QD	9 months (6–22)	Reduction in bleeding in 4/5 patients	No life-threatening bleeding or TEs
Escuriola Ettingshausen & Kreuz [24]	7	aPCC: 60–100 U/kg BID-TIW	6.9 years (0.8–17.1)	Mean annual number of joint bleeds – 1.5; mean annual number of muscle bleeds = 0.9	No AEs or TEs
Leissinger [27]	34	aPCC: 85 U/kg +/− 15% TIW	6 months	To be reported	No life-threatening bleeding or TEs

*Product-related.

QD = once daily; BID = twice daily; N/S = not specified; TE = thrombotic event; AE = adverse event; QOD = every other day; TIW = thrice weekly; QW = once weekly; BIW = twice weekly.

and two randomized controlled trials (RCTs) of BAP [25, 27] have been reported.

Long-term prophylaxis

Escuriola Ettingshausen and Kreuz are following six patients who started aPCC prophylaxis at the Frankfurt, Germany hemophilia treatment center immediately upon ITI failure (a seventh patient died from intrathoracic hemorrhage after discontinuing BAP) [24]. The prophylactic dosage ranges from 60 to 100 IU/kg, with the dosing interval individualized according to bleeding tendency. The patients began prophylaxis at a median age of 6.0 years (range, 1.5–11.8 years) and have continued to receive regular aPCC infusions for a median duration of 6.9 years (range,

0.8–17.1 years). The mean annual incidence of joint bleeding is 1.5 episodes per year (95% CI, 0.7–3.0 episodes/year), and the mean incidence of muscle bleeding is 0.9 episodes per year (CI, 0.6–1.2 episodes/year). No patient has experienced major joint damage during prophylaxis, and median Pettersson and orthopedic joint scores at last follow-up evaluation were 4 (range, 0–12) and 2 (range, 0–4), respectively. These findings support the value of early long-term prophylaxis for preserving joint function in inhibitor patients.

Short-term prophylaxis

Konkle et al. enrolled 38 patients in a trial of rFVIIa for short-term prophylaxis [25]. Of these patients, 22 satisfied the entry requirement for high baseline bleeding frequency (mean ≥ 4 bleeding episodes per month for 3 months) and were randomized to receive rFVIIa at a daily dose of 90 or 270 µg/kg for 3 months followed by a 3-month postprophylaxis period. Bleeding frequency was reduced by 45% during prophylaxis with the daily 90 µg/kg dose and by 59% with the daily 270 µg/kg dose ($P < 0.001$; no significant difference between the doses), and the majority of the reduction was sustained during the postprophylaxis period. The prophylactic effect was most pronounced for spontaneous joint bleeding, and patients reported significantly fewer hospital admissions and days absent from school or work during prophylaxis as compared with the preprophylaxis period.

Leissinger and colleagues evaluated short-term aPCC prophylaxis in a randomized, crossover study [27]. The treatment regimen consisted of 6 months of prophylaxis at a dose of 85 U/kg $\pm$ 15% administered three times weekly on nonconsecutive days followed by a 3-month wash-out period and 6 months on on-demand therapy (target dose: 85 U/kg $\pm$ 15%) or vice versa. A total of 36 patients >2 years of age with a history high-titer inhibitors (>5 BU), ≥ 6 relevant bleeds in the 6 months prior to study entry, and who were being treated with on-demand therapy were enrolled. Among the 34 subjects randomized, 23% were less than 12 years of age and 62% were older than 21. Total bleeding events were reduced by 62% and joint bleeding by 61% including bleeding into target joints.

Both RCTs demonstrate that BAP with rFVIIa or aPCC can reduce the number of hemorrhages in people who bleed frequently. Whether similar regimens will prove effective in patients who bleed less often remains uncertain.

Application of bypassing agent prophylaxis

As the ongoing study of early long-term aPCC prophylaxis indicates [24], secondary prophylaxis (Table 19.2) is possible in hemophilia patients with inhibitors. Nonetheless, the difficulty of controlling bleeding episodes in these individuals together with their heightened risk for severe joint disease means that many begin to exhibit some degree of arthropathy very soon after the development of an inhibitory antibody and before BAP is initiated. These patients may benefit from secondary prophylaxis. Secondary BAP cannot halt the progression of existing joint disease. However, data from hemophilia patients with and without inhibitors indicate that prophylaxis may reduce bleeding frequency [3,5,7,15–18,20–27], prevent joint disease in previously

unaffected joints [3,15], slow deterioration in previously affected joints [3,15], and improve QOL by permitting an increase in the activities of daily life [7].

When BAP is initiated, it may be continued long-term or applied to circumscribed time periods. Depending on the particular clinical circumstances, various prophylactic dosing regimens may be appropriate. Ideal body weight, as determined by lean body mass, should be used when calculating doses for obese patients.

Long-term use of bypassing agent prophylaxis

ITI, the process of eradicating inhibitors, involves frequent, continuing exposure to FVIII in order to achieve tolerance by antigen overload, thereby restoring replacement factor pharmacokinetics and allowing the use of FVIII concentrates to treat acute bleeding. ITI is unsuccessful in approximately 20% to 50% of hemophilia A patients with inhibitors, according to registry data. Other inhibitor patients are not candidates for or refuse ITI. Thus, inhibitors are entrenched in a substantial number of individuals, and they may benefit from long-term BAP, ideally started upon inhibitor diagnosis or immediately after ITI failure [24].

Bypassing agent prophylaxis during ITI

Approximately 2% of patients with severe hemophilia and inhibitors are currently receiving ITI therapy, according to prevalence estimates from the University Data Collection Program of the Centers for Disease Control and Prevention. ITI may protect against bleeding, but if clinically significant hemorrhage occurs, consideration should be given to initiating or reinstituting BAP. Both aPCC [12,14] and rFVIIa [26] have been shown to prevent intercurrent bleeding in patients at high-risk for bleeding undergoing ITI. To reduce the risk of thrombosis, a rare but potential complication of bypassing therapy, if aPCC is used for the management of acute hemorrhage as well as prophylaxis, the total daily dose should not exceed the manufacturer's recommendation of 200 U/kg daily. If rFVIIa is used for the control of acute hemorrhage in a patients receiving aPCC prophylaxis, aPCC and rFVIIa doses should be given at least 6 hours apart [28], unless the bleeding even is life-threatening.

In some inhibitor patients, ITI may be postponed to allow the antibody titer to decline to <10 BU, which the major registries have identified as a significant predictor of ITI success. During this interval, rFVIIa is recommended for prophylaxis and the management of acute bleeding because of the potential for anamnesis with aPCC.

Table 19.2 Prophylaxis definitions

Primary prophylaxis	Long-term, continuous* treatment initiated before 2 years of age and/or before the onset of joint damage (eg, no more than 1 hemarthrosis) [33]
Secondary prophylaxis	Long-term, continuous* treatment initiated after the onset of joint damage or other significant bleeding [33]
Episodic prophylaxis	Administration of prophylaxis before strenuous or high-risk activities that may cause bleeding [31]

*With the intent of treating 52 weeks per year up to adulthood and receiving treatment a minimum of 46 weeks per year.

Bypassing agent prophylaxis after severe or life-threatening bleeding

Secondary prophylaxis is advised following the acute treatment period for inhibitor patients treated for ICH, as recurrent central nervous system (CNS) hemorrhage is common after brain bleeding [29]. In a report by Antunes et al., six hemophilia patients without inhibitors who had suffered ICH experienced ten episodes of recurrent CNS bleeding [29]. The mean time between ICH and subsequent CNS hemorrhage was 1 year (range, 0.2–2.6 years), with 80% occurring within 1 year of the *de novo* hemorrhage. While the optimal duration of BAP following ICH is unclear, a duration of 1 to 6 months or longer is recommended [30].

Among inhibitor patients who have experienced limb-threatening bleeding (e.g., iliopsoas hemorrhage) and who are receiving intensive physical therapy after hematoma resolution, prophylactic coverage with aPCC or rFVIIa should continue for approximately 6 weeks [30].

Episodic bypassing agent prophylaxis

Episodic, limited, or intermittent prophylaxis is defined as a short period of factor replacement to prevent bleeding in specific situations [31]. Surgery is the prototypical use of episodic BAP. Other examples in which episodic BAP may be helpful include prior to participating in sports or other strenuous activities, during travel, particularly if the patient will not have rapid access to high-quality medical care, and before special events, such as college final exams or a wedding.

The goal of episodic prophylaxis is to completely prevent bleeding [31]. To this end, aggressive dosing may be required. For example, aPCC may be administered three or more times weekly at a dose of 50 U/kg, with the dosing regimen escalated to a maximum of 100 U/kg twice daily to suppress bleeding. rFVIIa may be given once or twice a day at doses of 90 to 270 µg/kg until bleeding is suppressed. A trial period of 4 to 12 weeks is recommended. Once bleeding is totally prevented, consideration should be given to reducing or discontinuing treatment [32].

Outcome measures

Clinical assessment at least every 3 months, and more often if complications develop, is key to monitoring the efficacy and safety of BAP. Other strategies for assessing prophylactic efficacy include reviewing the number and type of hemorrhages, the number of emergency room visits and hospital admissions, clinical joint evaluation, orthopedic joint score, periodic radiographs or magnetic resonance imaging (MRI), functional score, activity level, and QOL [2–5,7].

Measuring the FVIII inhibitor titer every 3 months for patients on ITI ensures that BAP is discontinued before the hemostatic system normalizes. A conservative approach is to stop prophylaxis when the inhibitor titer falls to 2 to 5 BU. When clinical signs are suggestive of disseminated intravascular coagulation or thrombosis, or when circumstances (e.g., dose escalation, sequential therapy) increase the likelihood of such complications, laboratory assessment of the platelet count, fibrinogen, D-dimers, and fibrin degradation byproducts is recommended. The development of CVAD-related complications or thromboembolic events may require CVAD removal and/or the discontinuation of BAP.

Conclusions

The established benefits of prophylaxis observed in patients with severe hemophilia A may be extended to patients with high-titer inhibitors through the use of prophylactic bypassing therapy. Case reports and the results from two randomized clinical trials indicate that both aPCC and rFVIIa may be used prophylactically in a variety of clinical settings and, depending on the particular circumstances, may be appropriate for long-term, short-term, and episodic administration.

References

1. Fischer K, van der Bom JG, Mauser-Bunschoten EP, Roosendaal G, Prejs R, Grobbee DE, et al. Changes in treatment strategies for severe haemophilia over the last 3 decades: effects on clotting factor consumption and arthropathy. Haemophilia 2001;7:446–52.
2. Lofqvist T, Nilsson IM, Berntorp E, Pettersson H. Haemophilia prophylaxis in young patients–a long-term follow-up. J Intern Med 1997;241:395–400.
3. Aledort LM, Haschmeyer RH, Pettersson H. A longitudinal study of orthopaedic outcomes for severe factor-VIII-deficient haemophiliacs. The Orthopaedic Outcome Study Group. J Intern Med 1994;236:391–9.
4. van den Berg HM, Fischer K, Mauser-Bunschoten EP, Beek FJ, Roosendaal G, van der Bom JG, et al. Long-term outcome of individualized prophylactic treatment of children with severe haemophilia. Br J Haematol 2001;112:561–5.
5. Manco-Johnson MJ, Abshire TC, Shapiro AD, Riske B, Hacker MR, Kilcoyne R, et al. Prophylaxis versus episodic treatment to prevent joint disease in boys with severe hemophilia. N Engl J Med 2007;357:535–44.
6. Shapiro AD, Donfield SM, Lynn HS, Cool VA, Stehbens JA, Hunsberger SL, et al. Defining the impact of hemophilia: the Academic Achievement in Children with Hemophilia Study. Pediatrics 2001;108:E105.
7. Panicker J, Warrier I, Thomas R, Lusher JM. The overall effectiveness of prophylaxis in severe haemophilia. Haemophilia 2003;9:272–8.
8. Brackmann HH, Wallny T. Immune tolerance: high-dose regimen. In: Rodriguez-Merchan EC, Lee CA, editors. Inhibitors in Patients With Hemophilia. Oxford, England: Blackwell Science; 2002. p. 45–8.
9. Lusher JM. Factor VIII inhibitors. Etiology, characterization, natural history, and management. Ann NY Acad Sci 1987;509:89–102.
10. Buchanan GR, Kevy SV. Use of prothrombin complex concentrates in hemophiliacs with inhibitors: clinical and laboratory studies. Pediatrics 1978;62:767–74.

11. Penner JA, Kelly PE. Management of patients with factor vIII or IX inhibitors. Semin Thromb Hemost 1975;1.

12. Brackmann HH, Gormsen J. Massive factor-VIII infusion in haemophiliac with factor-VIII inhibitor, high responder. Lancet 1977;2:933.

13. Brackmann HH, Oldenburg J, Schwaab R. Immune tolerance for the treatment of factor VIII inhibitors – twenty years' 'Bonn protocol'. Vox Sang 1996;70 Suppl 1:30–5.

14. Kreuz W, Escuriola-Ettingshausen C, Mentzer D. Factor VIII inhibitor bypass activity (FEIBA) for prophylaxis during immune tolerance induction (ITI) in patients with high-responding inhibitors [abstract]. Blood 2000;96:266a. Abstract 1141.

15. Hilgartner MW, Makipernaa A, DiMichele DM. Long-term FEIBA prophylaxis does not prevent progression of existing joint disease. Haemophilia 2003;9:261–8.

16. Schino L, Mancuso G, Morfini M, Piseddu G, Sbrighi P. APCC (FEIBA) home therapy retrospective survey in long-term secondary prophylaxis on 4 hemophilia A patients with factor VIII inhibitor. Poster presented at the XXVII International Congress for the World Federation of Hemophilia; May 21–25, 2006; Vancouver, Canada.

17. DiMichele D, Negrier C. A retrospective postlicensure survey of FEIBA efficacy and safety. Haemophilia 2006;12:352–62.

18. Cheng S-N, Chen Y-C, Chiag J-L. FEIBA prophylaxis in hemophilia A patient with inhibitors decrease bleeding episodes, maintain arthropathy and enhance quality of life. Haemophilia 2006;12:Abstract 14 PO 371.

19. Ewing N, DeGuzman C, Pullens L. Anamnesis in patients with hemophilia and inhibitors who receive activated prothrombin complex concentrates for prophylaxis. . J Thromb Haemost 2007;5 Abstract number P-T-158.

20. Leissinger CA, Becton DL, Ewing NP, Valentino LA. Prophylactic treatment with activated prothrombin complex concentrate (FEIBA) reduces the frequency of bleeding episodes in paediatric patients with haemophilia A and inhibitors. Haemophilia 2007;13:249–55.

21. Lambert T, Rothschild C, Goudemand J, Négrier C, Girault S, Moreau P, et al. Secondary prophylaxis with activated prothrombin complex concentrates (APCC) reduces bleeding frequency in haemophilia a patients with inhibitors. J Thromb Haemost 2009;7:Abstract PP-TH-593.

22. Valentino LA. The benefits of prophylactic treatment with APCC in patients with haemophilia and high-titre inhibitors: a retrospective case series. Haemophilia 2009;15:733–42.

23. Jimenez-Yuste V, Alvarez MT, Martin-Salces M, Quintana M, Rodriguez-Merchan C, Lopez-Cabarcos C, et al. Prophylaxis in 10 patients with severe haemophilia A and inhibitor: different approaches for different clinical situations. Haemophilia 2009;15:203–9.

24. Escuriola Ettingshausen C, Kreuz W. Early long-term FEIBA prophylaxis in haemophilia A patients with inhibitor after failing immune tolerance induction. A prospective clinical case series. Haemophilia 2010;16:90–100.

25. Konkle BA, Ebbesen LS, Erhardtsen E, Bianco RP, Lissitchkov T, Rusen L, et al. Randomized, prospective clinical trial of recombinant factor VIIa for secondary prophylaxis in hemophilia patients with inhibitors. J Thromb Haemost 2007;5:1904–13.

26. Morfini M, Auerswald G, Kobelt RA, Rivolta GF, Rodriguez-Martorell J, Scaraggi FA, et al. Prophylactic treatment of haemophilia patients with inhibitors: clinical experience with recombinant factor VIIa in European Haemophilia Centres. Haemophilia 2007;13:502–7.

27. Leissinger C, Negrier C, Berntorp E, Windyga J, Serban M, Antmen B, et al. A prospective, randomized, crossover study of an activated prothrombin complex concentrate for secondary prophylaxis in patients with hemophilia A and inhibitors (Pro-FEIBA): subject demographics and safety data. Poster presented at the Hemophilia World Congress 2010; World Federation of Hemophilia; July 10–14, 2010; Buenos Aires, Argentina. 2010.

28. Schneiderman J, Nugent DJ, Young G. Sequential therapy with activated prothrombin complex concentrate and recombinant factor VIIa in patients with severe haemophilia and inhibitors. Haemophilia 2004;10:347–51.

29. Antunes SV, Vicari P, Cavalheiro S, Bordin JO. Intracranial haemorrhage among a population of haemophilic patients in Brazil. Haemophilia 2003;9:573–7.

30. Teitel J, Berntorp E, Collins P, d'Oiron R, Ewenstein B, Gomperts E, et al. A systematic approach to controlling problem bleeds in patients with severe congenital haemophilia A and high-titre inhibitors. Haemophilia 2007;13:256–63.

31. Pipe SW, Valentino LA. Optimizing outcomes for patients with severe hemophilia A. Haemophilia 2007;13(suppl 4):1–16.

32. Perry D, Berntorp E, Tait C, Dolan G, Holme PA, Laffan M, et al. FEIBA prophylaxis in haemophilia patients: a clinical update and treatment recommendations. Haemophilia 2010;16:80–9.

33. Berntorp E, Astermark J, Bjorkman S, Blanchette VS, Fischer K, Giangrande PL, et al. Consensus perspectives on prophylactic therapy for haemophilia: summary statement. Haemophilia 2003;9(suppl 1):1–4.

20 Treatment of Bleeding in FVIII Inhibitor Patients

Paul L.F. Giangrande[1] and Jerome Teitel[2]

[1] Churchill Hospital, Oxford, UK
[2] St Michael's Hospital, Toronto, ON, Canada

Introduction

The development of factor VIII inhibitors in severe hemophilia patients generally does not affect the pattern, severity, or frequency of bleeding. Exceptions to this rule are patients with non-severe hemophilia who develop inhibitors, in whom the clinical phenotype usually becomes similar to that of patients with severe disease, and hemophilia B patients, in who inhibitors often cause unique complications. In all cases the development of an inhibitor profoundly affects treatment. The dual priorities in managing these patients are hemostatic therapy and inhibitor eradication. The available regimens for both these goals are incompletely effective and there is no consensus on optimal approaches.

Treatment of bleeding in FVIII inhibitor patients

In those patients in whom the current inhibitor titer is <3–5 BU, it may feasible to administer enough FVIII concentrate to achieve therapeutic plasma levels. Up to three times the standard dose may be required. It should be anticipated that FVIII levels will decline more rapidly than in patients without inhibitors. Furthermore, except in "low responder" patients the anamnestic response to FVIII will preclude therapy after a variable period, perhaps only a few days. If FVIII replacement fails to achieve therapeutic levels it should be abandoned quickly in favor of inhibitor bypassing therapy.

Inhibitor bypassing therapy

Plasma-derived prothrombin complex concentrates (PCC) were found to have efficacy in treating bleeding in FVIII inhibitor patients 30 years ago [1]. Although PCC still have a role in the treatment of active bleeding and possibly prophylaxis, activated derivatives (APCC) later proved to be more effective, and are much preferred where they are available. The alternative bypassing strategy is recombinant activated factor VII (rFVIIa) used in supra-physiologic concentrations. Neither agent fully normalizes thrombin generation. There is no validated method for laboratory monitoring of bypassing therapy, but thromboelastography (TEG) and thrombin generation assays may prove to be of value. There is considerable inter-individual variability in responses to the two agents [2]. There are also discrepant responses in individual patients as demonstrated in a prospective randomized crossover trial [3]. This variability validates the strategy of switching to the alternative bypassing agent in a patient whose response to the current therapy is suboptimal. Although conventionally used "on-demand" there is increasing interest in long-term prophylactic therapy with inhibitor bypassing agents [4,5].

APCC

Currently only one APCC (FEIBA®, Baxter) is available. APCC contain FVIIa but this is not the principle of its therapeutic effect. Doses of 50–100 inhibitor bypassing units/kg are effective in 50-90% of acute or surgical bleeding episodes. Thrombin generation declines with a half-life of 4 to 7 hours; where follow-up doses are necessary they may be administered at 6 to 12 hour intervals. APCC should not be given by continuous infusion. Cumulative daily doses should not exceed 200 units/kg. The production of APCC incorporates multiple viral exclusion and inactivation steps, and there have been no reports of pathogen transmission by this product. The major adverse effect of APCC is thrombosis, predominantly arterial, but this is rare when it is used as directed (4–8 events per 10^5 infusions) [6]. The safety of antifibrinolytic agents administered concomitantly with APCC has not been shown, although there have been anecdotal reports of their use. APCC contain small amounts of FVIII, and in some patients this induces an anamnestic rise in the inhibitor titer. This is rarely

Current and Future Issues in Hemophilia Care, First Edition. Edited by Emérito-Carlos Rodríguez-Merchán and Leonard A. Valentino.
© 2011 John Wiley & Sons, Ltd. Published 2011 by Blackwell Publishing Ltd.

a practical concern except in patients for whom an immune tolerance induction regimen is planned, in whom higher titers may delay its initiation or prejudice the outcome.

rFVIIa

rFVIIa (Novoseven®, Novo Nordisk) initiates hemostasis by activating FX at the platelet surface. The requirement for tissue factor in this pharmacological mechanism has been debated. rFVIIa is reported as effective in 70–100% of bleeding episodes. Its favorable characteristics include ease of reconstitution, small infusion volumes, stability at room temperature, its recombinant origin, and the absence of any plasma proteins during its manufacture. On the other hand, as rFVIIa has a short half life (2 to 3 hours in adults and 1.5 hours in children) frequent injections may be necessary to control major bleeding episodes. As for APCC, the major adverse effect of rFVIIa is thrombosis, but this occurs rarely ($\sim$ 4 per 10^5 infusions) [7]. The margin of safety is wide, and doses from 90 to 270 µg/kg are now commonly administered to inhibitor patients. rFVIIa has been given by continuous infusion but there are few data supporting the efficacy of this route of administration. As for APCC, there is no accepted method for laboratory monitoring of rFVIIa, pending validation of thrombin generation and TEG assays for this purpose. However, FVII activity levels typically rise several-fold above normal with corresponding reductions in the prothrombin time and INR. Concomitant use of antifibrinolytic agents is generally considered to be safe and is widely practiced.

Combination bypassing therapy

There is in vitro evidence that combining APCC and rFVIIa leads to synergistic thrombin generation, and there are limited clinical data supporting the efficacy and safety of their combined or sequential administration [8,9]. Clinicians have been understandably cautious about combining these agents owing to the potential for enhanced thrombogenicity. These strategies may be considered in patients with life threatening bleeding that is poorly responsive to either agent individually.

Other hemostatic approaches

As rFVIIa is believed to promote thrombin generation on the platelet surface, platelet transfusion might enhance its efficacy, especially in thrombocytopenic patients. Topical application of thrombin or "fibrin glue" products, and of absorbable collagen, gelatin or oxidized cellulose sponges may be helpful in controlling surface or accessible mucosal bleeding. Finally, the inhibitor titer can be lowered by immunoadsorption of patient plasma with an affinity matrix such as staphylococcal protein A, allowing the use of FVIII concentrate. This technology is not widely available.

Inhibitors in non-severe hemophilia A

Approximately 85% of patients with mild or moderate hemophilia A have missense mutations. Although only 5% of such patients develop inhibitors, several missense mutations in the A2 and C2 domains of FVIII are associated with inhibitor incidences in the range of 10–40% [10]. Inhibitor development in these patients often follows intensive FVIII treatment, frequently in the context of surgery or trauma. Inhibitors in non-severe hemophilia patients usually do not develop until adolescence or adulthood, and in some cases the clinical picture is reminiscent of acquired hemophilia, with ecchymoses, intramuscular hematomas, and gastrointestinal or urinary tract bleeding [11]. FVIII levels usually decline to undetectable levels, as most inhibitors neutralize the patient's endogenous FVIII. However, some inhibitors react only with non-mutated FVIII, in which case baseline levels do not fall. Spontaneous remission is common but anamnestic recurrences are frequent. Desmopressin is occasionally beneficial for mild bleeding episodes where the plasma FVIII activity is $\geq$0.05 IU/ml, and FVIII concentrate may be effective if the inhibitor titer is low. However, most patients will require inhibitor bypassing agents to control bleeding.

Treatment of bleeding in FIX inhibitor patients

Inhibitor development occurs in just 1–6% of in hemophilia B patients. In most cases, the molecular defect is a large gene deletion. Genotyping at diagnosis may help to identify patients who are particularly vulnerable. There is no suggestion that the incidence is higher amongst recipients of recombinant than plasma-derived FIX concentrates. Inhibitors in hemophilia B are typically high titer and appear soon after beginning treatment. These antibodies often fix complement, and serious allergic reactions may develop after infusions. An allergic reaction may be the first manifestation of inhibitor development and for this reason it is prudent to administer the first infusions of factor IX concentrate in hospital.

It is generally felt that rFVIIa is the best option for treatment of bleeding episodes in these patients. APCC are also effective but they should generally be avoided as they contain significant amounts of factor IX. However, they may be used in patients with a non-allergic phenotype and in whom an anamnestic rise in titer is acceptable. Desensitization to FIX may be successful in patients with allergic reactions.

Surgery in patients with inhibitors

Not so long ago, the consensus view was that the presence of FVIII or FIX inhibitors constituted a contraindication to elective surgery. This is no longer the case and a wealth of data published over the last two decades has shown that even major elective surgery may be undertaken with very good results [12–14].

Both APCC and rFVIIa may be used to cover surgical procedures in inhibitor patients. Published data suggest comparable safety and efficacy; the characteristics of both products are outlined above. The patient's clinical experience should be considered, and there should be a documented good response to the product chosen.

The challenges posed by elective orthopedic or other surgery in inhibitor patients are still formidable and should not be underestimated. Such operations should only be undertaken in comprehensive care centers which have the requisite multidisciplinary experience and facilities. Consideration must also be given to a number of practical points such as timing and staffing levels when planning elective procedures [15]. Surgery should ideally be scheduled for the morning of a day early in the week. Preoperative assessment of hemostasis should include the inhibitor titer as well as the platelet count and the prothrombin time. Levels of other coagulation factors should be assayed if there is impairment of liver function.

The overall cost of products to cover surgery in inhibitor patients is very high, typically in the order of US$ 500,000 [16,17]. This significant initial financial outlay often proves to be the major barrier to elective surgery in patients with inhibitors. However, it should be borne in mind that the costs may be recovered in due course through abolition of further bleeding episodes within the affected joint. Carrying out two procedures at the same time will help to reduce costs even more. This should only be considered if the patient is willing to comply with what is likely to be a longer stay and more demanding rehabilitation program after surgery.

Immune tolerance induction (ITI)

In most patients an attempt should be made to eradicate the FVIII inhibitor and restore a state of immune tolerance. The principle of ITI is the repeated administration of FVIII, often for many months, but the mechanisms by which this occurs are poorly understood. Therefore regimens have been devised empirically, and there is no universally accepted protocol. The optimal type of product, the dose and schedule, and the value of concomitant immunomodulatory therapy remain uncertain. The "Bonn protocol", reported in 1977, is the prototype high-dose ITI regimen. It incorporates FVIII given at 100 IU/kg twice daily plus inhibitor bypassing therapy until the inhibitor titer falls below 1 BU. Lower intensity regimens use FVIII 25–50 IU/kg daily or on alternate days. Low-dose regimens have the advantages of lower cost and less need for central venous line placement. However, they are associated with more frequent bleeding episodes during ITI, as was demonstrated by an international randomized trial which was stopped prematurely because of this complication. These considerations are relevant to outcome, as bacterial infections and the bleeding/inflammatory cycle may diminish the response rate to ITI. The Malmö protocol is another prototypical ITI regimen, which incorporates immunomodulation in the form of intravenous immune globulin, immunoadsorption where available, and cyclophosphamide, which is often considered problematic in young children.

Bleeding episodes during ITI should be treated with inhibitor bypassing agents. For patients who bleed frequently, prophylactic inhibitor bypassing therapy may be considered; optimal regimens have not been determined.

Based on registry data, the overall success rate of ITI in hemophilia A patients varies from 47–85%. There is no evidence that any of the above regimens is more effective than the others, although there may be differences in the time to achieve success. A complete response requires a negative Bethesda titer as well as

normal FVIII recovery and half-life. Partial success, with a negative inhibitor titer but abnormal FVIII pharmacokinetics, is often clinically valuable as this allows the patient to be treated with FVIII. Where ITI is successful it is usually achieved within 9 to 15 months, but 2 to 3 years may be required in some patients. However, it has been suggested that ITI may be discontinued after 6 to 9 months in patients who experience a rapid and profound rise in inhibitor titer shortly after starting the regimen. Low peak inhibitor titers and low titers at the initiation of ITI are the main variables which predict a successful outcome. Null mutations may predict not only a higher risk of inhibitor development but also a poorer response to ITI. It has been suggested that the success rate of ITI may be better with VWF-containing plasma-derived FVIII concentrate than with recombinant or highly purified FVIII [18] and that the inhibitor epitope profile may predict the success of ITI with VWF-containing concentrates [19]. This remains controversial, as is the assumption that VWF itself is the responsible substance.

It is recommended that patients be placed on prophylactic FVIII regimens for at least one year after successful ITI, and that surveillance continue for inhibitor recurrence. Inhibitors recur in about 15% of patients after successful ITI. Repeat or salvage regimens in such patients have poor rates of success. Recent data have suggested that depletion of CD20-positive B cells with rituximab, especially when given as adjunctive therapy with FVIII, may improve this response rate. This strategy is promising but it has not been tested prospectively, and the sustained response rate has varied widely, from 14–53% [20].

The success rate of ITI in patients with FIX inhibitors is much poorer than in hemophilia A, approximately 25% [21]. Patients with allergic reactions to FIX appear to have especially poor response rates, and they are also at risk for severe complications including nephrotic syndrome, presumably the result of immune-complex deposition in the kidneys. If ITI is contemplated in such patients it may be prudent to consider preceding this with a desensitization regimen to FIX.

ITI regimens are demanding for both families and treatment teams; they are resource-intensive, and available data to guide them are sparse and generally not of high quality. It is therefore recommended that these regimens be undertaken only in hemophilia treatment centers and that patients be enrolled in clinical trials or reported to registries.

Management of patients with inhibitors in the developing world

The high cost of the conventional products used to treat patients with inhibitors poses a formidable obstacle to treatment in countries with limited financial resources. This means in practice that in many developing countries specific therapy is only administered for the most severe bleeding episodes, and that minor bleeds are managed conservatively with analgesia and antifibrinolytic agents [22]. Donations of products may be solicited from organizations like the World Federation of Hemophilia (WFH) which operates an international humanitarian aid program. PCC may be used as relatively inexpensive inhibitor bypassing agents [23]. Radioactive or chemical synoviortheses are good therapeutic options for controlling recurrent joint bleeding in patients with inhibitors [24].

ITI is often simply not affordable and in some cases immunosuppressive drugs such as cyclophosphamide have been used in desperation. If the recent reports of the value of rituximab in ITI are confirmed, this may prove to be more cost-effective than repeated administration of products such as APCC and rFVIIa in developing countries.

New approaches to inhibitor treatment on the horizon

Pegylated rFVIIa has been developed with a view to prolonging the half-life of the current product. FVIIa was modified by the attachment of a 40 kDa polyethylene glycol group to the N-linked carbohydrate of rVIIa at positions Asn145 and Asn322. Preliminary data from clinical trials suggest that this may increase the half-life from around 3 to 16 hours. This very significant outcome could facilitate prophylactic treatment in patients with inhibitors. A more potent rFVIIa analog has also been developed in which three specific amino substitutions (V158D/E296V/M298Q) stabilize the molecule in its active conformation without tissue factor, resulting in increased activity on the surface of activated platelets [25]. In vitro data suggest that this novel agent has a faster onset of action as well as enhanced clot strength and stability.

Recombinant porcine FVIII is likely to become available in the next few years. This will be a replacement for the plasma-derived concentrate of porcine FVIII which was widely used in inhibitor patients until its withdrawal. The rationale for its use is that the structure of porcine FVIII is sufficiently similar to that of human FVIII to possess coagulant activity, yet sufficiently different to have limited cross-reactivity with anti-human FVIII inhibitor antibodies. One potential advantage of this product is that it should be possible to monitor plasma FVIII levels quite easily in the laboratory. The efficacy of porcine FVIII could be limited in patients whose inhibitors have a higher degree of cross reactivity. It may also induce a primary immune response leading to a limited period of efficacy.

It is likely that future treatment strategies will focus on immunomodulation rather than on bypassing therapy [26]. Memory B-lymphocytes are an obvious target for tolerance induction in patients who develop inhibitors, perhaps through such mechanisms as infusion of anti-idiotypic antibodies.

Conclusions

Hemostatic therapy is more problematic in patients with inhibitors than in other hemophilia patients. The available treat-
ments are generally less predictably efficacious, more costly, less amenable to long-term prophylactic administration, and cannot be reliably monitored by laboratory assays. Attempts to eradicate inhibitors by ITI are desirable in most patients. These intensive regimens are demanding of both patients and treaters, and they are expensive, lengthy, and only variably successful. Despite all these challenges and limitations, with diligent expert management most patients with inhibitors can expect similar longevity and little excess morbidity compared to hemophilia patients without inhibitors.

References

1. Lusher JM, Shapiro SS, Palascak JE, et al. Efficacy of prothrombin-complex concentrates in hemophiliacs with antibodies to factor VIII: a multicenter therapeutic trial. N Engl J Med 1980;303:421–425.
2. Berntorp E. Differential response to bypassing agents complicates treatment in patients with haemophilia and inhibitors. Haemophilia 2009;15:3–10.
3. Astermark J, Donfield SM, DiMichele DM, et al. A randomized comparison of bypassing agents in hemophilia complicated by an inhibitor: the FEIBA NovoSeven Comparative (FENOC) Study. Blood 2007;109:546–551.
4. Valentino LA. Assessing the benefits of FEIBA prophylaxis in haemophilia patients with inhibitors. Haemophilia 2010;16:263–271.
5. Konkle BA, Ebbesen LS, Erhardtsen E, et al. Randomized, prospective clinical trial of recombinant factor VIIa for secondary prophylaxis in hemophilia patients with inhibitors. J Thromb Haemost 2007;5:1904–1913.
6. Ehrlich HJ, Henzl MJ, Gomperts ED. Safety of factor VIII inhibitor bypass activity (FEIBA(R)): 10-year compilation of thrombotic adverse events. Haemophilia 2002;8:83–90.
7. Abshire T, Kenet G. Safety update on the use of recombinant factor VIIa and the treatment of congenital and acquired deficiency of factor VIII or IX with inhibitors. Haemophilia 2008;14:898–902.
8. Livnat T, Martinowitz U, Zivelin A, et al. Effects of factor VIII inhibitor bypassing activity (FEIBA), recombinant factor VIIa or both on thrombin generation in normal and haemophilia A plasma. Haemophilia 2008;14:782–786.
9. Schneiderman J, Rubin E, Nugent DJ, et al. Sequential therapy with activated prothrombin complex concentrates and recombinant FVIIa in patients with severe haemophilia and inhibitors: update of our previous experience. Haemophilia 2007;13:244–248.
10. Franchini M, Favaloro EJ, Lippi G. Mild hemophilia A. J Thromb Haemost 2010;8:421–432.
11. Hay CRM, Ludlam CA, Colvin BT, et al. Factor VIII inhibitors in mild and moderate-severity haemophilia. Thromb Haemost 1998;79:762–766.
12. Negrier C, Goudemand J, Sultan Y, et al. Multicenter retrospective study on the utilization of FEIBA in France in patients with factor VIII and factor IX inhibitors. Thromb Haemost 1997;77:1113–1119.
13. Obergfell A, Auvinen MK, Mathew P. Recombinant activated factor VII for haemophilia patients with inhibitors undergoing orthopaedic surgery: a review of the literature. Haemophilia 2008;14:233–241.

14. Hvid I, Rodriguez-Merchan EC. Orthopaedic surgery in haemophilic patients with inhibitors: an overview. Haemophilia 2002;8:288–291.

15. Giangrande PL, Wilde JT, Madan B, et al. Consensus protocol for the use of recombinant activated factor VII [eptacog alfa (activated); NovoSeven] in elective orthopaedic surgery in haemophilic patients with inhibitors. Haemophilia 2009;15:501–508.

16. Lyseng-Williamson KA, Plosker GL. Recombinant factor VIIa (Eptacog Alfa): A pharmacoeconomic review of its use in haemophilia in patients with inhibitors to clotting factors VIII or IX. Pharmacoeconomics 2007;25:1007–1029.

17. Bonnet PO, Yoon BS, Wong WY, et al. Cost minimization analysis to compare activated prothrombin complex concentrate (APCC) and recombinant factor VIIa for haemophilia patients with inhibitors undergoing major orthopaedic surgeries. Haemophilia 2009;15:1083–1089.

18. Kreuz W. The role of VWF for the success of immune tolerance induction. Thromb Res 2008;122 Suppl 2:S7–S12.

19. Greninger DA, Saint-Remy JM, Jacquemin M, et al. The use of factor VIII/von Willebrand factor concentrate for immune tolerance induction in haemophilia A patients with high-titre inhibitors: association of clinical outcome with inhibitor epitope profile. Haemophilia 2008;14:295–302.

20. Franchini M, Mengoli C, Lippi G, et al. Immune tolerance with rituximab in congenital haemophilia with inhibitors: a systematic literature review based on individual patients' analysis. Haemophilia 2008;14:903–912.

21. DiMichele D. The North American Immune Tolerance Registry: contributions to the thirty-year experience with immune tolerance therapy. Haemophilia 2009;15:320–328.

22. Mathews V, Nair SC, David S, et al. Management of hemophilia in patients with inhibitors: the perspective from developing countries. Semin Thromb Hemost 2009;35:820–826.

23. Berntorp E, Figueiredo S, Futema L, et al. A retrospective study of Octaplex in the treatment of bleeding in patients with haemophilia A complicated by inhibitors. Blood Coagul Fibrinolysis 2010;21:577–583.

24. Pasta G, Mancuso ME, Perfetto OS, et al. Synoviorthesis in haemophilia patients with inhibitors. Haemophilia 2008;14 Suppl 6:52–55.

25. Moss J, Scharling B, Ezban M, et al. Evaluation of the safety and pharmacokinetics of a fast-acting recombinant FVIIa analog, NN1731, in healthy male subjects. J Thromb Haemost 2009;7:299–305.

26. Saint-Remy JM. How to get rid of inhibitors. Haemophilia 2008;14 Suppl 3:33–35.

21 Discordancy of Bypassing Therapy

Jan Astermark

Skåne University Hospital, Malmö, Sweden

Introduction

The treatment of bleeding in patients with inhibitory antibodies is one of the most intriguing challenges in hemophilia care. In the case of low-responding inhibitors, the neutralizing effect can be overcome with saturating levels of the deficient factor. At higher inhibitor titer levels, however, bypassing agents, such as recombinant factor VIIa (rFVIIa) and factor eight bypassing activity (FEIBA) therapy are required to achieve hemostasis. The mechanism of action of these two drugs differs substantially, and a differential response in the treatment of bleeding has been suggested. Despite several available options and a growing knowledge of how to monitor the use of these agents, there are unfortunately no reliable in vitro measurements to predict the effects of the drugs. The aim of this review is to summarize the observations of differential responses in the clinical setting and to briefly discuss mechanisms that might contribute to variability in individual patients.

Mechanism of action

FEIBA is an activated prothrombin complex concentrate (aPCC) consisting of the vitamin K-dependent proteins FII, FVII, FIX and FX in the native as well as in the activated forms together with some minor anticoagulant activity [1]. The main contributors to the hemostatic activity are the complex formation of activated FX (FXa) and FII generating thrombin in the prothrombinase complex [1]. FVIIa in FEIBA enhances the hemostatic effect, but otherwise plays no major role in the mechanism of action.

RFVIIa enhances thrombin formation on the platelet surface by activating FX to FXa [2]. Importantly, high concentrations of rFVIIa have the ability to activate FX independent of tissue factor (TF). However, the presence of this cofactor will substantially improve the hemostatic potential.

Efficacy of bypassing therapy to control bleeding in hemophilia

A number of studies have evaluated the effects of FEIBA and rFVIIa on a variety of types of bleeding, but to date only two head-to-head comparison studies have been conducted. The first of these studies was the FEIBA NovoSeven Comparative (FENOC) study, in which the hemostatic effect of each drug was evaluated in a cross-over equivalence study design in 48 subjects with two consecutive joint bleeds [3,4]. The efficacy of each drug was evaluated by three different outcome measures up to 48 hours after onset of treatment, with the primary end-point at 6 hours. Using a dichotomous variable defined as effective or not effective, 80.1% of the bleeding events were effectively treated with FEIBA and 78.1% with rFVIIa at the primary endpoint. This was close to the pre-determined criteria for declaring equivalence. Using the self-reported pain scores on a visual analogue scale (VAS), statistical equivalence between the two drugs was shown at all time points. One of the main findings of the FENOC study, however, was that despite the high efficacy of both drugs, substantial within-individual variation with respect to ratings between the products was observed. At the two-hour time point, for example, 43.8% of the subjects rated one product effective and the other product not effective in its hemostatic effect without preference for either drug. At the primary endpoint at 6 hours, the corresponding figure was 31.9%. In an attempt to identify possible explanations for the high discordant rate, subgroup analyses were completed. These indicated that more frequent bleeding in the 12-month period before enrolment and the presence of target joints were associated with more frequent discordant ratings.

Current and Future Issues in Hemophilia Care, First Edition. Edited by Emérito-Carlos Rodríguez-Merchán and Leonard A. Valentino.
© 2011 John Wiley & Sons, Ltd. Published 2011 by Blackwell Publishing Ltd.

The second study by Young and coworkers consisted of three arms evaluating the effect after 9 hours of: three doses of 90 µg/kg rFVIIa administered every three hours; one dose of 270 µg/kg rFVIIa; and one dose of FEIBA 75 IU/kg, respectively [5]. No significant differences in the treatment responses were observed among the three arms using a global assessment score (54.5%, 37.5% and 27.3%, respectively) in 21 of the 42 randomized subjects. A significantly higher percentage of subjects, however, required additional hemostatics following the dose of FEIBA (36.4%) compared with the higher, but not the lower, dose of rFVIIa (8.3%).

In other studies, in which only one of the drugs has been evaluated for the treatment of bleeding, efficacy in the acute setting varies between 50 and 100% depending on the time interval between the onset of the bleeding and start of treatment, the dose, the dose interval, the number of doses given, the time of evaluation, as well as the location of the hemorrhage [6–18]. While both drugs have been shown to be highly effective in promoting hemostasis, it has also been shown that neither of them will induce an optimal hemostatic effect in all patients and for all type of bleeding. Unfortunately, there is currently no reliable method to predict the outcome of treatment in vitro; rather, one must rely on the clinical experience. Recent data comparing the effect of each drug in siblings have shown a significantly lower variation in the amount of thrombin formed within families compared with that between unrelated individuals [19]. This might reflect the important impact of other pro- and anticoagulant factors on the hemostatic effect of each drug, and that these are, at least to some extent, genetically determined.

Potential reasons for a differential response

The reasons why some patients experience a differential response to the bypassing agents are not clear, but several observations in vitro have been made and factors identified to at least partially explain this phenomenon. Some of these findings also suggest that the effect could vary from time to time and from location to location.

Phospholipids constitute one of these factors. They are known to be crucial for the activity of both drugs, and in a recent study the phospholipids present in FEIBA were shown to be sufficient to generate significant amounts of thrombin without any exogenous phospholipids. This was not the case for rFVIIa. In addition, a synergistic effect was seen with the combined use of the two drugs, the reason for which might be the phospholipid content of the FEIBA product [20]. A differential response by these agents may also be mediated by a different capacity to restore thrombin generation and activate FX, since these activities will potentially be important for regulating fibrinolysis and clot stability [21]. The amount of thrombin formed is also dependent on the surface on which the coagulation cascade will act, and in this context the platelets will constitute an important role [2,22]. In addition, platelets supply factors that further promote hemostasis. Hence,

the number of platelets, the degree to which they are activated, as well as platelet characteristics including platelet-binding proteins will likely have a major impact on the procoagulant activity of both drugs. The impact of platelets also suggests that the effect of the agents might differ from time to time and correlate with the inflammatory state. Another important fact is that the amount of FVIIa available to promote hemostasis differs dramatically between the two drugs. Tissue factor (TF) will, in the complex with factor VII/VIIa, exert both procoagulant and signaling activities, and therefore the interaction between these factors will certainly be of importance for the hemostatic effect [23]. In addition, the expression of TF is tissue-dependent, which suggests that the location of the hemorrhage might be important as well [24]. Patients with severe hemophilia and a mild bleeding phenotype have been found to have more thrombophilic markers present than those having a more severe phenotype [25]. Given that several different pro- and anticoagulant mechanisms are involved, the significance of these markers for the effect of bypassing agents is not obvious, but suggests another mechanism for evaluation. The FX and prothrombin concentrations have been found to influence thrombin generation in a cell-based model of hemophilia treated with rFVIIa [26]. At all concentrations of rFVIIa, increased prothrombin concentrations led to higher peak and rate of thrombin generation. This suggests that the level of prothrombotic factors besides FVIII and FIX will modulate the effects of the bypassing products and also implies a benefit of the combined use of the two drugs. Finally, cross-reacting antibodies towards rFVIIa have been described in patients with hemophilia A and in those with hemophilia B [27]. In strict biochemical terms, this is perhaps not unexpected in patients with hemophilia B, since FIX is structurally similar to the other vitamin K-dependent factors. In the case of hemophilia A, however, it is not as clear, although antibodies to FVIII have also been described in healthy subjects, and the formation of procoagulant complexes may create and provide new immunogenic epitopes [28].

Conclusions

Emerging data suggest that sequential and combined use of the two drugs at lower doses can be successful in the management of bleeding that is resistant to mono-therapy [29,30]. Based on the different mechanisms of action, this is indeed an attractive alternative. The risk of thrombotic side-effects, however, needs to be considered and more data are required before this approach can be used on a routine basis. An algorithm was recently suggested to help the physician in the management of resistant bleeding (Figure 21.1) [31]. In the near future, bypassing agents with higher procoagulant activity and longer half-lives will be available. In the longer term, this is presumably also true for alternative ways to bypass the deficient factor. To what extent these drugs will improve treatment of our patients with inhibitors, however, remains to be seen.

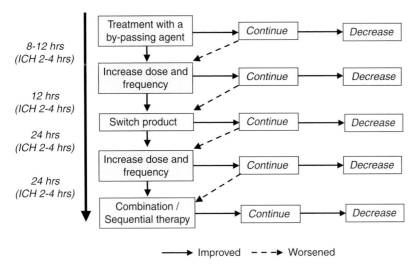

Figure 21.1 Modified algorithm for unresponsive severe hemorrhage according to Teitel et al. [31]. (Reproduced from Teitel J, Berntorp E, Collins P, D'Oiron R, Ewenstein B, Gomperts et al. A systematic approach to controlling problem bleeds in patients with severe congenital haemophilia A and high-titre inhibitors. Haemophilia. 2007;13(3):256–63.)

References

1. Turecek PL, Váradi K, Gritsch H, Schwarz HP. FEIBA: Mode of action. Haemophilia. 2004;10 Suppl 2:3–9.

2. Hedner U. Mechanism of action, development and clinical experience of recombinant FVIIa. J Biotechnol. 2006;124(4):747–57. Epub 2006 May 12.

3. Astermark J, Donfield SM, DiMichele DM, Gringeri A, Gilbert SA, Waters J, Berntorp E; FENOC Study Group. A randomized comparison of bypassing agents in hemophilia complicated by an inhibitor: the FEIBA NovoSeven Comparative (FENOC) Study. Blood. 2007;109(2):546–51. Epub 2006 Sep 21.

4. Donfield SM, Astermark J, Lail AE, Gilbert SA, Berntorp E; Fenoc Study Group. Value added: increasing the power to assess treatment outcome in joint haemorrhages. Haemophilia. 2008 Mar;14(2):276–80. Epub 2008 Jan 8.

5. Young G, Shafer FE, Rojas P, Seremetis S. Single 270 microg kg(-1)-dose rFVIIa vs. standard 90 microg kg(-1)-dose rFVIIa and APCC for home treatment of joint bleeds in haemophilia patients with inhibitors: a randomized comparison. Haemophilia. 2008;14(2):287–94. Epub 2007 Dec 10.

6. Sjamsoedin LJ, Heijnen L, Mauser-Bunschoten EP, van Geijlswijk JL, van Houwelingen H, van Asten P, Sixma JJ. The effect of activated prothrombin-complex concentrate (FEIBA) on joint and muscle bleeding in patients with hemophilia A and antibodies to factor VIII. A double-blind clinical trial. N Engl J Med. 1981;305(13): 717–21.

7. Hilgartner MW, Aledort L, Andes A, Gill J. FEIBA Study Group. Efficacy and safety of vapor-heated anti-inhibitor coagulant complex in hemophilia patients. Transfusion 1990;30:626–30.

8. Negrier C, Goudemand J, Sultan Y, Bertrand M, Rothschild C, Lauroua P, and the members of the French FEIBA study group. Multicenter retrospective study on the utilization of FEIBA in France in patients with factor VIII and factor IX inhibitors. Thromb Haemost 1997;77:1113–19.

9. Key NS, Aledort LM, Beardsley D, Cooper HA, Davignon G, Ewenstein BM et al. Home treatment of mild to moderate bleeding episodes using recombinant factor VIIa (Novoseven) in haemophiliacs with inhibitors. Thromb Haemost 1998;80(6):912–8.

10. Lusher JM, Roberts HR, Davignon G, Joist JH, Smith H, Shapiro A et al. A randomized, double-blind comparison of two dosage levels of recombinant factor VIIa in the treatment of joint, muscle and mucocutaneous haemorrhages in persons with haemophilia A and B, with and without inhibitors. rFVIIa Study Group. Haemophilia. 1998;4(6):790–8.

11. Arkin S, Blei F, Fetten J, Foulke R, Gilchrist GS, Heisel MA et al. Human coagulation factor FVIIa (recombinant) in the management of limb-threatening bleeds unresponsive to alternative therapies: results from the NovoSeven emergency-use programme in patients with severe haemophilia or with acquired inhibitors. Blood Coagul Fibrinolysis. 2000;11(3):255–9.

12. Lusher JM. Acute hemarthroses: the benefits of early versus late treatment with recombinant activated factor VII. Blood Coagul Fibrinolysis. 2000;11 Suppl 1:S45–9.

13. Shirahata A, Kamiya T, Takamatsu J, Kojima T, Fukutake K, Arai M et al. Clinical trial to investigate the pharmacokinetics, pharmacodynamics, safety, and efficacy of recombinant factor VIIa in Japanese patients with hemophilia with inhibitors. Int J Hematol. 2001;73(4):517–25.

14. Dimichele D, Négrier C. A retrospective post licensure survey of FEIBA efficacy and safety. Haemophilia. 2006;12(4):352–62.

15. Parameswaran R, Shapiro AD, Gill JC, Kessler CM; HTRS Registry Investigators. Dose effect and efficacy of rFVIIa in the treatment of haemophilia patients with inhibitors: analysis from the Hemophilia and Thrombosis Research Society Registry. Haemophilia 2005;11(2):100–6.

16. Kavakli K, Makris M, Zulfikar B, Erhardtsen E, Abrams ZS, Kenet G; NovoSeven trial (F7HAEM-1510) investigators. Home treatment of haemarthroses using a single dose regimen of recombinant activated factor VII in patients with haemophilia and inhibitors. A multicentre, randomised, double-blind, cross-over trial. Thromb Haemost. 2006;95(4):600–5.

17. Santagostino E, Mancuso ME, Rocino A, Mancuso G, Scaraggi F, Mannucci PM. A prospective randomized trial of high and standard dosages of recombinant factor VIIa for treatment of haemarthroses in hemophiliacs with inhibitors. J Thromb Haemost 2006;4(2):367–71.

18. Holme PA, Glomstein A, Grønhaug S, Tjønnfjord GE. Home treatment with bypassing products in inhibitor patients: a 7.5-year experience. Haemophilia. 2009;15(3):727–32.

19. Klintman J, Berntorp E, Astermark J; on behalf of the MIBS Study Group. Thrombin generation in vitro in the presence of bypassing agents in siblings with severe haemophilia A. Haemophilia. 2010;16(1):e210–5.

20. Livnat T, Martinowitz U, Zivelin A, Seligsohn U. Effects of factor VIII inhibitor bypassing activity (FEIBA), recombinant factor VIIa or both on thrombin generation in normal and haemophilia A plasma. Haemophilia. 2008;14(4):782–6.

21. Bolliger D, Szlam F, Molinaro RJ, Escobar MA, Levy JH, Tanaka KA. Thrombin generation and fibrinolysis in anti-factor IX treated blood and plasma spiked with factor VIII inhibitor bypassing activity or recombinant factor VIIa. Haemophilia. 2010;16:510-17.

22. Monroe DM, Hoffman M, Roberts HR. Platelets and thrombin generation. Arterioscler Thromb Vasc Biol. 2002;22(9):1381–9.

23. Mackman N. The many faces of tissue factor. J Thromb Haemost. 2009;7 Suppl 1:136–9.

24. Drake TA, Morrissey JH, Edgington TS. Selective cellular expression of tissue factor in human tissues. Implications for disorders of hemostasis and thrombosis. Am J Pathol. 1989;134(5):1087–97.

25. Shetty S, Vora S, Kulkarni B, Mota L, Vijapurkar M, Quadros L, Ghosh K. Contribution of natural anticoagulant and fibrinolytic factors in modulating the clinical severity of haemophilia patients. Br J Haematol. 2007;138(4):541–4.

26. Allen GA, Hoffman M, Roberts HR, Monroe DM. Manipulation of prothrombin concentration improves response to high-dose factor VIIa in a cell-based model of haemophilia. Br J Haematol. 2006;134(3):314–9.

27. Astermark J, Ekman M, Berntorp E. Antibodies to factor VIIa in patients with haemophilia and high-responding inhibitors. Br J Haematol. 2002;119(2):342–7.

28. Gilles JG, Saint-Remy JM. Healthy subjects produce both anti-factor VIII and specific anti-idiotypic antibodies. J Clin Invest. 1994;94(4):1496–505.

29. Schneiderman J, Rubin E, Nugent DJ, Young G. Sequential therapy with activated prothrombin complex concentrates and recombinant FVIIa in patients with severe haemophilia and inhibitors: update of our previous experience. Haemophilia. 2007;13(3):244–8.

30. Martinowitz U, Livnat T, Zivelin A, Kenet G. Concomitant infusion of low doses of rFVIIa and FEIBA in haemophilia patients with inhibitors. Haemophilia. 2009;15(4):904–10.

31. Teitel J, Berntorp E, Collins P, D'Oiron R, Ewenstein B, Gomperts et al. A systematic approach to controlling problem bleeds in patients with severe congenital haemophilia A and high-titre inhibitors. Haemophilia. 2007;13(3):256–63.

5 Joint Health and Disease

22 Experimental Studies on Hemarthrosis, Synovitis and Arthropathy

Leonard A. Valentino and Narine Hakobyan

Rush University Medical Center, Chicago, IL USA

Introduction

Joint bleeding (hemarthrosis) accounts for more than 90% of all serious bleeding events in patients with severe hemophilia [1]. Recurrent bleeding into the same joint (a target joint) causes progressive structural damage to muscle, cartilage and bone, resulting in pain, deformity, disability and poor quality of life.

This chapter provides an overview of what is known about the mechanisms by which joint bleeding induces arthropathy and highlights potential new areas for investigation.

Joint components

All joint structures, including the synovium, cartilage, bone, and the vascular system within the joint, are potential targets of hemarthrosis. Synovial joints are free-moving and are lubricated by synovial fluid, which primarily consists of high concentrations of hyaluronic acid, albumin, and phagocytes. The bones that conjoin to create a synovial joint are encased in a thin (2 mm) layer of smooth hyaline or articular cartilage that is surrounded by a fibrous sheath consisting of dense connective tissue (Figure 22.1).

Articular cartilage

Articular cartilage is impacted by mechanical (load and motion), chemical (enzymatic), and immunological (cytokines) processes that cause fibrosis of the synovial lining and disintegration of the hyaline cartilage. The inciting event(s) leading to blood-induced joint disease (BIJD) remain unknown but likely involve iron-catalyzed reactive oxygen intermediates (ROIs) that cause chondrocyte apoptosis [2]. The presence of certain biomarkers, such as cartilage oligomeric matrix protein (COMP) and type II collagen telopeptides, suggest that articular is cartilage an early target BIJD.

Following a joint bleeding episode, macrophages ingest iron in blood, converting it to hemosiderin. Inflammatory mediators are then produced within the synovium, creating an intra-articular cytokine storm that damages both cartilage and bone. Next, connective tissue proteinases released from the hypertrophic synovium, chondrocytes, and pannus tissue degrade the cartilage matrix.

Changes in the composition of the articular cartilage matrix, prominent in hemophilic arthropathy, alter the viscoelastic properties of the matrix [3] and result in abnormal forces transmitted to bone. When cartilage is cultured in vitro in the presence of whole blood, mononuclear cells, and added erythrocytes or with monocytes/macrophages and added erythrocytes, proteoglycan synthesis is inhibited [4]. This same effect, which can be reversed by using dimethylsulphoxide to remove the ROIs, can be produced using hemolysed erythrocytes in combination with interleukin (IL)-1B, suggesting that extravasation of erythrocytes into the joint space is an early event in BIJD [4].

Synovial membrane

Recurrent joint bleeding and the deposition of iron in the synovium causes synovial hypertrophy and chronic inflammation [5]. The resultant production of tumor necrosis factor (TNF)-a, interferon gamma, IL-1, and IL-6 promotes receptor activator of nuclear factor-kappa B ligand (RANKL) expression [6]. Iron induces C-Myc expression by synovial fibroblasts [7]. In mice, joint bleeding increases the expression of MDM2, the p53 binding protein [8] which may limit apoptosis further causing proliferation of synovial membrane.

Blood vessels

Vascular development and angiogenesis are likely required for the synovium to expand beyond several millimeters in size [9]. Pericytes, which are formed from differentiated intimal/subintimal smooth muscle cells, ensure vascular integrity [10] and contribute

Current and Future Issues in Hemophilia Care, First Edition. Edited by Emérito-Carlos Rodríguez-Merchán and Leonard A. Valentino.
© 2011 John Wiley & Sons, Ltd. Published 2011 by Blackwell Publishing Ltd.

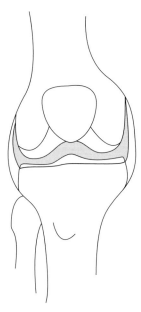

Figure 22.1 Diagram of a normal synovial joint. Synovial joints allow movement of articulating bones. The articular cartilage covers the bone epiphyses and provides a cushion to resist the load of weight bearing. A fibrous capsule that is continuous with the periosteum of bone contains many nerve fibers but lacks blood and lymph vessels, encases the articulating surfaces. A clear, viscous, non-Newtonian fluid lubricates the joint and reduces friction. The synovial fluid consists of hyaluronic acid, lubricin, proteinases, and collagenases. The synovial membrane, which covers the non-cartilaginous surfaces within joints, is composed of two layers, a subintimal and intimal layer. Fibroblast cells within the intimal layer have a synthetic function while macrophages provide a scavenger function removing blood and other deleterious substances from the joint space. Beneath the intima there is a rich network of delicate blood vessels to provide oxygen, nutrients and growth factors to the synovium and the avascular cartilage.

to ongoing blood vessel formation by fibrinolysis and proteolytic degradation of the extracellular matrix [11]. The impact of iron on blood vessels may result from an increase in synovial cell mitotic activity and pinocytosis by endothelial cells and from enhanced collagen synthesis. Blood may also act directly on blood vessels, increasing their vascular permeability because of the effects of platelets.

Bone cells

Progression of BIJD is marked by bone remodeling with osteoclastic (but not osteoblastic) activity due to increasing levels of the biomarkers N-terminal cross-linking telopeptide of collagen type I and tartrate-resistant acid phosphatase isoform-5b. This leads to a decrease in bone mineral density and subsequent osteoporosis, both associated with hemophilic arthropathy.

Pathophysiology of joint disease

The stimulus: blood constituents
See Box 22.1.

> **Box 22.1 Blood constituents potentially responsible for hemophilic arthropathy. Plasma and cellular components of blood may play roles in the development of blood-induced joint disease.** MMP = matrix metalloproteinase; PG = proteoglycan; IL = interleukin; TNFα = tumor necrosis factor-alfa; VEGF = vascular endothelial growth factor; TIMP = tissue inhibitor of metalloproteinase.
>
> - Plasma components
>   - Enzymes
>   - MMP-1, -3, -13
>   - Thrombin
>   - Tryptase/chymase
>   - Plasmin
>   - "PG-degrading activity"
>   - Cytokines
>   - TNFα
>   - IL6
>   - Growth factors
>   - VEGF
> - Cellular components
>   - Erythrocytes
>   - Hemoglobin
>   - Iron
>   - Leukocytes
>   - Monocytes/macrophages
>   - TIMP-1
>   - CD-3—T-cells
>   - Platelets
>   - Growth factors

Severe or recurrent joint bleeding results in the deposition of large amounts of hemosiderin into the synovial membrane [12]. The accumulation of iron alters the metabolic properties of the synovium, likely triggering the development BIJD [13].

Plasma enzymes, cytokines, chemokines, and growth factors
Circulating factors, such as plasma enzymes, cytokines, chemokines, and growth factors, are believed to play key roles in the development of BIJD by promoting cell proliferation and inducing proteoglycan release from cartilage. The link between thrombin, a mitogen for synovial fibroblast-like cells, and synovial hyperplasia as well as the influence of fibrin on the inflammatory response are areas requiring further study. Synovial cells, the neutral proteinases they produce (e.g., elastase), and other enzymes may degrade cartilage, thereby reducing its proteoglycan content [14–16].

Increased iron uptake by synovial cells leads to a vicious cycle of bleeding-synovitis-bleeding. In hemophilic mice, bloody synovial fluid contains increased concentrations of IL-1β, IL-6, keratinocyte-derived chemokine, and MCP-1 [17,18]. The presence of these cytokines escalates the uptake of transferrin- and nontransferrin-bound iron into monocytes and increases transferrin-bound iron uptake by synovial fibroblasts [19], perpetuating the cycle of bleeding and synovitis.

Vascular endothelial growth factor (VEGF), involved in angiogenesis and chondrocyte metabolism [20], may have similar activity in hemophilic arthropathy, although further research is needed to confirm this.

Signals from blood for joint destruction
Exactly how blood in the joint space causes cartilage and bone destruction is unclear, but members of the TNF receptor superfamily of cytokines, which include RANK; its ligand, RANKL; and its

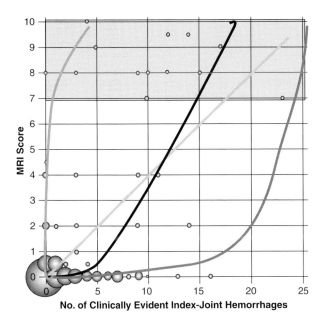

No. of Clinically Evident Index-Joint Hemorrhages

Figure 22.2 Clinically evident joint hemorrhages in the US Joint Outcome Study. The grey center line indicates that in some subjects there was a direct relationship between the number of joint hemorrhages and the MRI score and in others there was a threshold number of hemarthroses needed to cause joint damage (black line). The far left hand line indicates the MRI score of subjects with radiographic evidence of joint damage by age 6 years but who had no or only a few clinically evident hemarthroses and the far right hand line those subjects with a normal MRI score despite many clinically evident episodes of hemarthrosis. Original figure from Marilyn J. Manco-Johnson, Thomas C. Abshire, Amy D. Shapiro et al. Prophylaxis versus Episodic Treatment to Prevent Joint Disease in Boys with Severe Hemophilia. N Engl J Med. 2007;357:535–544. Reproduced with permission, copyright © 2007 Massachusetts Medical Society. All rights reserved.

natural decoy receptor, osteoprotegrin (OPG), may be prominently involved [21]. The balance of these proteins regulates osteoclast formation and activity, and they are the final effector proteins of osteoclastic bone resorption [22].

The process of BIJD begins with inflammatory synovitis [23], which leads to cartilage and bone destruction. The inflammatory milieu combined with local hypoxia promotes blood vessel formation and synovial membrane angiogenesis [24–27]. These nascent blood vessels are of poor quality and their increased permeability [28] predisposes to bleeding, perpetuating the bleeding–inflammation–bleeding cycle. The increased expression of RANK by normal neutrophils and RANKL by both normal and inflammatory neutrophils together with a decrease in OPG expression favor osteoclast differentiation and bone resorption [29]. Arthropathy results from a disruption of the dynamic equilibrium between osteoclastic bone resorption and osteoblastic bone formation [30–32].

Conclusions

The structural joint damage, pain, deformity, and disability that characterize hemophilic arthropathy may occur after only a few

(or no) bleeding episodes in persons predisposed to arthropathy. Alternatively, BIJD may only develop after numerous hemarthroses in those individuals whose joints are protected from the adverse effects of blood (Figure 22.2). Data generated from research into the pathophysiology of OA and RA combined with accumulating data in humans and from animal models of hemophilia suggests that multiple blood constituents trigger the arthropathic process, and that several joint components are the targets. Further study is needed to understand the precise mechanisms by which bleeding induces hemophilic joint damage. Once elucidated, therapeutics might be designed to counter the effects of blood in the joint.

References

1. Pergantou H, Matsinos G, Papadopoulos A, Platokouki H, Aronis S. Comparative study of validity of clinical, X-ray and magnetic resonance imaging scores in evaluation and management of haemophilic arthropathy in children. Haemophilia. 2006 May;12(3): 241–7.

2. Roosendaal G, Lafeber FP. Pathogenesis of haemophilic arthropathy. Haemophilia. 2006 Jul;12(Suppl 3):117–21.

3. Cohen NP, Foster RJ, Mow VC. Composition and dynamics of articular cartilage: structure, function, and maintaining healthy state. J Orthop Sports Phys Ther. 1998 Oct;28(4):203–15.

4. Hooiveld MJ, Roosendaal G, van den Berg HM, Bijlsma JW, Lafeber FP. Haemoglobin-derived iron-dependent hydroxyl radical formation in blood-induced joint damage: an in vitro study. Rheumatology (Oxford). 2003 Jun;42(6):784–90.

5. Nishiya K. Stimulation of human synovial cell DNA synthesis by iron. J Rheumatol. 1994 Oct;21(10):1802–7.

6. Hashizume M, Hayakawa N, Mihara M. IL-6 trans-signalling directly induces RANKL on fibroblast-like synovial cells and is involved in RANKL induction by TNF-alpha and IL-17. Rheumatology (Oxford). 2008 Nov;47(11):1635–40.

7. Wen FQ, Jabbar AA, Chen YX, Kazarian T, Patel DA, Valentino LA. c-myc proto-oncogene expression in hemophilic synovitis: in vitro studies of the effects of iron and ceramide. Blood. 2002 Aug 1;100(3): 912–6.

8. Hakobyan N, Kazarian T, Jabbar AA, Jabbar KJ, Valentino LA. Pathobiology of hemophilic synovitis I: overexpression of mdm2 oncogene. Blood. 2004 Oct 1;104(7):2060–4.

9. Paleolog EM, Miotla JM. Angiogenesis in arthritis: role in disease pathogenesis and as a potential therapeutic target. Angiogenesis. 1998; 2(4):295–307.

10. Israely T, Dafni H, Granot D, Nevo N, Tsafriri A, Neeman M. Vascular remodeling and angiogenesis in ectopic ovarian transplants: a crucial role of pericytes and vascular smooth muscle cells in maintenance of ovarian grafts. Biol Reprod. 2003 Jun;68(6):2055–64.

11. Nehls V, Schuchardt E, Drenckhahn D. The effect of fibroblasts, vascular smooth muscle cells, and pericytes on sprout formation of endothelial cells in a fibrin gel angiogenesis system. Microvasc Res. 1994 Nov;48(3):349–63.

12. Dryll A, Lansaman J, Bardin T, Ryckewaert A. [Hemopigmented villonodular synovitis: ultrastructural study and a comparison with hemophiliac synovitis]. Rev Rhum Mal Osteoartic. 1983 Feb;50(2): 87–93.

13. Roosendaal G, Vianen ME, Wenting MJ, van Rinsum AC, van den Berg HM, Lafeber FP, et al. Iron deposits and catabolic properties of synovial tissue from patients with haemophilia. J Bone Joint Surg Br. 1998 May;80(3):540–5.

14. Furmaniak-Kazmierczak E, Cooke TD, Manuel R, Scudamore A, Hoogendorn H, Giles AR, et al. Studies of thrombin-induced proteoglycan release in the degradation of human and bovine cartilage. J Clin Invest. 1994 Aug;94(2):472–80.

15. Saklatvala J, Barrett AJ. Identification of proteinases in rheumatoid synovium. Detection of leukocyte elastase cathepsin G and another serine proteinase. Biochim Biophys Acta. 1980 Sep 9;615(1):167–77.

16. Roosendaal G, Mauser-Bunschoten EP, De Kleijn P, Heijnen L, van den Berg HM, van Rinsum AC, et al. Synovium in haemophilic arthropathy. Haemophilia. 1998 Jul;4(4):502–5.

17. Ovlisen K, Kristensen AT, Jensen AL, Tranholm M. IL-1 beta, IL-6, KC and MCP-1 are elevated in synovial fluid from haemophilic mice with experimentally induced haemarthrosis. Haemophilia. 2009 May;15(3):802–10.

18. Ovlisen K, Kristensen AT, Tranholm M. In vivo models of haemophilia – status on current knowledge of clinical phenotypes and therapeutic interventions. Haemophilia. 2008 Mar;14(2):248–59.

19. Telfer JF, Brock JH. Proinflammatory cytokines increase iron uptake into human monocytes and synovial fibroblasts from patients with rheumatoid arthritis. Med Sci Monit. 2004 Apr;10(4):BR91–5.

20. Murata M, Yudoh K, Masuko K. The potential role of vascular endothelial growth factor (VEGF) in cartilage: how the angiogenic factor could be involved in the pathogenesis of osteoarthritis? Osteoarthritis Cartilage. 2008 Mar;16(3):279–86.

21. Boyce BF, Xing L. Biology of RANK, RANKL, and osteoprotegerin. Arthritis Res Ther. 2007;9(Suppl 1):S1.

22. Anandarajah AP. Role of RANKL in bone diseases. Trends Endocrinol Metab. 2009 Mar;20(2):88–94.

23. Hakobyan N, Kazarian T, Valentino LA. Synovitis in a murine model of human factor VIII deficiency. Haemophilia. 2005 May;11(3):227–32.

24. Taylor PC, Sivakumar B. Hypoxia and angiogenesis in rheumatoid arthritis. Curr Opin Rheumatol. 2005 May;17(3):293–8.

25. Bosco MC, Delfino S, Ferlito F, Puppo M, Gregorio A, Gambini C, et al. The hypoxic synovial environment regulates expression of vascular endothelial growth factor and osteopontin in juvenile idiopathic arthritis. J Rheumatol. 2009 Jun;36(6):1318–29.

26. Dhaouadi T, Sfar I, Abelmoula L, Jendoubi-Ayed S, Aouadi H, Ben Abdellah T, et al. Role of immune system, apoptosis and angiogenesis in pathogenesis of rheumatoid arthritis and joint destruction, a systematic review. Tunis Med. 2007 Dec;85(12):991–8.

27. Gonzalez LM, Querol F, Gallach JE, Gomis M, Aznar VA. Force fluctuations during the maximum isometric voluntary contraction of the quadriceps femoris in haemophilic patients. Haemophilia. 2007 Jan;13(1):65–70.

28. Bignold LP. Importance of platelets in increased vascular permeability evoked by experimental haemarthrosis in synovium of the rat. Pathology. 1980 Apr;12(2):169–79.

29. Gravallese EM. Bone destruction in arthritis. Ann Rheum Dis. 2002 Nov;61(Suppl 2):ii84–6.

30. Manolagas SC. Cell number versus cell vigor – what really matters to a regenerating skeleton? Endocrinology. 1999 Oct;140(10):4377–81.

31. Manolagas SC. Birth and death of bone cells: basic regulatory mechanisms and implications for the pathogenesis and treatment of osteoporosis. Endocr Rev. 2000 Apr;21(2):115–37.

32. Katagiri T, Takahashi N. Regulatory mechanisms of osteoblast and osteoclast differentiation. Oral Dis. 2002 May;8(3):147–59.

23 Assessment of Joint Involvement in Hemophilia

Erik Berntorp

Skåne University Hospital, Malmö, Sweden

Introduction

Although brain hemorrhage and bleeding into internal organs constitute major threats to the life of the person with hemophilia (PWH), bleeding into the joints is the principal health problem and prevention of joint disease is the primary goal of hemophilia treatment. Repeated joint bleeds cause arthropathy.

Physical examination

Physical examination is the traditional method for measuring joint impairment caused by bleeding in hemophilia. The need for a reproducible scoring system became evident some time ago, as long term follow-up is necessary for the evaluation of hemophilia treatment. The Orthopedic Advisory Committee of the World Federation of Hemophilia (WFH) endorsed a scoring system in 1985 [12]. In this scoring system the six major joints particularly impacted by hemophilia, i.e. elbows, knees and ankles, are examined. Each joint is assigned a score of 0–12 with 0 for a normal joint and 12 for most affected, then the scores for each joint are summed. An (S) is added after the number if chronic synovitis is diagnosed clinically. The guidelines for scoring are shown in Table 23.1.

For the joint evaluation (of a non-bleeding joint), an indicator for pain can be added where 0 = no pain, no functional deficit and no use of analgesics; 1 = mild pain which does not interfere with occupation nor with activities of daily living; 2 = moderate pain which means partial or occasional interference with occupation or ADL, use of non-narcotic medications but may require occasional narcotics and 3 = severe pain which interferes with occupation or ADL. An indicator for bleeding per year is also included in the original description for clinical evaluation of joints where

0 = none; 1 = no major, 1–3 minor; 2 = 1–2 major or 4–6 minor; 3 = 3 or more major or 7 or more minor hemarthroses.

This scoring system has been used at a number of hemophilia treatment centers as part of routine clinical follow-up and in some of the major studies of prophylaxis in which orthopedic outcome was assessed, e.g., in the Swedish report on 25 years experience of prophylaxis [6] and in the Orthopaedic Outcome Study [13].

The WFH score was developed during a time when few patients were treated with prophylaxis and before the era of primary prophylaxis, i.e., initiated at young age prior to demonstrable joint disease and sometimes prior to any bleeding [14]. As treatment became more wide spread and intense, the occurrence of joint disease became less frequent and less advanced. The WFH score was not designed for evaluation of these patients and many received scores of "0", despite the obvious presence of joint disease upon clinical examination. Consequently, the scoring system was updated and amended by several authors [15,16] and made applicable for use in children. These scoring systems were combined and further evaluated by a group within the IPSG. A new score was produced: the Hemophilia Joint Health Score [17]. The HJHS is an 11-item scoring tool for assessing joint impairment in children ages 4–18 years. The most significant similarities to and adaptations of the previous scales are as follows: joint instability was retained from the WFH score but reduced to 1 point in order to capture more significant changes as opposed to normal variations in children. From the Colorado versions [16] the 3-point scale for swelling, gait and strength was retained and the more age-appropriate tasks (e.g. gait) for the developing child were maintained. From the Stockholm instrument [15] duration of swelling (to capture chronic synovitis) and degrees lost (not percentage) for range of motion were retained. This score was validated and found reliable with an inter-observer coefficient of 0.83 and a test-retest of 0.89. The HJHS measures, in addition to the WFH score, strength and gait and the scores for single joints have been made more sensitive for

Current and Future Issues in Hemophilia Care, First Edition. Edited by Emérito-Carlos Rodríguez-Merchán and Leonard A. Valentino.
© 2011 John Wiley & Sons, Ltd. Published 2011 by Blackwell Publishing Ltd.

Physical finding	Score	Scoring key
Swelling	0 or 2 + (S)	0 = Not present 2 = Present (S) = Added after score if chronic synovitis is present
Muscle atrophy	0–1	0 = None or minimal (<1 cm) 1 = Present
Axial deformity (measured at ankle or knee)	0–2	Knee 0 = Normal = 0–7° valgus 1 = 8–15° valgus or 0–5° varus 2 = > 15° valgus or > 5° varus Ankle 0 = No deformity 1 = Up to 10° valgus or up to 5° varus 2 = > 10° valgus or > 5° varus
Crepitus on motion	0–1	0 = None 1 = Present
Range of motion	0–2	0 = Loss of 10% of total full range of motion (FROM) 1 = Loss of 10–33 1/3% of total FROM 2 = Loss of > 33 1/3% of total FROM
Flexion contracture (measured at hip, knee, or ankle)	0–2	0 = <15° FFC (fixed flexion contracture) 2 = 15° or greater FFC at hip or knee or equines at ankle
Instability	0–2	0 = None 1 = Noted on examination but neither interferes with function nor requires bracing 2 = Instability that creates a functional deficit or requires bracing

Table 23.1 Guidelines for the WFH physical examination score. (Reproduced from Pettersson H, Gilbert M, editors. Classification of the hemophilic arthropathy. New York: Springer-Verlag; 1985.)

early changes and account for normal development. This score may also be used in adults, although it cannot be directly compared with earlier examination and scoring using the WFH scale, and requires further validation in larger studies of both children and adults. The HJHS has, for example, replaced the WFH score at the Malmö Center with good results (personal communication).

Radiologic scores

X-ray

The score named after Pettersson [18] is a score based on X-ray examination of ankles, knees and elbows and is an additive score, i.e., the sum of scores for each joint (Table 23.2). This contrasts to the Arnold and Hilgartner score [19] which is a progressive scale with a classification of joint changes into five stages. The Pettersson score was incorporated in the scoring systems endorsed by WFH [12] and has been used in several large studies investigating long-term outcome of hemophilia therapy [6,13,20].

The radiologic score is more sensitive than the orthopedic score. In the cohort described by Nilsson et al. [6], the most intensively treated group, aged 3–12 years (born 1979–88) started treatment at 1–2 years of age and in large doses ranging from 2000 to 9000 IU FVIII/IX kg^{-1} body weight per year. The patients had virtually no joint bleeding and the entire group (n = 15) had orthopedic and radiologic joint scores of 0. In the less intensively treated but still young group aged 13 to 17 years (n = 20), however, the orthopedic joint scores ranged from 0 to 7, and the radiologic scores from 0 to 22. Fourteen patients had orthopedic joint scores of 0, and 11 had radiologic scores of 0. In the two oldest groups, aged 18 to 32 years, scores were generally higher. This study showed that it was possible to keep some patients free of joint disease, as measured by the WFH-endorsed orthopedic score as well as a radiologic score, but that the radiologic scores were higher with fewer patients having scores of 0. It should be kept in mind that the score as such does not necessarily reflect the performance and well-being of the patient. The scoring systems have greater utility for research than for clinical evaluation of individual patients.

MRI

Improvement of therapy has led to the need for more refined systems to monitor subtle changes in joint health. Radiography does not permit sensitive evaluation of soft tissues; therefore the pathologic process is often underestimated. This was underscored by the findings in a study recently published by Manco-Johnson et al. [10]. In this study, 65 patients were randomized to prophylaxis (n = 32) or enhanced episodic therapy (n = 33). Of these, 27 and 22 completed the protocol in their respective study arms. The mean period of participation in the study was 49

Table 23.2 Radiologic evaluation recommended by the Orthopedic Advisory Committee of the World Federation of Hemophilia, the Pettersson score. (Reproduced with permission from Pettersson H, Ahlberg A, Nilsson IM. A radiologic classification of hemophilic arthropathy. Clin Orthop Relat Res. 1980 Jun(149):153–9.)

Type of change	Finding	Score (points)
Osteoporosis	Absent	0
	Present	1
Enlarged epiphysis	Absent	0
	Present	1
Irregular subchondral surface	Absent	0
	Partially involved	1
	Totally involved	2
Narrowing of joint space	Absent	0
	Joint space > 1 mm	1
	Joint space ≤ 1 mm	2
Subchondral cyst formation	Absent	0
	1 cyst	1
	> 1 cyst	2
Erosions of joint margins	Absent	0
	Present	1
Gross incongruence of articulating bone ends	Absent	0
	Slight	1
	Pronounced	2
Joint deformity (angulation and/or displacement between articulating bones)	Absent	0
	Slight	1
	Pronounced	2

months. Primary outcome data for both MRI and radiographic studies were obtained for 50 of 65 participants (77%). A total of 18 abnormal joints (13 ankles, 3 elbows, and 2 knees) were detected in 15 children – two in the prophylaxis group and 13 in the episodic therapy group. Six of the abnormalities were detected both by MRI and radiography, seven by MRI alone, and one by radiography alone. Some joints had abnormal MRI scores but no hemarthroses, and some had normal MRI scores despite many hemarthroses. Thus, it was obvious that radiography is less sensitive than MRI but also that additional research must be done to understand the pathologic process that initiates arthropathy in hemophilia. There is broad individual variation with respect to the number of hemarthroses required to start the process. The MRI scale used in this study, the Denver scale, was developed by Nuss and colleagues [21]. It is a progressive scale, in which the most severe damage determines the score. In Europe, a new scoring method has been developed by Lundin et al. [22]. This scale, like the Petterson radiographic scale, uses an additive approach. With the goal of creating a universal MRI scale, the International MRI Working Group developed a Compatible MRI scoring system for assessment of hemophilic arthropathy [23]. This scale has a progressive component taken from the Denver scale and an additive component taken from the European scale. The reliability and

validity of the scale have been studied [24], and it was found to perform better for early discrimination of osteoarticular changes. Further use of this instrument in prospective clinical studies and trials will determine its ability to quantify the perceived benefit of interventions and allow for refinement of the instrument.

Ultrasonography

Sonography can be a useful complementary modality in the evaluation of hemophilic arthropathy. It is readily available, does not require sedation, and is an easy examination for small children. The technique is especially promising for detecting soft tissue changes which are the earliest findings in hemophilic arthropathy. A systematic protocol for its use has been proposed, but further assessment in clinical trials is needed [25,26].

Conclusions

The most affected joints are elbows, knees and ankles. It is not known how many hemorrhages into a joint are required to initiate progressive cartilage and joint destruction but it is likely that only a small number are necessary to start the pathologic process [1,2]. As hemarthroses can occur as frequently as 20–30 times per year [3,4] in the severe form of the disease, it is easy to understand that the PWH is at high risk for developing pronounced joint disease. In the United States, 36% of patients with severe hemophilia tracked as part of the Centers for Disease Control and Prevention (CDC) Universal Data Collection (UDC) database reported a need for mobility assistance, and 30% miss school or work due to upper or lower extremity joint problems [5]. Cohort studies and a recent prospective randomized study have clearly shown that long term prophylaxis, starting early in life, can prevent most arthropathic development, increase quality of life and diminish the burden on the health care [6–10] system. A significant observation is that children who do not report clinically overt bleeds can have signs of joint disease detected by MRI examination [10]. Obviously, it is clinically important to use tools that are able to detect early joint disease – this is essential when measurements are being performed in the context of research to develop efficacious prophylaxis protocols. Assessment of joint disease in hemophilia is primarily based on physical examination, radiologic examination and MRI. Ultrasonography is a promising technique that is very early in its development. Scoring systems have been formulated, and the goal is to come to international consensus regarding the use of these systems. In recent years this work has, to a large extent, been promoted within the frame of the International Prophylaxis Study Group (IPSG) [11].

References

1. Roosendaal G, Lafeber FP. Blood-induced joint damage in hemophilia. Semin Thromb Hemost. 2003 Feb;29(1):37–42.
2. Funk M, Schmidt H, Escuriola-Ettingshausen C, Pons S, Dzinaj T, Weimer C, et al. Radiological and orthopedic score in pediatric hemophilic patients with early and late prophylaxis. Ann Hematol. 1998 Oct;77(4):171–4.

3. Ramgren O. Haemophilia in Sweden. III. Symptomatology, with special reference to differences between haemophilia A and B. Acta Med Scand. 1962 Feb;171:237–42.

4. Ahlberg A. Haemophilia in Sweden. VII. Incidence, treatment and prophylaxis of arthropathy and other musculo-skeletal manifestations of haemophilia A and B. Acta Orthop Scand Suppl. 1965: Suppl 77: 3–132.

5. CDC. Summary Report of UDC Activity National: Treatment and Outcome by Severity (Hemophilia). In: Prevention DoHaHSCfDCa, editor. Atlanta; 2008.

6. Nilsson IM, Berntorp E, Lofqvist T, Pettersson H. Twenty-five years' experience of prophylactic treatment in severe haemophilia A and B. J Intern Med. 1992 Jul;232(1):25–32.

7. Steen Carlsson K, Hojgard S, Glomstein A, Lethagen S, Schulman S, Tengborn L, et al. On-demand vs. prophylactic treatment for severe haemophilia in Norway and Sweden: differences in treatment characteristics and outcome. Haemophilia. 2003 Sep;9(5): 555–66.

8. Schramm W, Royal S, Kroner B, Berntorp E, Giangrande P, Ludlam C, et al. Clinical outcomes and resource utilization associated with haemophilia care in Europe. Haemophilia. 2002 Jan;8(1):33–43.

9. Miners AH, Sabin CA, Tolley KH, Lee CA. Primary prophylaxis for individuals with severe haemophilia: how many hospital visits could treatment prevent? J Intern Med. 2000 Apr;247(4):493–9.

10. Manco-Johnson MJ, Abshire TC, Shapiro AD, Riske B, Hacker MR, Kilcoyne R, et al. Prophylaxis versus episodic treatment to prevent joint disease in boys with severe hemophilia. N Engl J Med. 2007 Aug 9;357(6):535–44.

11. Feldman BM, Funk S, Lundin B, Doria AS, Ljung R, Blanchette V. Musculoskeletal measurement tools from the International Prophylaxis Study Group (IPSG). Haemophilia. 2008 Jul;14Suppl 3:162–9.

12. Pettersson H, Gilbert M, editors. Classification of the hemophilic arthropathy. New York: Springer-Verlag; 1985.

13. Aledort LM, Haschmeyer RH, Pettersson H. A longitudinal study of orthopaedic outcomes for severe factor-VIII-deficient haemophiliacs. The Orthopaedic Outcome Study Group. J Intern Med. 1994 Oct;236(4):391–9.

14. Donadel-Claeyssens S. Current co-ordinated activities of the PED-NET (European Paediatric Network for Haemophilia Management). Haemophilia. 2006 Mar;12(2):124–7.

15. Hill FG, Ljung R. Third and fourth Workshops of the European Paediatric Network for Haemophilia Management. Haemophilia. 2003 Mar;9(2):223–8.

16. Manco-Johnson MJ, Nuss R, Funk S, Murphy J. Joint evaluation instruments for children and adults with haemophilia. Haemophilia. 2000 Nov;6(6):649–57.

17. Hilliard P, Funk S, Zourikian N, Bergstrom BM, Bradley CS, McLimont M, et al. Hemophilia joint health score reliability study. Haemophilia. 2006 Sep;12(5):518–25.

18. Pettersson H, Ahlberg A, Nilsson IM. A radiologic classification of hemophilic arthropathy. Clin Orthop Relat Res. 1980 Jun(149): 153–9.

19. Arnold WD, Hilgartner MW. Hemophilic arthropathy. Current concepts of pathogenesis and management. J Bone Joint Surg Am. 1977 Apr;59(3):287–305.

20. Fischer K, Astermark J, van der Bom JG, Ljung R, Berntorp E, Grobbee DE, et al. Prophylactic treatment for severe haemophilia: comparison of an intermediate-dose to a high-dose regimen. Haemophilia. 2002 Nov;8(6):753–60.

21. Nuss R, Kilcoyne RF, Geraghty S, Shroyer AL, Rosky JW, Mawhinney S, et al. MRI findings in haemophilic joints treated with radiosynoviorthesis with development of an MRI scale of joint damage. Haemophilia. 2000 May;6(3):162–9.

22. Lundin B, Pettersson H, Ljung R. A new magnetic resonance imaging scoring method for assessment of haemophilic arthropathy. Haemophilia. 2004 Jul;10(4):383–9.

23. Lundin B, Babyn P, Doria AS, Kilcoyne R, Ljung R, Miller S, et al. Compatible scales for progressive and additive MRI assessments of haemophilic arthropathy. Haemophilia. 2005 Mar;11(2):109–15.

24. Doria AS, Babyn PS, Lundin B, Kilcoyne RF, Miller S, Rivard GE, et al. Reliability and construct validity of the compatible MRI scoring system for evaluation of haemophilic knees and ankles of haemophilic children. Expert MRI working group of the international prophylaxis study group. Haemophilia. 2006 Sep;12(5):503–13.

25. Keshava S, Gibikote S, Mohanta A, Doria AS. Refinement of a sonographic protocol for assessment of haemophilic arthropathy. Haemophilia. 2009 Sep;15(5):1168–71.

26. Zukotynski K, Jarrin J, Babyn PS, Carcao M, Pazmino-Canizares J, Stain AM, et al. Sonography for assessment of haemophilic arthropathy in children: a systematic protocol. Haemophilia. 2007 May;13(3):293–304.

24 Imaging of the Hemophilic Joint

Carmen Martin-Hervás and Emérito-Carlos Rodríguez-Merchán

La Paz University Hospital, Madrid, Spain

Introduction

The diagnosis of hemophilia is based on clinical data and laboratory tests, and radiologic imaging is used to evaluate complications of the disease. Recurrent joint bleeds results in progressive arthropathy. Ankles, knees and elbows are the joints most frequently involved [1]. It is important to diagnose, and monitoring joint changes in order to make therapeutic decisions. The radiological findings of hemophilic arthropathy (HA) depend on the stage of disease, the age of the patient at onset and the joint involved. These findings include joint effusion, soft tissue swelling, epiphyseal overgrowth, subchondral cysts, osseous erosion and secondary degenerative changes [2]. Imaging modalities such as conventional radiography (X-ray), ultrasonography (US), and magnetic resonance imaging (MRI), may be useful for the evaluating patients with HA [3].

Radiography

X-ray has been successfully used for decades to objectively evaluate and stage HA [4]. Findings of HA demonstrated on X-ray include osteoporosis, osteonecrosis, epiphyseal overgrowth, widening of the intercondylar notch of the knee, bone cysts, joint-space irregularity and narrowing, angulations of the knee and ankle and bony fusion [1]. Soft-tissue swelling can be suggested, but is often not clearly delineated (Figure 24.1). However, although radiography visualizes primarily bone lesions, it is insensitive to the early changes of HA and to the less advanced joint damage seen in patients receiving prophylactic treatment [5]. The earliest changes in HA are to the synovium, and these soft-tissue changes are poorly demonstrated on X-ray [4]. Osseous changes due to hemorrhage only appear late in the disease. Cartilage destruc-

tion cannot be visualized directly, but only inferred from changes, such as loss of joint space and an irregular subchondral surface. Assessment of joint-space loss is difficult in children, particularly if comparison films are not available [6]. There are two main classification systems in use for grading HA on X-ray. These are the Arnold–Hilgartner scale, described in 1977 [7], and the Pettersson score, described in 1980 [4]. The Arnold–Hilgartner system is a progressive scale for the assessment of HA, the worst imaging finding reflecting the stage of the arthropathy. The Pettersson score is an additive scale. Each abnormality is graded from 0 to 1 or 2, and abnormalities due to different stages of the disease will all be included. The highest score for an individual joint is 13, which indicates a totally destroyed joint [4] (Figure 24.2). There are differences between the two scoring systems. The progressive one is simple and easy to use by everyone. The additive one is more meticulous, but discriminates better between different stages of HA.

One study assessing both intra- and interobserver variability of the two scoring systems demonstrated generally good correlation if there is minimal or maximal joint disease, but poor levels of agreement if there is mild or moderate HA [8]. The World Federation of Hemophilia recommends the Pettersson score for universal use [9].

Once radiographic changes are present, the clinical course of the arthropathy is usually progressive and irreversible. Improved therapy has lead to the need for more sensitive tools for the assessment of the degree of joint damage, which can evaluate the subtle joint changes not seen on plain film. However, once the disease is advanced, it can usually be monitored with X-ray alone [5].

Ultrasonography

US is an imaging technique with a progressive and extensive use in the musculoskeletal system as it is readily available and does not require the child to be sedated. It can be a useful complementary

Current and Future Issues in Hemophilia Care, First Edition. Edited by Emérito-Carlos Rodríguez-Merchán and Leonard A. Valentino.

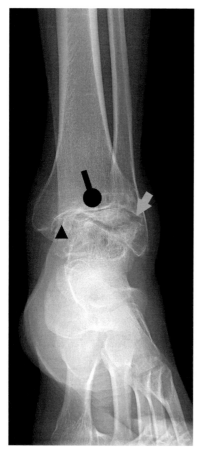

Figure 24.1 X-ray: Anteroposterior (AP) view of the ankle demonstrating soft tissue swelling (white arrow), osteoporosis, epiphyseal overgrowth, subchondral bone cysts (round arrow), and significantly narrowed joint space (arrowhead).

technique in the evaluation of HA. US has some other potential advantages, including lack of ionizing radiation, cost-and time-effectiveness, accessibility, real time and dynamic examinations. In this way, US can be used as a first diagnostic imaging procedure instead of MRI. The major disadvantage of US is its operator dependence, requiring a long learning curve and a limited value of images for orthopaedic surgeons and physicians that prefer a more anatomical imaging modality, such as MRI [10].

Linear high-resolution (7–17 MHz) US probes are typically used for assessing HA [11], enabling the visualization of superficial musculoskeletal structures such as synovium, tendons, musculature and the cartilage/osteochondral interface at the edge of the joints on grey-scale sonograms. US can also be used to follow the progression or regression of soft tissue hematomas and pseudotumors [2].

US can be used to assess joint effusions in acute episodes. US as a diagnostic technique in the initial stages of hemophilia permit the differentiation between effusion and synovial thickening (Figure 24.3). A selective compression with the US probe may help to distinguish both entities; the fluid will be displaced out, while the synovium remains incompressible [10,12]. A hemarthrosis may demonstrate a different echogenicity, depending on the stage of degradation of the blood products [11]. The normal synovium is a thin membrane. When it becomes inflamed, diffuse or nodular thickening of the membrane is seen, which may show increased vascular flow on Doppler US. Differentiation between hemarthrosis and synovial hypertrophy helps to determine when factor replacement is necessary for patients treated on demand [5]. The selective implementation of prophylaxis would require the availability of a more sensitive tool to monitor for the development of synovitis than is currently possible with clinical surveillance or X-ray. MRI is such a tool and is utilized for the evaluation of HA [13]. However, MRI is expensive, and requires sedation in younger children, precluding its utility for monitoring synovitis [14].

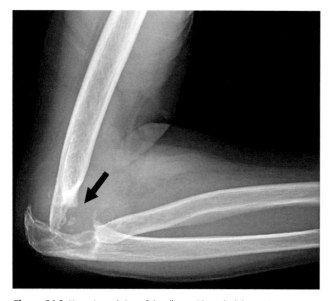

Figure 24.2 X-ray: Lateral view of the elbow with marked destruction, subluxation and disorganization of the joint (arrow).

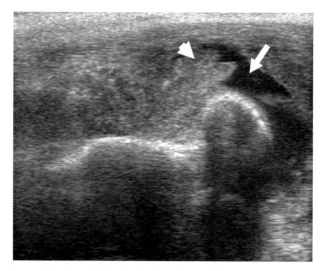

Figure 24.3 Elbow. US: Longitudinal view of the radial head with joint effusion (arrow) and severe synovial thickening (arrowhead), demonstrated as a hypoechoic tissue.

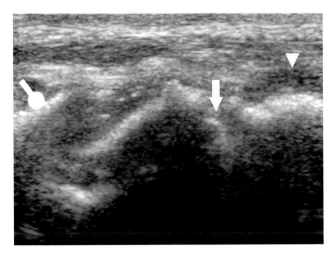

Figure 24.4 Ankle. US: Longitudinal view over the anterior tibiotalar joint showing narrowing of the joint space, a tibial bony spur (round arrow), mild synovial hyperplasia (arrowhead), irregularity of the hyaline cartilage and subchondral plate of the talar dome (arrow).

US with power Doppler has been used to detect and quantify vascularity in other arthritides [15], and has the capability of evaluating synovial vascularity in hemophilic joints. A recent study [16] showed a strong correlation between Doppler and dynamic contrast-enhanced MRI measurements in hemophilic knees, elbows and ankles. In fact, contrast-enhanced US may be comparable to MRI in estimating synovial vascularity for the diagnosis of active synovitis as seen with rheumatoid arthritis [17]. US also reveals early cartilaginous involvement and partial visualization of the joints [17] (Figure 24.4).

Previous studies evaluated the US findings of HA [11,18], and described a systematic protocol for data acquisition of US findings in hemophilic joints [12,19]. Nevertheless, the value of this technique for the assessment of HA in comparison with MRI and physical examination has not been fully evaluated thus far. As a result, this technique has been underutilized in clinical practice. Another challenge of US relates to the interpretation of images and comparison with other diagnostic tests.

Magnetic resonance imaging

MRI was introduced as a medical imaging modality in the 1980s and it uses radiowaves and magnetic fields [3].

MRI has been shown to more accurately assess HA than radiography. MRI has obvious advantages, including the increased level of detail of soft tissue and cartilage changes and lack of ionizing radiation, but it is more costly, less accessible, more time consuming and requires sedation in younger children [6,14].

MRI provides information on all aspects of HA, demonstrating early arthropathic changes such as hemarthrosis, effusion, synovial hypertrophy, hemosiderin deposition and small focal carti-

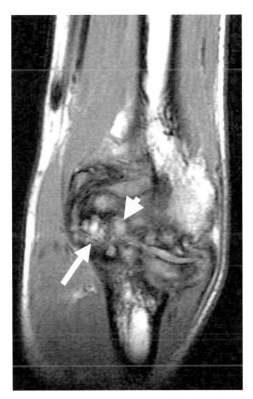

Figure 24.5 T1-weighted MRI coronal view of an elbow showing erosions, subchondral cysts (arrowhead) and cartilage destruction with joint space narrowing (arrow).

lage defects without joint space narrowing, which cannot be delineated by X-ray imaging. Moreover, MRI can provide information about more advanced changes, such as erosions, subchondral cysts and cartilage destruction with joint space narrowing [5,17] (Figure 24.5).

A high correlation between the presence of osseous changes on X-ray and the presence of synovial or cartilaginous changes on MRI, especially in the advanced stages of the disease has been demonstrated. The sensitivity of MRI to detect the changes of early HA is high [21], but is lower for the elbow compared to the knee or ankle [5].

Exact recommendations of the sequences to be performed in HA have not been established [6]. A T1-weighted sequence is always useful to demonstrate anatomy and osteochondral lesions. A short T1 inversion recovery (STIR) sequence is very sensitive for demonstrating bone oedema (Figure 24.6), and gradient-echo (GRE) sequences improves the visualization of cartilage, synovium, and hemosiderin [17,20]. T2* GRE sequence result in enhanced visibility of blood products in the acute stage (deoxyhemoglobin) and the chronic stage (hemosiderin), and can identify even the smallest amount of hemosiderin deposition in a joint [20] (Figure 24.7). However, when there is a significant amount of hemosiderin in the joint, the degree of artefact may be too great to enable interpretation.

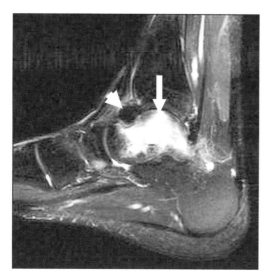

Figure 24.6 Sagital STIR image of the ankle, demonstrating bone edema of talar dome (arrow) and synovial hypertrophy with iron deposits in the tibiotalar joint (arrowhead).

Detailed images of cartilage can be obtained with either a proton density fat-saturated sequence or a fat-suppressed, three-dimensional, spoiled-gradient echo sequence [20].

Synovial hypertrophy is usually best visualized with an intermediate signal on T1- and T2-weighted images, enabling differentiation from fluid within the joint. However, active synovitis may show signal characteristics similar to that of fluid [5]. Enhancement of the synovium with intravenous contrast media may theoretically help distinguish active synovitis from

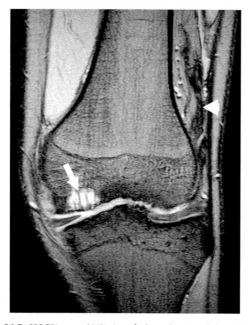

Figure 24.7 GRE T2* coronal MRI view of a knee showing subchondral cysts (arrow) and mild hemosiderin deposits (arrowhead) intensely black.

Table 24.1 The Denver MRI scale of hemophilic arthropathy. (Reproduced from Nuss R, Kilcoyne R, Geraghty F, et al. Haemophilia, 2000;6:162–169.)

Scale	Findings
0	Normal joint
Effusion/hemarthrosis	
1	Small
2	Moderate
3	Large
Synovial hyperplasia/hemosiderin	
4	Small
5	Moderate
6	Large
Cysts/erosions	
7	1 cyst or partial surface erosion
8	>1 cyst or full surface erosion
Cartilage loss	
9	<50% cartilage loss
10	>50% cartilage loss

fibrotic synovium [6]. However, the presence of fibrosis and hemosiderin within the proliferative synovium in HA limits the degree of visible enhancement. Therefore, intravenous contrast medium is not routinely recommended in the evaluation of HA; it also increases the invasiveness and the cost of the examination [6,20,21–23].

MR is a powerful tool in the diagnosis, staging and treatment of patients with HA. To measure arthropathic changes in clinical practice and in clinical research trials, tentative hemophilic arthropathy scales based on MRI findings have been developed in the last decade [13,21,24,25].

The first MRI staging system reported was the Denver scale from Nuss et al. in 2000 [13] (Table 24.1). This is a progressive scoring system, modelled on the Arnold and Hilgartner scale, with the worst finding determining the score in a particular joint. However, as it measures only the depth of the cartilage, it is less discriminating between different degrees of cartilaginous change [5].

The European score is a more detailed additive score that was modelled on the Pettersson score [24] (Table 24.2). This additive system is more complex than the Denver scale. However, it does allow the separate evaluation of osteochondral and soft-tissue changes. It assesses both the depth and width of cartilage changes. Its greatest value is in the evaluation of moderate to severe joint changes, but it is also reported to be better than the Denver scale at discriminating between early and advanced arthropathy [25].

Several other MRI grading systems have also been suggested [20,21,23]. The development of many different MRI scoring systems threatens to hamper the comparison of results from different centers. In an attempt to standardize the MRI interpretation of HA, the International Prophylaxis Study Group developed the

Table 24.2 The European Score. (Reproduced from Lundin B, Pettersson H, Ljung R. Haemophilia 2004;10:383–389.)

Subchondral cysts	Present in at least one bone
	Present in at least two bones
	More than three cysts In at least one bone
	More than three cysts In at least two bones
	Largest size more than 4 mm in at least one bone
	Largest size more than 4 mm in at least two bones
Irregularity/erosion of subchondral cortex	Present in at least one bone
	Present in at least two bones
	Involves more than half of joint surface in at least one bone
	Involves more than half of joint surface in at least two bones
Chondral destruction	Present in at least one bone
	Present in at least two bones
	Full-thickness defect in at least one bone
	Full-thickness defect in at least two bones
	Full-thickness defect involves over > 1/3 of joint surface in at least one bone
	Full-thickness defect involves > 1/3 of joint surface in at least two bones
Effusion/hemarthrosis (e)	Hypertrophic synovium

Compatible MRI Scale [25] (Table 24.3). This scale combines a 10-step progressive component based on the Denver Scale and a 20-step additive component based on the European score, with identical definitions of mutual steps. The Compatible MRI scale is highly reproducible, is excellent in deciding the presence or absence of HA, but performs relatively poorly at discriminating mild disease from moderate and severe disease [5,26].

Other imaging techniques

Computed tomography (CT)

Both MRI and contrast-enhanced CT are useful in determining the thickness of the wall and the extent of hemophilic pseudotumors, more consistently than US [2]. They usually destroy adjacent bone, [13] and may be visualized with CT.

Nuclear medicine

Radiosynovectomy is effective in improving the function of hemophiliac joints [27]. In spite of the potential value of scintigraphy for evaluating post-therapy joint changes, the limited spatial resolution of this imaging modality for the assessment of osteochondral abnormalities and its radiation-bearing potential has limited its use for follow-up of arthropathic changes, instead of US and MRI.

Table 24.3 The Compatible MRI Scale. (Reproduced From Lundin B, Pettersson H, Ljung R. Haemophilia 2004;10:383–389.)

	Progressive scale (P)	Additive scale (A)
Effusion/hemarthrosis		
Small	1	
Moderate	2	
Large	3	
Synovial hypertrophy		
Small	4	1
Moderate	5	2
Large	6	3
Hemosiderin		1
Small	4	
Moderate	5	
Large	6	
Changes of subchondral bone or joint margins		
Any surface erosion	7	1
Any surface erosion in at least two bones		1
Half or more of the articular surface eroded in at least one bone	8	1
Half or more of the articular surface eroded in at least two bones		1
At least one subchondral cyst	7	1
More than one subchondral cyst	8	1
Subchondral cysts in at least two bones		1
Multiple subchondral cysts in at least two bones		1
Cartilage loss		
Any loss of joint cartilage height	9	1
Any loss of cartilage height in at least two bones		1
Any loss of joint cartilage height involving more than one third of the joint surface in at least one bone		1
Any loss of joint cartilage height involving more than one-third of the joint surface in at least two bones		1
Full-thickness loss of joint cartilage in at least some area in at least one bone	10	1
Full-thickness loss of joint cartilage in at least some area in at least two bones		1
Full-thickness loss of joint cartilage involves at least one-third of the joint surface in at least one bone		1
Full-thickness loss of joint cartilage involves at least one-third of the joint surface in at least two bones		1
Scores	Highest number	

Positron emission tomography (PET)

PET is a technique that uses molecules labeled with isotopes that emit positrons from their nucleus. The most commonly used tracer is 2-deoxy-2-(18F) fluoro-*p*-deoxyglucose (FDG) [28]. After intravenous injection, FDG is taken up by the cells according to their level of glucose metabolism. Preliminary results demonstrated that the increased glucose metabolism of many inflammatory cell types and the FDG uptake by inflammatory tissues are the basis for the potential use of FDG-PET in the detection and monitoring of chronic HA in hemophilia [17].

Conclusions

Diagnostic imaging is used to objectively evaluate and stage HA. X-ray is useful to monitor advanced stages of the disease once considerable cartilage and/or bone damage has occurred in the joint. US can be used as a complementary technique to assess and follow up the soft-tissue changes of the arthropathy. MRI, with its excellent soft-tissue contrast, can accurately evaluate the early changes and the less advanced joint damage seen in patients receiving prophylactic therapy. MRI is the imaging method of choice for detecting the abnormalities of HA, staging their severity, and following the effects of treatment.

References

1. Resnick D. Diagnosis of Bone and Joint Disorders, 4th edn. Philadelphia: Saunders, 2002.
2. Kerr R. Imaging of musculoskeletal complications of hemophilia. Semin Musculoskelet Radiol 2003;7:127–136.
3. Doria AS, Lundin B. Imaging modalities for assessment of hemophilic arthropathy. In: Textbook of Hemophilia, 2nd edn. Lee CA, Berntorp EE, Hoots WK. Wiley-Blackwell, Oxford, 2010: 191–199.
4. Petterson H, Ahlberg A, Nilsson IM. A radiologic classification of haemophilic arthropathy. Clin Orthop Relat Res 1980;149:153–159.
5. Jelbert A, Vaidya S, Fotiadis N. Imaging and staging of haemophilic arthropathy. Clin Radiol 2009;64:1119–1128.
6. Kilcoyne RF, Lundin B, Pettersson H. Evolution of the imaging tests in haemophilia with emphasis on radiography and magnetic resonance imaging. Acta Radiol 2006;47:287–296.
7. Arnold WD, Hilgartner MW. Haemophilic arthropathy. Current concepts of pathogenesis and management. J Bone Joint Surg Am 1977;59:287–305.
8. Silva M, Lucky JV, Quon D, et al. Inter- and intra-observer reliability of radiographic scores commonly used for the evaluation of haemophilic arthropathy. Haemophilia 2008;14:504–512.
9. Nuss R, Kilcoyne RF. Diagnosis by imaging of haemophilic joints. In E.C. Rodríguez-Merchán, Ed. The Haemophilic Joints. New Perspectives. Blackwell Publishing, Oxford, 2003: 24–29.
10. Bernabeu-Taboada D, Martin-Hervás C. Sonography of haemophilic joints. In Rodríguez-Merchán EC, Ed. The Haemophilic Joints. New Perspectives. Blackwell Publishing, Oxford, 2003: 30–35.
11. Zukotynski K, Jarrin J, Babyn PS, et al. Sonography for assessment of haemophilic arthropathy in children: a systematic protocol. Haemophilia 2007;13:293–304.
12. Merchan ECR, De Orbe A, Gago J. Ultrasound in the diagnosis of the early stages of hemophilic arthropathy of the knee. Acta Orthop Belg 1992;58:122–125.
13. Nuss R, Kilcoyne R, Geraghty F, et al. MRI findings in haemophilic joints treated with radiosynoviorthesis with development of an MRI scale of joint damage. Haemophilia 2000;6:162–169.
14. Acharya SS. Hemophilic joint disease – current perspective and potential future strategies. Transfusion and Apheresis Science 2008; 38:49–55.
15. DiMichele DM. The potential role of power Doppler ultrasound in the diagnosis of haemophilic arthropathy. Haemophilia 2010;16(Suppl. 3):67–68.
16. Acharya SS, Schloss, R, Dyke JP, et al. Power Doppler sonography in the diagnosis of hemophilic synovitis – a promising tool. J Thrombosis Haemostasis 2008;6:2055–2061.
17. Doria AS, State-of-the-art imaging techniques for the evaluation of haemophilic arthropathy: present and future. Haemophilia 2010;16 (Suppl. 5): 107–114.
18. Bernabeu D, Hidalgo P, Martín C, et al. Ultrasound evaluation of haemophilic arthropathy involving the elbow and ankle. Haemophilia 2002;8 (Suppl 4): 469–481.
19. Keshava S, Gibikote S, Mohanta A, et al. Refinement of a sonographic protocol for assessment of haemophilic arthropathy. Haemophilia 2009;15:1168–1171.
20. Rand T, Trattnig S, Male CH, et al. Magnetic resonance imaging in hemophilic children: value of Gradient Echo and contrast-enhanced imaging. Magnetic Resonante Imaging 1999;17:199–205.
21. Funk MB, Schmidt H, Becker S, et al. Modified magnetic resonance imaging score compared with orthopaedic and radiological scores for the evaluation of haemophilic arthropathy. Haemophilia 2002;8:98–103.
22. Nuss R, Kilcoyne R, Geraghty S, et al. Utility of magnetic resonance imaging for management of hemophilic arthropathy in children. J Pediatr 1993;123:388–392.
23. Doria AS, Lundin B, Miller S, et al. Reliability and construct validity of the compatible MRI scoring system for evaluation of elbows in haemophilic children. Haemophilia 2008;14:303–314.
24. Lundin B, Pettersson H, Ljung R. A new magnetic resonance imaging scoring method for assessment of haemophilic arthropathy. Haemophilia 2004;10:383–389.
25. Lundin B, Babyn P, Doria AS, et al. Compatible scales for progressive and additive MRI assessments of haemophilic arthropathy. Haemophilia 2005;11:109–115.
26. Fotiadis N, Economou I, Haritanti A, et al. The compatible MRI scoring system for staging of haemophilic arthropathy. Haemophilia 2008;14:866–867.
27. Manco-Johnson MJ, Nuss R, Lear J, et al. 32P Radiosynoviorthesis in children with hemophilia. J Pediatr Hematol Oncol 2002;24:534–539.
28. Ribbens C, Hustinx R. Nuclear (Scintigraphic) methods and FDG-PET in rheumatoid arthritis and osteoarthritis, Chapter 7. In: Bruno MA, Mosher TJ, Gold GE, eds. Arthritis in Color, Advanced Imaging of Arthritis. Philadelphia, PA: Saunders, Elsevier, 2009;138–149.

25

Initial and Advanced Stages of Hemophilic Arthropathy, and Other Musculo-Skeletal Problems: The Role of Orthopedic Surgery

Emérito-Carlos Rodríguez-Merchán[1], Victor Jimenez-Yuste[1], and Nicholas J. Goddard[2]

[1] La Paz University Hospital, Madrid, Spain
[2] Royal Free Hospital, London, UK

Introduction

Intra-articular hemorrhage (hemarthrosis) is the most common complication in the patient with hemophilia. Recurrent hemarthroses start at a very early age in the patient's life, sometimes as early as 2 years old, when the child begins to walk. The joints most commonly affected, in order of decreasing frequency are the knees, elbows and ankles.

After a small number of hemarthrosis, a state of hypertrophic synovitis will result due to the lack of ability of normal synovium to reabsorb an excessive quantity of blood within the joint. This hypertrophic synovium is hyperemic and richly vascularized, resulting in asymmetrical growth of the epiphyses, giving the form of angular deformities and leg length discrepancies during childhood [1].

If chronic hemophilic synovitis is left untreated a vicious cycle of bleeding–synovitis–bleeding will result. Later on, the articular cartilage will also become involved. The exact mechanisms of such articular changes still remain poorly understood. They will eventually lead to hemophilic arthropathy, a particular type of degenerative osteoarthritis [2,3] (Figure 25.1).

Intramuscular hemorrhages are also common in hemophilia, and may be severe enough to necessitate the intervention of an orthopedic surgeon. Some intramuscular hematomas can cause severe neurological complications, such as a sural nerve palsy following an iliopsoas hematoma or a compartment syndrome of the forearm (Volkman paralysis) (Figure 25.2).

However, the most dangerous complication of a deep intramuscular hematoma is its slow transformation into what is termed a hemophilic pseudotumor. An incomplete treatment of the initial hematoma, with continuous partial resorption and recurrences is commonly the source of the pseudotumor. In the late stages cortical bone can be involved, and pathological fractures may occur.

Prophylactic treatment of the disorder from cradle to college theoretically eliminates the orthopedic complications of hemophilia. This is achieved by the regular administration of factor VIII or factor IX concentrates, prophylaxis.

This chapter focuses on the diagnosis, evaluation and treatment of the most important early and advanced articular problems of the hemophiliac.

Initial stages of hemophilic arthropathy

Some experimental studies have shown a blood-induced joint damage in hemophilic joints [3]. Blood breakdown products have been reported to affect the chondrocytes. Roosendaal et al. [4] investigated the harmful effect of blood components on human cartilage "in vitro".

The role of iron deposition in the pathophysiology of hemophilic synovitis has not been established fully. Stein and Duthie [5] described well-defined cytoplasmic deposits of iron, termed siderosomes, in synovial cells, subsynovial tissue, and in chondrocytes in the superficial layers of articular cartilage. The hemosiderin staining of the synovium and cartilage bears testimony to the destructive elements of the proteolytic enzymes.

Hemarthrosis: the role of arthrocentesis

An arthrocentesis usually is a very single and efficient procedure that many times can be carried out at the outpatient clinic or at the patient's bedside for the elbows, knees and ankles. However, puncture of shoulders and hips requires an image intensifier and certain orthopedic knowledge to be correctly performed, and to avoid potential complications such as the extra-articular puncture or iatrogenic neurovascular injuries. Moreover, they

Current and Future Issues in Hemophilia Care, First Edition. Edited by Emérito-Carlos Rodríguez-Merchán and Leonard A. Valentino.

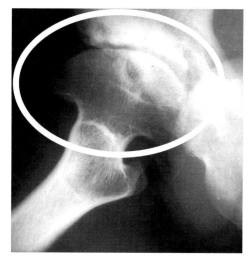

Figure 25.1 X-rays of a hip joint showing the final stage of hemophilic arthropathy (circle).

should be carried out in an operating theater under anesthesia. Therefore, shoulder and hip punctures should be strictly considered as orthopedic procedures. We usually perform articular punctures for the evacuation of acute and voluminous hemarthroses.

Hypertrophic hemophilic synovitis

When a joint fails to fully recover between bleeding episodes, the synovium hyperthrophies, and the articulation remains permanently warm and swollen. Chronic hemophilic synovitis is caused by recurrent hemarthroses into a joint, but the exact mechanism involved in the process is not well-understood. The pathogenesis is thought to be multifactorial, including general and local physical factors, chemical factors, and inflammatory factors [6,7].

Recurrent bleeding has a destructive effect on cartilage and bone. The recurrent hemarthroses stimulate the synovium which

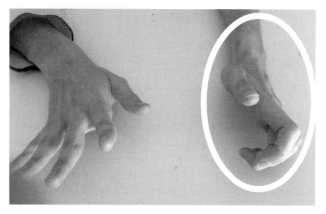

Figure 25.2 Some intramuscular hematomas can cause a compartment syndrome (circle) of the forearm (Volkman's paralysis). Compare with the contralateral non-affected upper limb.

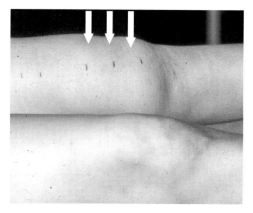

Figure 25.3 Clinical view of knee joint with intense hemophilic synovitis (arrows); compare with the healthy contralateral knee.

hypertrophies within the joint. This hypertrophied tissue occupies space and is likely to be injured and cause additional bleeding. This process initiates, and is responsible for, the chronic synovitis within joints of hemophiliacs (Figures 25.3 and 25.4).

Arnold and Hilgartner [8] found that hydrolytic enzymes increase in hemophilic synovium and joint fluid. Acid phosphatase and cathepsin D may play a role in maintaining a chronically inflamed synovium. The released enzymes responsible for the breakdown of protein have a destructive effect not only on free blood, but also on the synovium, cartilage, and bone.

On the other hand, synovitis causes painful movements. As the synovium increasingly becomes scarred, there is a gradual conversion from friable hyperemic tissue to fibrotic scar tissue. This process is the natural evolution of hemophilic synovitis. Increased intraarticular pressure, from the hemarthrosis and flexion deformity, may contribute to damage to the synovium and articular cartilage. In the hemophilic joint, the nutrition of the articular cartilage may be affected by the abnormal synovial fluid, immobilization of the joint, and the presence of fibrous adhesions.

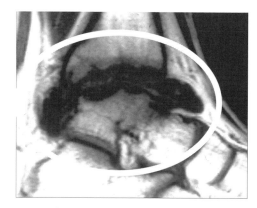

Figure 25.4 MRI of an ankle joint showing an intense degree of hemophilic synovitis (arrows).

Radiosynovectomy, chemical synovectomy and arthroscopic synovectomy

There are two basic types of procedures for synovial control: medical synovectomy and surgical synovectomy (open or arthroscopic). A medical synovectomy consists of the intra-articular injection of a certain material with the aim of stabilizing the synovial membrane of a joint. It is commonly accepted today that medical synovectomy is the procedure of choice, and that surgical synovectomy should be performed only if a number of consecutive medical synovectomies fail to stop or diminish the frequency of recurrent hemarthrosis. The main indication of medical synovectomy is chronic hypertrophic synovitis associated with recurrent hemarthroses that does not respond to hematological treatment. Medical synovectomy should be performed under factor coverage to avoid the risk of re-bleeding during the procedure. In patients with inhibitors, medical synovectomy can also be performed with minimal risk. In fact, the procedure is especially indicated in patients with inhibitors due to its ease of performance and low rate of complications.

Chronic hypertrophic synovitis is not associated with as much pain. The synovium is palpable as a soft tissue firmness whereas a hemarthrosis will have a fluid characteristic.

Before making the recommendation for a medical synovectomy, the diagnosis should be confirmed by radiographs, ultrasonography and/or MRI (Figure 25.4). The differential diagnosis between synovitis and hemarthrosis can be determined by ultrasonography and MRI. Radiographs should also be obtained in order to assess the degree of hemophilic arthropathy at the time of diagnosis. In many situations, synovitis and hemarthrosis occur together. At the knee, ultrasonography is very specific and reliable.

There are two basic types of medical synovectomies: chemical and radioactive. The materials most commonly used for chemical synovectomy are rifampicin and oxytetracycline. The radioisotopes currently used for radiosynovectomy are ^{90}Y, ^{186}Rhe and ^{32}P. Radiosynovectomy is the method of choice because it appears to be more efficacious than chemical synovectomy.

On average, radiosynovectomy has a 75–80% satisfactory outcome in the long term. From the clinical standpoint, such efficacy can be measured by the decrease in the number of hemarthroses, with complete cessation for several years in some cases. One should bear in mind that in 20–25% of cases, radiosynovectomy fails to control hemarthroses. In such cases, it can be repeated.

It is commonly accepted that the more severe the degree of synovitis, the more difficult it will be to remove the synovium by means of a radiosynovectomy. In fact, in cases where marked hypertrophy is present, it may be necessary to perform multiple consecutive radiosynovectomies, or even a surgical synovectomy. Chemical synovectomy with rifampicin can be repeated 10–15 times at weekly intervals. With radiosynovectomy, no more than three injections are advised at 3-month intervals. When repeated radiosynovectomy fail, a surgical synovectomy may be indicated.

The main complication of a radiosynovectomy is a cutaneous burn if the radioactive material is injected out of the joint. Another potential complication is an inflammatory reaction after injection; in such a case, rest and NSAIDs (COX-2) will control these symptoms.

The safety of radiosynovectomy still remains a cause for concern. Although several chromosomal studies demonstrated the possibility of transitory damage without malignant transformation [9,10], two cases of acute lymphocytic leukemia related to radiosynovectomy have been reported so far in children with hemophilia [11].

Radiosynovectomy is a very effective procedure that decreases both the frequency and the intensity of recurrent intra-articular bleeds related to joint synovitis. The procedure should be performed as soon as possible to minimize the degree of articular cartilage damage. It can also be used in patients with inhibitors with minimal risk of complications [12].

Surgical synovectomy may be done through an open technique or preferably by arthroscopic means. Arthroscopic synovectomy should be carried out through three or more portals in order to perform a "complete" synovectomy.

Articular contractures

Articular contractures in patients with hemophilia are the result of recurrent intra-articular and intra-muscular bleeding episodes. Approximately 50% of severe hemophiliacs have articular contractures angular deformity of $>10°$. The management of an articular contracture in a patient with hemophilia represents a major challenge. The problems that arise are complex, and require a range of knowledge from an understanding of basic biological events to fine details of surgical technique [13].

The treatments available are physiotherapy, orthotics and corrective devices, and surgical procedures. End-stage arthropathy of the knee is the most frequent cause of severe pain and disability in hemophiliacs. Some patients have such severe arthropathy that a total joint arthroplasty is required.

Advanced hemophilic arthropathy

Angular deformities

During childhood, the hyperemia produced by the hypervascularity of the synovium, commonly results in an asymmetrical growth of the epiphyses. At the knee it frequently results in a valgus deformity. At the elbow a hypertrophic radial head is typical, as is a valgus joint deformity at the ankle. Therefore, the hemophilic patient will present with a flexed and valgus knee, a valgus ankle with equinus position, and a flexed elbow.

Theoretically, osteotomies around the knee and ankle could correct these angular deformities. However, to date, these procedures have not been frequently reported in the hemophilia literature. In the authors' opinion, the attending physician should perform a

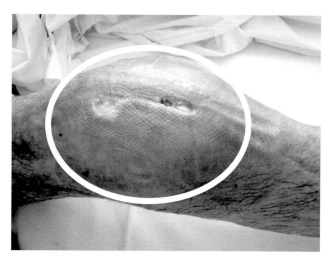

Figure 25.5 Clinical view (circle) of an infected total knee arthroplasty.

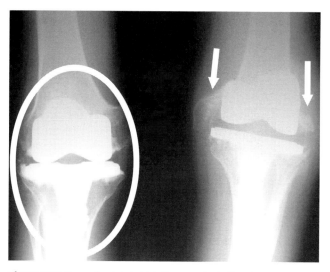

Figure 25.6 X-rays of an infected total knee prosthesis. Note the severe osteolysis of the femoral condyles (arrows) that caused loosening of the implant. Compare with the contralateral non-infected knee prosthesis (circle).

supramalleolar osteotomy (ankle) or a supracondylar osteotomy (elbow and knee), to prevent the degenerative changes that articular misalignment will produce in the future. Bone fixation of the osteotomy should be related to the patient's age (staples, wires, or a blade-plate).

Hemophilic arthropathy

The most important difference between hemophilic arthropathy and idiopathic osteoarthritis is the lack of correlation between pain and the radiographic signs. Many hemophilic patients will present with severe joint destruction over many years with little or no pain. The surgical treatment of hemophilic arthropathy is always symptomatic, and will depend on the degree of pain and functional impairment.

In its final stages in adult patients, a total joint arthroplasty should be performed especially at the shoulder, elbow, hip and knee [14–18] (Figures 25.5 and 25.6). At the ankle, arthrodesis should be recommended. Sometimes, multiple surgical procedures may be done in a single operative session. In young adults and adolescents there are some surgical techniques that can be performed other than total joint replacement including: resection of the radial head and partial synovectomy to improve painful elbow pronation-supination; knee joint debridement to delay a total knee replacement; osteotomies around the knee or the ankle for varus or valgus misalignments; and curettage and bone filling, with cancellous bone and fibrin seal, of some large subchondral cysts.

Other musculo-skeletal problems of hemophilia

Intramuscular hematomas

Muscle hematomas can occur in any part of the body; however the most common sites are the iliopsoas muscle [19] and the flexor compartment of the forearm. The former is commonly associated with a crural nerve palsy, the later with a compartment syndrome. An iliopsoas hematoma of the right side can mimic appendicitis

and care must be taken to avoid this misdiagnosis. Crural nerve palsy will be discussed below. CT scans and ultrasonography are the best ways to diagnose and to follow up an iliopsoas hematoma to full recovery.

With appropriate hematological treatment, the hematoma will be reabsorbed but there is a tendency for recurrence. Thus, treatment should be maintained for several weeks until the physician is assured of its total disappearance. Generally speaking any hematoma should be monitored and treated long-term with factor coverage. It is paramount to make sure that complete reabsorption has occurred to avoid the risk of the development of a pseudotumor. Another risk in immuno-compromised patients is hematogenous spontaneous infection of the hematoma.

Pseudotumors

Pseudotumor is a serious, but very rare, complication; it is a progressive cystic swelling involving muscle, produced by recurrent bleeding and accompanied by radiographic evidence of bone involvement (Figure 25.7).

Most pseudotumors are seen in adults and occur near the large bones of the proximal skeleton. However, a number develop distal to the wrist and ankle in younger patients before reaching skeletal maturity.

If untreated, proximal pseudotumors will destroy soft tissues, erode bone and produce vascular or neurological lesions. Surgical removal is the treatment of choice, but carries a mortality rate of 20%. Regression, but not a true cure, may occur with long-term replacement therapy and immobilization; this conservative treatment is not recommended except in patients with high-titer inhibitors in whom intervention is not feasible. In such cases, percutaneous evacuation of the pseudotumor and filling with a fibrin seal or cancellous bone, depending on the size of the cavity, may be carried out.

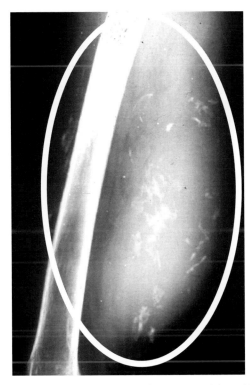

Figure 25.7 Pseudotumor of the thigh (circle) in a patient with hemophilia.

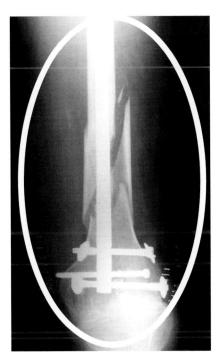

Figure 25.8 Femoral fracture of a hemophilic patient treated by means of a retrograde intramedullary locked nail (circle) with a satisfactory result.

Distal pseudotumors should be treated primarily with long-term factor replacement and cast immobilization as they may respond to many modalities of conservative management. The presence of one or more progressively enlarging masses in the limbs or pelvis of a person with hemophilia should raise the suspicion of a pseudotumor, although chondrosarcoma and liposarcoma have occurred in such patients. Ultrasonography, CT scan, MRI and vascular injections should be undertaken, but preoperative biopsy is contraindicated.

Fractures

Prompt recognition and treatment of fractures in hemophilic patients improves the chances of a successful outcome. The majority of fractures are caused by high energy trauma and are located at the supracondylar area of the femur. The early administration of factor concentrate in a quantity and duration sufficient to insure healing is important in the management of bone fractures in hemophilia. Correction of the hemostatic defect will allow an optimal orthopedic treatment which should follow common guidelines for the treatment of fractures in a non-hemophilic population (Figure 25.8).

Conclusions

Primary prophylaxis is paramount to try to avoid the development of hemophilic synovitis and arthropathy. The best treatment for synovitis is radiosynovectomy (rhenium-186 for ankle and elbows,

yttrium-90 for knees). With both methods (prophylaxis and radiosynovectomy) the development of severe hemophilic arthropathy can be delayed. In the final stages of hemophilic arthropathy in adult patients, a total joint arthroplasty should be performed especially at the hip and knee. Muscle hematomas can occur in any part of the body. Any muscle hematoma should be monitored and treated long-term with factor coverage to make sure that complete reabsorption has occurred to avoid the risk of the development of a pseudotumor.

References

1. Rodriguez-Merchan EC. Effects of hemophilia on articulations of children and adults. Clin Orthop Relat Res 1996;328:7–13.
2. Rodriguez-Merchan EC, Ribbans WJ. Editorial Comment. Symposium. Prevention and treatment of chronic hemophilic synovitis. Clin Orthop Relat Res 1997;343:2.
3. Valentino LA, Hakobyan N, Rodriguez N, Hoots WK. Pathogenesis of haemophilic synovitis: experimental studies on blood-induced joint damage, Haemophilia 2007;13(Suppl.3):10–3.
4. Roosendaal G, Vianen ME, van der Berg HM, et al. Cartilage damage as a result of hemarthrosis in a human in vitro model. J Rheumatol 1997;24:1350–4.
5. Stein H, Duthie RB. The pathogenesis of chronic haemophilic synovitis. J Bone Joint Surg (Br) 1981;63-B:601–9.
6. Rodriguez-Merchan EC. The destructive capabilities of the synovium in the haemophilic joint. Haemophilia 1998;4:506–51.
7. Rodriguez-Merchan EC. Effects of hemophilia on articulations of children and adults. Clin Orthop Relat Res 1996;328:7–13.

8. Arnold WD, Hilgartner MW. Hemophilic arthropathy. J Bone Joint Surg (Am) 1977;59-A:287–305.

9. Fernandez-Palazzi F. Treatment of acute and chronic synovitis by non-surgical means. Haemophilia 1998;4:518–23.

10. Dunn AL, Busch MT, Wyly JB, Abshire TC. Radionuclide synovectomy for hemophilic arthropathy: a comprehensive review of safety and efficacy and recommendation for a standardized treatment protocol. Thromb Haemost 2002;87:383–93.

11. Dunn AL, Manco-Johnson M, Busch MT, Balark KL, Abshire TC. Leukemia and P32 radionuclide synovectomy for hemophilic arthropathy. J Thromb Haemost 2005;3:41–2.

12. Rodriguez-Merchan EC. Synoviorthesis in hemophilia. In: Textbook of Hemophilia. 2nd edition. Lee CA, Berntorp EE, Hoots WK, eds. Wiley-Blackwell 2010, Oxford, UK, pp. 182–186.

13. Rodriguez-Merchan EC. Therapeutic options in the management of articular contractures in haemophiliacs. Haemophilia 1999;5 (Suppl. 1):5–9.

14. Löfqvist T, Sanzen L, Petersson C, et al. Total hip replacement in patients with hemophilia. 13 hips in 11 patients followed for 1–16 years. Acta Orthop Scand 1996;67:321–4.

15. Kelley SK, Lachiewicz PF, Gilbert MS, et al. Hip arthroplasty in hemophilic arthropathy. J Bone Joint Surg Am 1995;77-A:828–34.

16. Rodriguez-Merchan EC. Total knee replacement in haemophilic arthropathy, J Bone Joint Surg Br 2007;89-B:186–8.

17. Miles J, Rodriguez-Merchan EC, Goddard NJ. The impact of haemophilia on the success of total hip arthroplasty. Haemophilia 2008;14:81–4.

18. Rodriguez-Merchan EC. Total joint arthroplasty: the final solution for the knee and hip when synovitis could not be controlled. Haemophilia 2007;13(Suppl. 3):49–58.

19. Fernandez-Palazzi F, Rivas-Hernandez S, De Bosch NB, et al. Hematomas within the iliopsoas muscles in hemophilic patients. The Latin American experience. Clin Orthop Relat Res 1996;328: 19–24.

26 Perioperative Thromboprophylaxis for Persons with Hemophilia Undergoing Orthopedic Surgery

Gerard Dolan[1], Donna M. DiMichele[2], and Emérito-Carlos Rodríguez-Merchán[3]

[1]Nottingham University Hospitals, Nottingham, UK
[2]Weill Cornell Medical College, New York, NY, USA
[3]La Paz University Hospital, Madrid, Spain

Introduction

Severe hemophilia is characterised by hemarthroses. Although ankles, knees and elbows are most frequently affected, attention is now also being focused on the manifestations of hip arthropathy in this population [1]. Recurrent hemarthroses lead to chronic hemophilic arthropathy and may necessitate major orthopedic surgery including joint replacement at a relatively young age [2]. A recently published national experience documented that knee and hip arthroplasty accounted for 97% of such orthopedic procedures performed in persons with hemophilia [3].

In the non-hemophilic population, major orthopedic surgery is associated with a substantial risk of venous thromboembolism (VTE) [4]. This may have serious consequences and it has been estimated that such hospital-acquired venous thrombosis is the second most common medical complication of surgery, is a leading cause of prolonged stay in hospital, and is an important cause of increased mortality [4]. There is a large body of evidence that demonstrates that thromboprophylaxis substantially reduces the risk of deep vein thrombosis (DVT), pulmonary embolism (PE), including fatal PE, and consequently reduces the risk of short and long term morbidity and mortality [4,5]. This evidence has led to the widespread introduction of effective strategies to prevent VTE [4,6]. The applicability of such strategies during high risk orthopedic surgery in persons with hemophilia remains a matter of clinical uncertainty. Consequently, standards of practice vary among centers that specialize in the care of this unique population. This chapter discusses the scope of the problem of VTE in persons with hemophilia undergoing orthopedic surgery relative to the same in individuals without a hemorrhagic diathesis; reviews the published approaches to the use of prophylactic anticoagulation in the setting of an underlying severe bleeding disorder; and advocates for prospective data collection to better facilitate evidence-based decision making in this setting.

General prevalence of VTE after orthopedic surgery

Venous injury, venous stasis resulting from reduced mobility and hypercoagulability are among the factors cited as causing venous thrombosis after major orthopedic surgery. Deep vein thrombosis may start during surgery or may occur in the days or weeks following surgery [4,6]. The majority of thrombi are clinically silent and resolve spontaneously without treatment. Those that do present symptomatically usually do so within 3 months of surgery, but the majority present after discharge from hospital. VTE following surgery is one of the commonest reasons for readmission [4]. Since there is no accurate way of predicting which non-hemophilic individuals will develop symptomatic clots, thromboprophylaxis is recommended for all individuals undergoing major joint surgery.

Those individuals undergoing major joint surgery may also have additional risk factors for VTE and this may influence they type and duration of thromboprophylaxis. Such risk factors include advanced age and obesity. Therefore, a full clinical assessment is recommended before surgery [4,6] (Table 26.1).

Current and Future Issues in Hemophilia Care, First Edition. Edited by Emérito-Carlos Rodríguez-Merchán and Leonard A. Valentino.
© 2011 John Wiley & Sons, Ltd. Published 2011 by Blackwell Publishing Ltd.

Table 26.1 Reports of clinical episodes of venous thromboembolism in patients with hemophilia undergoing surgery

Report	No of surgical procedures	Outcome	Reference
Kasper et al. 1973	72	No clinical VTE	22
Djulbegovic et al. 1995	27	No clinical VTE	23
Manchini et al. 2004	93	No clinical VTE	24
Rodriguez-Merchan 2004	35	No clinical VTE	25
Miles et al. 2008	34	No clinical VTE	26

General principles of orthopedic thromboprophylaxis

There are various interventions that may reduce the risk of VTE. It is important to avoid dehydration and mobilise the patient as soon as possible after surgery. Mechanical methods include Graduated Compression Stockings (GCS), foot impulse devices and intermittent pneumatic compression (IPC) devices. These can be effective but the evidence for this is not as strong as for pharmacological treatment [4,6]. The choice of mechanical method should be based on the clinical situation and specific patient characteristics [6]. Currently, the most commonly recommended forms of anticoagulant prophylaxis are low molecular weight heparin (LMWH) and fondaparinux. Unfractionated heparin may be used in renal failure and several new anticoagulants demonstrate efficacy in preventing VTE [4,6].

In the absence of thromboprophylaxis, hip surgery is associated with a high risk of asymptomatic (40–60%) and symptomatic (2–5%) DVT [4,6]. The risk of fatal pulmonary embolism is 1:300. For hip surgery, prophylactic anticoagulation is recommended [4,6] There is less evidence for efficacy of non-anticoagulant methods such as GCS or IPC, and they are not recommended as the sole means of thromboprophylaxis for major hip surgery, except for individuals with a high risk of bleeding [4].

The risk of VTE with total knee replacement (TKR) is 40–84%, higher than with hip surgery [4,6]; however, the risk of proximal DVT is lower and the duration of VTE risk is shorter following surgery [4]. Pharmacologic anticoagulant thromboprophylaxis is recommended for TKR, but there is evidence for the efficacy of IPC as an effective alternative to anticoagulants in patients at high risk of bleeding [4,6]. The risk of VTE with arthroscopic knee surgery is considered low and, in the absence of other risk factors, anticoagulation is not generally recommended, However, if additional clinical risk factors are present, low molecular weight heparin or the equivalent should be considered [2].

There are fewer data on the risks of VTE associated with distal lower limb surgery including ankle surgery. The risk of VTE appears lower in this setting, with additional risk factors for VTE appearing to be advanced age and obesity. Studies have reported an incidence of between 0.52% in one population, some of whom may have received thromboprophylaxis, and 3.5% in another group

---

Box 26.1 Risk for VTE in surgical patients

Regard surgical patients and patients with trauma as being at increased risk of VTE if they meet one of the following criteria:

- Surgical procedure with a total anesthetic and surgical time of more than 90 minutes, or 60 minutes if the surgery involves the pelvis or lower limb
- Acute surgical admission with inflammatory or intra-abdominal condition
- Expected significant reduction in mobility
- Active cancer or cancer treatment
- Age over 60 years
- Critical care admission
- Dehydration
- Known thrombophilias
- Obesity (body mass index [BMI] over 30 kg/m^2)
- One or more significant medical comorbidities (for example: heart disease; metabolic, endocrine or respiratory pathologies; acute infectious diseases; inflammatory conditions)
- Personal history or first-degree relative with a history of VTE
- Use of hormone replacement therapy
- Use of estrogen-containing contraceptive therapy
- Varicose veins with phlebitis

CG92 Venous Thromboembolism – reducing the risk. National Institute for Health and Clinical Excellence.2010. http://guidance.nice.org.uk/CG92/Guidance.

---

that received none [7,8]. At this time, the benefit of thromboprophylaxis in the absence of other risk factors is not clear and it is not routinely recommended by some authorities. Elbow and upper limb arthroplasty may carry a risk of both upper limb and lower limb VTE. Again, risks depend on the type of surgery and concurrent risk factors [4,6].

VTE in persons with congenital bleeding disorders: considerations in the surgical setting

Individuals with inherited bleeding disorders are considered to have protection against VTE by virtue of their coagulation factor deficiency, and reports of spontaneous venous thromboembolism are rare [9,10]. However, there have been reports of VTE in association with surgery. In this setting, it has been postulated that the protection against VTE is mitigated by the administration of clotting factor concentrate, [9,11]. In patients without hemophilia, high Factor VIII (FVIII) levels are associated with a risk of VTE [12]. Furthermore, in non-hemophilic individuals, FVIII levels have been shown to double from baseline within 24 hours of surgery, with high FVIII levels persisting for several days [13].However for patients with hemophilia A, FVIII levels are usually carefully controlled, are not generally permitted to increase to levels noted in non-hemophilic subjects, and are not maintained in a high range for long periods of time. Before the advent of highly purified factor IX concentrate, individuals with hemophilia B were treated with prothrombin complex concentrates (PCCs) or activated PCCs (APCC). During this period, thromboembolic complications were frequently seen, particularly during surgery and in individuals with liver disease. In these cases, thrombosis was linked to the presence of activated clotting factors, particularly FIXa [9,14]. The introduction of highly purified and recombinant FIX concentrates was associated with a significant reduction in risk of thrombosis and since then, there have been very few cases of VTE associated with hemophilia B [14].

There are few data on the influence of various additional factors listed in Table 26.1 on the risk of VTE with hemophilia. Since underlying thrombophilia is listed as a risk factor for VTE in the general population, there has been interest as to whether the acquisition or inheritance of thrombophilia markers increases the risk of thrombosis for hemophilia. Several groups have studied the potential influence of markers such as factor V Leiden in ameliorating the bleeding phenotype of severe hemophilia, and have postulated that these markers may also increase the risk of thrombosis by "removing" any protection afforded by the coagulation factor deficiency [9,15]. Some small published series of patients found a milder clinical phenotype with less bleeding in patients who had inherited thrombophilic abnormalities [16,17]. However, this was not a consistent finding and other groups have found no similar significant effect [18]. There have been reports of thrombosis occurring in individuals with hemophilia and abnormalities such as factor V Leiden undergoing major joint surgery, but these events are rare and their significance is far from clear [19]. There have also been some suggestions that screening for thrombophilic abnormalities should be part of the preoperative assessment of hemophiliacs, but there is insufficient evidence to support this and much larger studies would be needed to clarify the value of this approach [19]. An increased risk for VTE has been reported for individuals with HIV infection [20] and recurrent VTE has been reported in an individual with severe hemophilia and HIV infection [21]. The mechanism for this increased risk is not clear but many potential explanations have been proposed. As such HIV infection should be considered in pre-operative risk assessment of such patients.

There have been reassuring data from several publications of the surgical experience with mostly major orthopedic surgery in primarily severe hemophilia A without inhibitors in which no evidence of clinical VTE was found [22–27]. These studies did not screen for asymptomatic VTE. Kasper et al. [22] reported a cohort of 72 hemophilic subjects undergoing a variety of major surgical procedures with no evidence of VTE; Dulbegovic [23] found no VTE in a series of 27 individuals undergoing orthopedic surgery. Manchini et al. [24] also found no evidence of VTE in 93 individuals with bleeding disorders after major orthopedic surgery, nor did Rodriguez-Merchan et al. [25] who reported their series of 35 individuals undergoing knee arthroplasty without clinical VTE. The study of Miles et al. [26] was the only one to report the perioperative use of mechanical thromboprophylaxis (GCS), and no VTE was found in 34 individuals post hip surgery. More recently Hermans et al. [27] reported their series of 29 major orthopedic procedures in which they used Doppler ultrasound to screen for VTE. Although no clinical VTE was observed, three patients (10%) were found to have distal DVTs upon screening. Two of these individuals had severe hemophilia A; no treatment was given and the DVTs did not progress. The third subject had mild hemophilia B and was treated with a short course of low dose LMWH. Additionally, an international survey of 160 hemophilia treatment centers was conducted to determine the incidence of VTE associated with the use of coagulation factor concentrates. Of 14,125 hemophilia patients treated, apart from the report of thrombophlebitis associated with central venous catheter (CVC) placement, only two cases of VTE were reported and only one was associated with orthopedic surgery [28]. This confirms the low risk of symptomatic VTE in persons with hemophilia who are undergoing surgery. More adolescents are now undergoing joint arthroplasty. Although their risk of VTE would not be expected to be increased compared with that of older adults in the absence of additional high risk factors unrelated to hemophilia, no specific published data exist to corroborate that assumption.

VTE in persons with hemophilia and inhibitors

The risk of VTE for persons with hemophilia and inhibitors undergoing orthopedic surgery deserves special consideration The use of bypassing agents in the non-surgical treatment of congenital hemophilia with inhibitors has been associated with thrombosis, including VTE [9]. In a review compiling the published reports of thrombosis associated with the use of the currently licensed APCC, Ehrlich et al. [29] reported an incidence of four thrombotic events per 100,000 infusions. This included three venous thrombotic events, one of which was associated with an indwelling central venous catheter. Other risk factors were found in the majority of patients experiencing thrombosis and high doses of the APCC appeared to be a particular risk. This report only included published reports of thrombosis but suggests that the risk of VTE with the currently licensed APCC is low. VTE has also been reported with recombinant activated factor VII (rVIIa). In a study of more than 6500 patients receiving rVIIa, only six cases of VTE were found. Some of these occurred in association with CVC use, or in the presence of other risks such as concurrent use of PCC or underlying pro-inflammatory conditions [9].

In the last several years there has been growing advocacy for the wider adoption of bypass therapy prophylaxis to prevent the crippling arthropathy associated with the long-term manifestation of inhibitors in individuals with hemophilia A and B and the use of joint arthroplasty as a "last resort" [30,31]. Nonetheless, with the availability of bypassing hemostatic agents, orthopedic surgery is now frequently considered in the case of severe arthropathy, and has been shown to be both safe and effective when managed by an experienced team of hematologists and orthopedic surgeons [32–35]. Most papers have focused on efficacy and the methods, if any, used for thromboprophylaxis are inconsistently described. VTE other than local thrombophlebitis [34] are also not reported. Once again, specific published experience in adolescents is lacking.

Thromboprophylaxis in hemophilic surgical patients: current practice

All candidates for major surgery should have a careful risk assessment in which the potential benefits of thromboprophylaxis should be balanced against any risks. A significant consideration is the risk of bleeding with anticoagulation, and most guidelines list bleeding disorders such as hemophilia as a relative or absolute contraindication to pharmacologic thromboprophylaxis [4,6]. Certainly, the administration of drugs that may cause bleeding to an individual already at risk of surgical bleeding may not be advisable. However, in modern clinical practice, individuals with congenital bleeding disorders are carefully managed to avoid low plasma levels of coagulation factors during and after surgery and so, the bleeding risks of administering prophylactic doses of anticoagulants may not be high. Consequently, this risk should be weighed against the person with hemophilia's risk of VTE in the setting of orthopedic surgery. In those that may be considered at very high risk of VTE, practical guidance as to which anticoagulant and timing of administration is very useful. Most existing guidelines concentrate on VTE risk assessment and management. This approach may not be applicable to patients with hemophilia and other bleeding disorders for whom, in the absence of other factors, the overall risk of thrombosis may be low and mechanical thromboprophylaxis may offer a better risk: benefit profile. Alternatively, for those individuals with multiple risk factors, coagulation factor deficiency may not protect against VTE, especially in the situation of surgery where therapeutic correction of coagulation occurs. Thus a detailed risk analysis for each individual patient is warranted.

There is currently a lack of consensus and no clear guidelines for thromboprophylaxis for persons with hemophilia without inhibitors. This is shown in three surveys of current practice in hemophilia centers. Hermans et al., in a multicenter European survey found that 50% of centers reported using anticoagulant prophylaxis after major orthopedic surgery [36]. Zakarija and Aledort reported that in 19 adult centers in the USA, 47% used postoperative thromboprophylaxis with either LMWH or fondaparinux [37]. Pradhan et al. surveyed 60 hemophilia centers in the USA and found that 67% of centers determined that hip and knee arthroplasty in persons with hemophilia warranted the use of thromboprophylaxis; of these, 55% reported that they provided such treatment. The majority used prophylaxis in defined circumstances, i.e. when plasma factor VIII/IX levels were above 1 U/dL. In this survey, among centers using thromboprophylaxis, 67% employed mechanical methods and 33% used anticoagulant or antiplatelet pharmacotherapy [38].

National consensus guidelines exist in the United Kingdom (UK) and Canada for the hemostatic management of orthopedic surgery using bypass therapy for persons with hemophilia and inhibitors [39,40]. Although all other aspects of surgical management are addressed in detail, there is no consensus opinion rendered on the approach to VTE prophylaxis in this setting [39].

The Canadian guidance document recommends that patients with inhibitors not be routinely given postoperative thromboprophylaxis, which could otherwise be considered for individuals with VTE risk factors in addition to the surgery itself (level 2C evidence) [40]. Whether this recommendation includes mechanical prophylaxis is unclear.

Conclusions

The published literature suggests that VTE is an uncommon occurrence in persons with hemophilia with or without inhibitors who undergo orthopedic surgery. Consequently, few adaptive guidelines exist for thromboprophylaxis in this setting. However, an interesting feature of the reports of absence of VTE in hemophilia has been that many patients undergoing major joint surgery are of a relatively young age. Age is a significant risk factor for VTE and the hemophilia population is aging. In future, there will be many more older individuals undergoing orthopedic surgery as a result of hemophilic arthropathy, and many will live long enough to need revision surgery. It is also likely that more surgical procedures will be performed in this aging population for degenerative arthropathy such as osteoarthritis. There is therefore an urgent need to understand more about the risk of VTE in hemophilia and other bleeding disorders and to establish risk assessment tools applicable to this population. It is also important to establish the most effective and safest way to manage any risk and it is likely this will only be achieved through prospective observational studies requiring wide collaboration.

References

1. Mann HA, Choudhury MZ, Allen DJ, Lee CA, Goddard NJ. Current approaches in haemophilic arthropathy of the hip. Haemophilia. 2009 May; 15(3):659–64. Epub 2009 Feb 27.
2. Rodriguez-Merchan EC. Management of musculoskeletal complications of Hemophilia. Seminars in Thrombosis and Hemostasis 2003;29:87–96.
3. Tagariello G, Iorio A, Santagostino E, Morfini M, Bisson R, Innocenti M, Mancuso ME, Mazzucconi MG, Pasta GL, Radossi P, Rodorigo G, Santoro C, Sartori R, Scaraggi A, Solimeno LP, Mannucci PM; Italian Association Hemophilia Centre (AICE). Comparison of the rates of joint arthroplasty in patients with severe factor VIII and IX deficiency: an index of different clinical severity of the 2 coagulation disorders. Blood 2009 Jul 23; 114(4): 779–84. Epub 2009 Apr 8.
4. Geerts WH, Bergqvist D, Pineo GF, Heit JA, Samama CM, Lassen MR, Colwell CW. Prevention of Venous Thromboembolism: American College of Chest Physicians Evidence-Based Clinical Practice Guidelines (8th Edition). Chest 2008;133:381S–453S.
5. Zhan C, Miller MR. Excess length of stay, charges and mortality attributable to medical injuries during hospitalization. JAMA 2003;290:1868–1874.

6. CG92 Venous thromboembolism – reducing the risk. National Institute for Health and Clinical Excellence. 2010. http://guidance.nice.org.uk/CG92/Guidance.

7. Mayle RE, DiGiovanni CW, Lin SS, Tabrizi P, Chou LB. Current Concepts Review: Venous Thromboembolic Disease in Foot and Ankle Surgery. Foot and Ankle International 2007;28;11:1207–1216.

8. Martin SL, Hardy MA. Venous thromboembolism prophylaxis in foot and ankle surgery: A literature review. Foot and Ankle J 2008;1;5: 4–13.

9. Franchini M. Thrombotic complications in patients with hereditary bleeding disorders. Thrombosis & Haemostasis 2004;92:298–304.

10. Stewart AJ, Manson LM, Dennis R, Allan PL, Ludlam CA. Thrombosis in a duplicated superficial femoral vein in a patient with haemophilia A. Haemophilia 2000;6:47–49.

11. Ritchie B, Woodman RC, Poon MC. Deep venous thrombosis in haemophilia A. American Journal of Medicine 1992;93:699–700.

12. O'Donnell J, Tuddenham EG, Manning R, Kemball-Cook G, Johnson D, Laffan M. High prevalence of elevated factor VIII levels in patients referred for thrombophilia screening: role of increased synthesis and relationship to acute phase reaction. Thrombosis and Haemostasis 1997;77:825–828.

13. Hermanides J, Huijgen R, Henny CP, Mohammed NH, Hoekstra JBL, Levi M, DeVries JH. Hip surgery sequentially induces stress hyperglycaemia and activates coagulation. Netherlands Journal of Medicine 2009;67:6:226–229.

14. Lowe GDO. Factor IX and thrombosis. British Journal of Haematology 2001;115:507–513.

15. Dargaud Y, Meunier S, Negrier C. Haemophilia and thrombophilia: an unexpected association! Haemophilia 2004;10:319–326.

16. Nichols WC, Amano K, Cacheris PM et al. Moderation of haemophilia A phenotype by the factor V R506Q mutation. Blood 1996;88:1183–1187.

17. Lee DH, Walker IR, Teitel J et al. Effect of the factor V Leiden mutation on the clinical expression of severe hemophilia A. Thrombosis and Haemostasis 2000;83:387–391.

18. Arbini AA, Mannucci PM, Bauer KA. Low prevalence of the factor V Leiden mutation among "severe" hemophiliacs with a 'milder' bleeding diathesis. Thrombosis and Haemostasis 1995;74:1255–1258.

19. Pruthi RK, Heit JA, Green MM, Emiliusen LM, Nichols JL, Wilke JL, Gastineau DA. Venous thromboembolism after hip fracture surgery in a patient with haemophilia B and factor V Arg506Gln (factor V Leiden). Haemophilia 2000;6:631–634.

20. Saber AA, Aboolian A, LaRaja RD et al. HIV/AIDS and the risk of deep vein thrombosis: a study of 45 patients with lower limb extremity involvement. American Journal of Surgery 2001;67:645–647.

21. De Gaetano Donati K, Tacconelli E, Scoppettuolo G, De Stefano V, Cauda R, Tumbarello M. Recurrent venous thrombosis in a patient with haemophilia A and HIV infection. Haematological 2002;87:(01)ECR04.

22. Kasper CK. Postoperative thrombosis in hemophilia B. New England Journal of Medicine 1973;2889:160.

23. Djulgobevic B. Lack of prophylactic anticoagulant therapy is not associated with clinical thrombotic complications in patients with hemophilia who undergo orthopaedic surgical procedures. American Journal of Hematology 1995;50;229–230.

24. Franchini M, Tagliaferri A, Rosetti G, Pattacini C, Pozzoli D, Lorenz C, Gandini G. Absence of thromboembolic complications in patients with hereditary bleeding disorders undergoing major orthopaedic surgery without antithrombotic prophylaxis. Thrombosis and Haemostasis 2004;91:1053–1055.

25. Rodriguez-Merchan EC. Total knee replacement in hemophilic arthropathy. Journal of Bone and Joint Surgery 2007;89:186–188.

26. Miles J, Rodriguez-Merchan EC, Goddard NJ. The impact of haemophilia on the success of total hip arthroplasty. Haemophilia 2008;14;81–84.

27. Hermans C, Hammer F, Lobet S, Lambert C. Subclinical deep venous thrombosis observed in 10% of haemophilic patients undergoing major orthopaedic surgery. Journal of Thrombosis and Haemostasis 2010;8:1138–1140.

28. Mannucci PM. Venous Thromboembolism in Von Willebrand Disease. Thrombosis and Haemostasis 2002;88:378–379.

29. Ehrlich HJ, Henzl MJ, Gomperts ED. Safety of factor VIII bypass activity (FEIBA): 10-year compilation of thrombotic adverse events. Haemophilia 2002;8:83–90.

30. Santagostino E, Morfini M, Auerswald GK, Benson GM, Salek SZ, Lambert T, Salaj P, Jimenez-Yuste V, Ljung RC. Paediatric haemophilia with inhibitors: existing management options, treatment gaps and unmet needs. Haemophilia. 2009 Sep; 15(5):983–9.

31. Rodriguez-Merchan EC, Quintana M, Jimenez-Yuste V. Orthopaedic surgery in haemophilia patients with inhibitors as the last resort. Haemophilia. 2008 Nov; 14(Suppl 6):56–67.

32. DiMichele D, Négrier C. A retrospective post-licensure survey of FEIBA efficacy and safety. Haemophilia. 2006 Jul; 12(4):352–62

33. Rodriguez-Merchan EC, Quintana M, Jimenez-Yuste V, Hernández-Navarro F. Orthopaedic surgery for inhibitor patients: a series of 27 procedures (25 patients). Haemophilia. 2007 Sep; 13(5):613–9.

34. Obergfell A, Auvinen MK, Mathew P. Recombinant activated factor VII for haemophilia patients with inhibitors undergoing orthopaedic surgery: a review of the literature. Haemophilia. 2008 Mar;14(2):233–41. Epub 2007 Dec 12.

35. Hedner U, Lee CA. First 20 years with recombinant FVIIa (NovoSeven). Haemophilia. 2011;17(1):e172–82.

36. Hermans C, Altisent C, Batorova A, Chambost H, de Mooerloose P, Karafolidou A, Klmaroth R, Richards M, White B, Dolan G. Replacement therapy for invasive procedures in patients with haemophilia: literature review, European survey and recommendations. Haemophilia 2009;15:639–658.

37. Zakarija A, Aledort L. How we treat: Venous Thromboembolism prevention in haemophilia patients undergoing major orthopaedic surgery. Haemophilia 2009;15:1308–1310.

38. Pradhan SM, Key NS, Boggio L, Pruthi R. Venous thrombosis prophylaxis in haemophiliacs undergoing major orthopaedic surgery: a survey of haemophilia treatment centres. Haemophilia 2009;15:1327–1353.

39. Giangrande PL, Wilde JT, Madan B, Ludlam CA, Tuddenham EG, Goddard NJ, Dolan G, Ingerslev J. Consensus protocol for the use of recombinant activated factor VII [eptacog alfa (activated); NovoSeven] in elective orthopaedic surgery in haemophilic patients with inhibitors. Haemophilia. 2009 Mar; 15(2):501–8. Epub 2009 Feb 1.

40. Teitel JM, Carcao M, Lillicrap D, Mulder K, Rivard GE, St-Louis J, Smith F, Walker I, Zourikian N. Orthopaedic surgery in haemophilia patients with inhibitors: a practical guide to haemostatic, surgical and rehabilitative care. Haemophilia. 2009 Jan;15(1):227–39. Epub 2008 Aug 25.

6   New Developments

27 New Technologies for the Pharmacokinetic Improvement of Coagulation Factor Proteins

Leonard A. Valentino

Rush University Medical Center, Chicago, IL, USA

Introduction

The control of bleeding in persons with hemophilia requires replacement of the deficient coagulation protein: factor (F) VIII for hemophilia A and FIX for hemophilia B. Purified plasma-derived (pd) FVIII and FIX concentrates became available in the United States in the early 1970s and 1992, respectively, and the first recombinant (r) FVIII and FIX products reached the US market in 1992 and 1999, respectively (Table 27.1). Existing treatment with FVIII and FIX concentrates effectively controls at least 90–95% of bleeding episodes in hemophilia patients (Table 27.1). Nonetheless, factor replacement therapy is complicated by inhibitor formation and the relatively short duration of hemostatic activity.

A key focus of current hemophilia research is the creation of bioengineered clotting factors that are less immunogenic and have increased protein expression, greater bioactivity, and longer biologic half-lives.

Less immunogenic drugs

Approximately 30% of patients with severe hemophilia A [1] and 3% of those with severe hemophilia B [2] develop alloantibodies that bind to functional domains on the FVIII or FIX molecule and inhibit or neutralize its function. Inhibitors are considered the most serious complication associated with the treatment of hemophilia because hemorrhages no longer respond to standard therapy [3]. Consequently, patients with inhibitory antibodies are at increased risk for serious bleeding and disability, particularly severe joint disease.

A variety of genetic and environmental factors are associated with inhibitor development. Whether the choice of factor con-

centrate contributes to the development of inhibitory antibodies remains unclear.

B-domain-deleted FVIII

Approximately 25 years ago, it was observed that removal of the B-domain of the FVIII molecule increased manufacturing yield without compromising biologic activity [4]. The first B-domain-deleted (BDD)-rFVIII concentrate was introduced to the US market in 2000, and both of the currently available products (Table 27.1) are produced using Chinese hamster ovary (CHO) cells. Use of a human cell line for the commercial production of BDD-rFVIII may reduce FVIII immunogenicity by virtue of its human pattern of posttranslational modifications, including glycosylation.

A BDD-rFVIII produced in a human cell line is now in clinical development [5]. Preclinical studies in animals found no toxic effects and normal in vivo FVIII survival and recovery. Characterization of protein function showed normal von Willebrand factor (VWF) and phospholipid binding, thrombin activation and generation, and activated FX (FXa) generation, and ratios of FVIII potency measured by 1-stage clotting and chromogenic assays were comparable to that of full-length rFVIII concentrates. Interestingly, the affinity of the human cell line-produced BDD-rFVIII for VWF appears to be approximately 40% higher than that of other rFVIII molecules. This characteristic may translate into a longer half-life for the investigational formulation.

Recombinant activated FVII

One proposed strategy for reducing inhibitor risk is to preferentially use recombinant activated FVII (rFVIIa), currently indicated for hemostasis in the presence of high-titer alloantibodies, to treat bleeding episodes in patients with hemophilia A or B without inhibitors. A pilot project by Rivard and colleagues prospectively evaluated the ability of rFVIIa (90 µg every 2 hours) to postpone FVIII exposure in infants with severe hemophilia A until after

Current and Future Issues in Hemophilia Care, First Edition. Edited by Emérito-Carlos Rodríguez-Merchán and Leonard A. Valentino.
© 2011 John Wiley & Sons, Ltd. Published 2011 by Blackwell Publishing Ltd.

Table 27.1 FVIII and FIX concentrates and bypassing agents available in the United States (Adapted from: Brooker M. Registry of clotting factor concentrates. Eighth edition. World Federation of Hemophilia. April 2008, number 6. © World Federation of Hemophilia, 2008.)

Product	Manufacturer/manufacturing site
pdFVIII concentrates	
Alphanate	Grifols; Los Angeles, CA
Hemofil M AHF	Baxter BioScience, Los Angeles, CA
Humate P	CSL Behring; Marburg, Germany
Koate CVI	Talecris; Clayton, NC
Kogenate FS	Bayer; Berkeley, CA
Helixate FS	Bayer; Berkeley, CA
Monoclate P	CSL Behring; Kankakee, IL
rFVIII concentrates	
Advate rAHF PFM	Baxter BioScience; Neuchatel, Switzerland
Helixate FS	Bayer; Berkeley, CA
Kogenate FS	Bayer; Berkeley, CA
Recombinate rAHF	Baxter BioScience; Thousand Oaks, CA
ReFacto*	Wyeth; Stockholm, Sweden
Xyntha*	Wyeth; Stockholm, Sweden
pdFIX concentrates	
AlphaNine SD	Grifols; Los Angeles, CA
Mononine	CSL Behring, Kankakee, IL
rFIX concentrates	
BeneFIX	Wyeth; Andover, MA

*B-domain-deleted rFVIII.

2 years of age, when the risk of inhibitor development may decline [6]. While the investigators found this approach to be successful in only three of 11 children, they speculated that outcomes may be improved with higher rFVIIa doses. New rFVIIa formulations that increase thrombin generation and have a longer half-life may provide a more effective and less immunogenic hemophilia therapy.

More potent, longer-acting FVIII and FIX concentrates

The half-life of FVIII and FIX ranges from 15.3 to19.7 hours [7] and 16.4 to 20.8 hours [8], respectively. The availability of more potent, longer-acting drugs would reduce the number of infusions needed to treat acute bleeding episodes and extend the time between prophylactic infusions.

PEGylation

Chemical modification by polyethylene glycol derivatives (PE-Gylation) is an established method for improving the pharmacokinetic (PK) and pharmacodynamic (PD) properties of therapeutic proteins. PEGylation enhances the biologic half-life of these proteins by (1) increasing their molecular size, (2) reduc-

ing their susceptibility to proteolytic cleavage and degradation, and (3) changing their surface-charge properties to interfere with receptor-mediated clearance processes [9,10]. Targets for PEGylation include amine groups of lysine residues and sulfhydryl groups of cysteine residues.

PEGylated rFVIII

In laboratory experiments, increasing the amount of PEG covalently bound by amine coupling to FVIII lysine residues resulted in a decrease in specific activity but had no impact on the biochemical and functional properties of the molecule [10]. Specifically, compared with unmodified FVIII, PEG-rFVIII had equivalent functionality in FXa activity assays, and electrophoretic analysis showed a similar pattern of bands: heavy chain fragments of 180 kDa and 120 kDa and a light chain fragment of 80 kDa.

A notable difference between the two FVIII formulations was that PEG-rFVIII was more slowly inactivated by thrombin than was unmodified rFVIII [10]. PK studies performed in hemophilic mice found the terminal half-life of PEG-rFVIII was more than twice that of unmodified rFVIII (4.9 hours vs. 1.9 hours), and the area under the curve (AUC) increased nearly 2-fold with the PEG-rFVIII formulation. In other animal experiments, infusion of PEG-rFVIII into mice deficient in both VWF and FVIII increased FVIII half-life to 8.3 hours compared with 2.3 hours for FVIII co-administered with VWF [11]. This finding suggests that PEGylation interferes with clearance mechanisms and may substitute for the formation of the VWF/FVIII complex.

Studies in mice and rabbits found that site-specific linkage of PEG extended the circulating half-life of BDD-rFVIII approximately 2-fold compared with wild type BDD FVIII [12]. While activation of the PEG-BDD-rFVIII was determined by the site of PEGylation, thrombin generation was normal.

In other experiments, covalent attachment of PEG to cysteine residues on rFVIII using a coupling strategy that specifically and homogeneously modified the molecule produced a conjugate structure similar to native rFVIII (Bayer Healthcare unpublished data). Administration of this PEG-rFVIII formulation to FVIII-deficient mice resulted in an increase in FVIII half-life and AUC compared with unmodified rFVIII. In tail-vein transection assays, a dose-dependent improvement in survival was observed in mice given the investigational agent, even when infusion occurred 96 hours prior to tail injury.

The effects of PEGylation on FVIII immunogenicity are unclear. While PEG itself is not antigenic, anti-PEG antibodies are generated when the linking chemistry results in bulky aromatic or heterocyclic groups in the PEGylated conjugate [13]. This finding suggests that the B-domain may be a potentially less immunogenic target for PEGylation.

PEGylated rFIX

Selective attachment of PEG to N-glycans of the activation peptide of rFIX has been shown to extend circulating half-life 5-fold compared with unmodified rFIX (76 ± 3 h vs. 16 ± 5 h). This observation suggests the possibility of once weekly dosing for patients on FIX prophylactic regimens [14].

PEGylated rFVIIa

A major drawback to the use of rFVIIa during acute bleeding events is the need to infuse every 2 to 3 hours when standard US doses of 90 µg/kg are used. Mean rFVIIa residence time was increased and higher levels persisted for several hours in rats injected with a liposome-encapsulated PEGylated rFVIIa molecule [15]. Furthermore, thromboelastography showed the PEG-rFVIIa induced faster clot formation and had higher clot stability than did commercially-available rFVIIa.

In other studies, PEG-rFVIIa was as effective as unmodified rFVIIa in activating FX in the absence of tissue factor (TF), and no significant differences were observed between the two products in TF-dependent FX activation at saturating concentrations [16]. At lower concentrations, PEG-rFVIIa activated FX at a slightly lower rate than did unmodified rFVIIa, but this decreased affinity for TF may not affect TF-driven FXa generation.

Polysialic acid

Chemical modification by polysialic acid (PSA) is another technique for enhancing the PK and PD properties of drugs. PSA is an anionic moiety that adds multiple negative charges to a protein, thereby changing its size, surface charge, and binding capabilities. As applied to FVIII, PSA modification may extend half-life without compromising functional activity [11], and it may protect FVIII from neutralizing antibodies [17]. Preclinical evaluation of a PSA-rFVIII compound is underway.

Albumin fusion

Albumin is the most abundant naturally-occurring protein in blood and has a circulating half-life exceeding 20 days [18]. Because albumin is not immunogenic, its fusion with a coagulation factor may be a viable technology for extending zymogen half-life without increasing inhibitor risk.

Constructs of the genetic fusion of rFIX and rFVIIa to albumin were expressed in mammalian cells and characterized after purification. In animals given rFIX-fusion protein (FP), in vivo FIX recovery, AUC, and terminal half-life were increased compared with unmodified rFIX, and in vivo activity was similar for both formulations [19]. In rats given rFVIIa-FP, half-life was extended 6- to 7-fold compared with wild-type rFVIIa. In vivo efficacy assessments in rats depleted of vitamin K-dependent coagulation factors showed near-equivalent results for rFVIIa-FP and rFVIIa immediately after drug injection [20]. When testing was delayed for 16 hours, however, rFVIIa-FP was more effective in correcting the clotting time.

Fragment crystallizable (Fc) fusion

Another strategy for improving the PK of coagulation factors is construction of fragment crystallizable (Fc) chimeric proteins. This process involves genetic fusion of the constant region of the immunoglobulin G (IgG) protein to a targeted protein [21].

In animal studies, the administration of rFIX genetically conjugated to the Fc domain of IgG_1 (rFIX-Fc) was associated with a longer circulating half-life than that of unmodified rFIX, with both formulations having comparable procoagulant activity [22]. In FIX-deficient mice and hemophilic dogs given rFIX-Fc, terminal plasma half-life was markedly increased compared with unmodified rFIX, and bleeding was prevented for an extended period of time. A phase I clinical trial of rFIX-Fc has been completed and phase II/III trials are underway.

Increased catalytic activity

Increasing the catalytic activity of a clotting factor molecule may extend its coagulation activity and biologic lifetime. In hemophilic dogs, a chimeric FIX made by replacing the first epidermal growth factor-like domain of canine FIX with that of FVII resulted in at least a 2-fold increase in clotting activity and a biological half-life equivalent to rFIX [23]. In other experiments, changing residue 338 in human FIX from arginine to alanine produced a molecule with approximately three times more clotting activity than that of wild-type FIX [24].

Aptamers

Chemically synthesized aptamers, selected nucleic acid binding species that have affinity and specificity for protein targets, have been shown to improve protein stability and PK properties [25, 26]. The first aptamer therapeutic approved for use in humans was pegaptanib, a targeted antivascular endothelial growth factor developed for ocular disease [27]. An aptamer antagonist of TF pathway inhibitor [28] is currently in preclinical development for use in hemophilia A [29].

Biosuperior molecules

A strategy known as DNA shuffling was used to develop a rFVIIa variant with enhanced ability to activate FX in the absence of TF, thus resulting in a more potent enzyme [30]. Modifications were then introduced to improve rFVIIa binding to platelets via the Gla-domain and to reduce rFVIIa thrombogenicity. Additionally, the number of N-glycosylations was increased with the goal of prolonging circulating half-life. In animal studies, one candidate molecule demonstrated significantly heightened TF-independent activity and improved PK parameters (e.g., longer half-life, larger AUC) and a greater in vitro thrombin burst than did commercially available rFVIIa. A phase I trial in hemophilia A and B patients with inhibitors is planned.

Also in development is a fast-acting rFVIIa analog with three amino acid substitutions that stabilize the molecule in its active conformation in the absence of TF, resulting in increased activity on the surface of activated platelets. Preclinical data indicate that compared with rFVIIa, the analog has a faster onset of action, forms a stronger clot that is more resistant to fibrinolysis, and exhibits an improved therapeutic window [31–33]. The first clinical trial of the analog administered to 24 healthy human subjects showed an increase in thrombin generation with a concomitant reduction in prothrombin time and activated partial thromboplastin time; plasma fibrinogen concentration was unchanged [34]. No serious adverse events, including thromboembolic events, occurred with the study drug, and no subject developed inhibitors.

Conclusions

The ultimate goal of hemophilia care is correction of the underlying genetic defect(s) through gene transfer or repair, but this goal is unlikely to be reached for many years. In the meantime, the development of bioengineered factor concentrates that are less immunogenic, more potent, and longer lasting than currently available products will represent a significant step forward in hemophilia management and will be welcomed by patients, their families and caregivers, and treating physicians.

References

1. Brackmann HH, Wallny T. Immune tolerance: high-dose regimen. In: Rodriguez-Merchan EC, Lee CA, editors. Inhibitors in Patients With Hemophilia. Oxford: Blackwell Science; 2002. p. 45–8.

2. Kessler CM. New perspectives in hemophilia treatment. Hematology/The Education Program of the American Society of Hematology. American Society of Hematology. 2005;429–35.

3. Leissinger CA. Prevention of bleeds in hemophilia patients with inhibitors: emerging data and clinical direction. Am J Hematol. 2004 Oct;77(2):187–93.

4. Toole JJ, Pittman DD, Orr EC, Murtha P, Wasley LC, Kaufman RJ. A large region (approximately equal to 95 kDa) of human factor VIII is dispensable for in vitro procoagulant activity. Proc Natl Acad Sci USA. 1986 Aug;83(16):5939–42.

5. Sandberg H, Agerkvist I, Lindner E, Martinelle K, Winge S. A novel recombinant B-domain-deleted factor VIII expressed in a human cell line. J Thromb Haemost. 2007;5(suppl 2): Abstract number P-T-027.

6. Rivard GE, Lillicrap D, Poon MC, Demers C, Lepine M, St-Louis J, et al. Can activated recombinant factor VII be used to postpone the exposure of infants to factor VIII until after 2 years of age? Haemophilia. 2005 Jul;11(4):335–9.

7. Vlot AJ, Mauser-Bunschoten EP, Zarkova AG, Haan E, Kruitwagen CL, Sixma JJ, et al. The half-life of infused factor VIII is shorter in hemophiliac patients with blood group O than in those with blood group A. Thromb Haemost. 2000 Jan;83(1):65–9.

8. Poon MC, Aledort LM, Anderle K, Kunschak M, Morfini M. Comparison of the recovery and half-life of a high-purity factor IX concentrate with those of a factor IX complex concentrate. Factor IX Study Group. Transfusion. 1995 Apr;35(4):319–23.

9. Turecek P, Scheifflinger F, Siekmann J, Váradi K, Matthiessen H, Weber A, et al. Biochemical and functional characterization of PEGylated rVWF. Blood. 2006;108(11): Abstract 1021.

10. Turecek P, Siekmann J, Gritsch H, Váradi K, Ahmad R-U, Muchitsch E-M, et al. In vitro and in vivo characterization of full-length rFVIII modified with PEG via coupling to primary amino groups. Blood. 2007;110(11): Abstract 3147.

11. Rottensteiner H, Turecek PL, Pendu R, Meijer AB, Lenting P, Mertens K, et al. PEGylation or polysialylation reduces FVIII binding to LRP resulting in prolonged half-life in murine models. Blood. 2007; 110(11): Abstract 3150.

12. Regan L, Jiang X, Ramsey P, Severs J, Sompalli S, Samuels N, et al. Biological activity of pegylated factor VIII. J Thromb Haemost. 2007;5(supplement 2): Abstract P-T-026.

13. Bailon P, Won CY. PEG-modified biopharmaceuticals. Expert Opin Drug Deliv. 2009 Jan;6(1):1–16.

14. Hansen L, Ostergaard H, Tranholm M, Agersoe H. The pharmacokinetics of a long-acting factor IX (40K PEG-RFIX) in minipigs suggests at least a once-weekly dosing regime. J Thromb Haemost. 2009;7(suppl 2): Abstract OC-MO-085.

15. Yatuv R, Dayan I, Carmel-Goren L, Robinson M, Aviv I, Goldenberg-Furmanov M, et al. Enhancement of factor VIIa haemostatic efficacy by formulation with PEGylated liposomes. Haemophilia. 2008 May;14(3):476–83.

16. Ghosh S, Sen P, Ezban M, Pendurthi UR, Mohan Rao LV. Activity and regulation of long-acting factor VIIa analogs. Blood. 2007;110(11): Abstract 3141.

17. Saenko EL, Pipe SW. Strategies towards a longer acting factor VIII. Haemophilia. 2006 Jul;12 Suppl 3:42–51.

18. Sterling K. The turnover rate of serum albumin in man as measured by I131-tagged albumin. J Clin Invest. 1951 Nov;30(11):1228–37.

19. Metzner HJ, Weimer T, Kronthaler U, Lang W, Schulte S. Genetic fusion to albumin improves the pharmacokinetic properties of factor IX. Thromb Haemost. 2009 Oct;102(4):634–44.

20. Weimer T, Wormsbacher W, Kronthaler U, Lang W, Liebing U, Schulte S. Prolonged in-vivo half-life of factor VIIa by fusion to albumin. Thromb Haemost. 2008 Apr;99(4):659–67.

21. Jazayeri JA, Carroll GJ. Fc-based cytokines : prospects for engineering superior therapeutics. BioDrugs. 2008;22(1):11–26.

22. Peters RT, Low SC, Kamphaus GD, Dumont JA, Amari JV, Lu Q, et al. Prolonged activity of factor IX as a monomeric Fc fusion protein. Blood. 2010 Mar 11;115(10):2057–64.

23. Chang JY, Monroe DM, Stafford DW, Brinkhous KM, Roberts HR. Replacing the first epidermal growth factor-like domain of factor IX with that of factor VII enhances activity in vitro and in canine hemophilia B. J Clin Invest. 1997 Aug 15;100(4):886–92.

24. Chang J, Jin J, Lollar P, Bode W, Brandstetter H, Hamaguchi N, et al. Changing residue 338 in human factor IX from arginine to alanine causes an increase in catalytic activity. J Biol Chem. 1998 May 15;273(20):12089–94.

25. Lee JF, Stovall GM, Ellington AD. Aptamer therapeutics advance. Curr Opin Chem Biol. 2006 Jun;10(3):282–9.

26. Yan AC, Levy M. Aptamers and aptamer targeted delivery. RNA Biol. 2009 Jul;6(3):316–20.

27. Ng EW, Shima DT, Calias P, Cunningham ET, Jr., Guyer DR, Adamis AP. Pegaptanib, a targeted anti-VEGF aptamer for ocular vascular disease. Nat Rev Drug Discov. 2006 Feb;5(2):123–32.

28. Waters E, Kurz J, Genga R, Nelson J, McGinness K, Schaub R. An aptamer antagonist of tissue factor pathway improves coagulation in hemophilia A and FVIII antibody-treated plasma. Blood. 2009;114: Abstract 544.

29. U.S. National Institutes of Health. First-in-human and proof-of-mechanism study of ARC19499 administered to hemophilia patients. Available at: http://www.clinicaltrials.gov/ct2/results?term= NCT01191372. Accessed: November 29, 2010.

30. Bornaes C, Jensen RB, Röpke M, Breinholt VM, Nygaard FB, Halkier T, et al. Improved procoagulant and pharmacokinetic properties of two novel recombinant human factor VIIa variants prepared

by directed molecular evoluation and rational design. J Thromb Haemostas. 2007;5(S2): Abstract O-W-038.

31. Holmberg HL, Lauritzen B, Tranholm M, Ezban M. Faster onset of effect and greater efficacy of NN1731 compared with rFVIIa, aPCC and FVIII in tail bleeding in hemophilic mice. J Thromb Haemost. 2009 Sep;7(9):1517–22.

32. Sorensen B, Persson E, Ingerslev J. Factor VIIa analogue (V158D/E296V/M298Q-FVIIa) normalises clot formation in whole blood from patients with severe haemophilia A. British journal of haematology. 2007 Apr;137(2):158–65.

33. Allen GA, Persson E, Campbell RA, Ezban M, Hedner U, Wolberg AS. A variant of recombinant factor VIIa with enhanced procoagulant and antifibrinolytic activities in an in vitro model of hemophilia. Arterioscler Thromb Vasc Biol. 2007 Mar;27(3):683–9.

34. Moss J, Scharling B, Ezban M, Moller Sorensen T. Evaluation of the safety and pharmacokinetics of a fast-acting recombinant FVIIa analogue, NN1731, in healthy male subjects. J Thromb Haemost. 2009 Feb;7(2):299–305.

35. Brooker M. Registry of clotting factor concentrates. Eighth edition. World Federation of Hemophilia. April 2008, number 6.

28 Current and Future Approaches to Gene Therapy in Patients with Hemophilia

Maria-Teresa Alvarez-Román, Monica Martín-Salces, Victor Jiménez-Yuste, and Emérito-Carlos Rodríguez-Merchán

La Paz University Hospital, Madrid, Spain

Introduction

Hemophilia treatment consists in replacing the missing coagulation factor (concentrates of clotting FVIII for hemophilia A and clotting FIX for hemophilia B). Current products used to treat patients with hemophilia are effective and safe. However, there are some disadvantages such as the requirement of frequent intravenous administration, the development of an immune response to FVIII or FIX (it occurs in about 20–30% in hemophilia A and 1–2% hemophilia B) and lingering concerns about potential viral contamination and transmission of other infectious agents. Besides, treatment is very expensive and there is a limited availability of these products to only 30% of the hemophilia population worldwide.

Gene therapy would allow continuous synthesis of FVIII or FIX proteins, eliminating the need for FVIII or FIX replacement therapy to correct the deficiency [1,2]. So, it could be an attractive alternative for the treatment of hemophilia and it may mean the cure for these patients.

The main challenges in this field are to maintain long-term therapeutic levels of clotting factor from the transgene and to avoid immune response against the transgene product.

Several vectors have been used in gene therapy such as virus (retrovirus, adenovirus and adeno-associated virus), plasmids and naked DNA. Numerous clinical trials have tested the safety and efficacy of these vectors in different animal models using mice, dogs and monkeys, but no sustained protein levels in human patients have been achieved.

Gene transfer vectors

In this section we will review the main viral vectors and the most important non-viral vectors.

Viral vectors

Currently, viral vectors provide the most effective means to deliver transgenes to recipient cells. Viral vectors are generated by deleting some or all viral coding sequences and replacing them with a promoter, which directly transcribes in the appropriate cell type, and by FVIII or FIX coding sequence. Currently there are a number of promising clinical trials that use viral vectors, nevertheless, the most important disadvantage of this approach is the toxicity of viruses [3].

Three types of viral vectors have been studied for hemophilia gene transfer purposes: two forms of retrovirus (the classical oncoretroviruses like Moloney murine leukemia virus and lentiviruses like HIV1), adenovirus and adeno-associated virus (AAV).

Retrovirus vectors

Retroviruses use reverse transcriptase to convert RNA into double-stranded DNA. The DNA is subsequently integrated into the genome of the host cell, which results in long-term expression, but it has some risk of insertional mutagenesis.

The surface of retroviruses consists of a lipid bilayer with membrane proteins, GP41 and GP120, both encoded by the *env* gene. The cells targeted by the virus are determined by these surface proteins. For gene therapy vectors, is common to replace the retroviral *env* gene with other sequences that change the tropism of the vector.

Oncoretroviruses and lentiviruses belong to retrovirus family and are widely used vectors for gene therapy in hemophilia.

Oncoretroviruses

Vectors derived from the Moloney strain of murine leukemia virus (MoMLV) were the first retroviral vectors used for gene transfer. The main advantage of these viruses is an efficient transduction and a genomic integration with persistent expression. However, MoMLV only transduces dividing cells, which is an important

Current and Future Issues in Hemophilia Care, First Edition. Edited by Emérito-Carlos Rodríguez-Merchán and Leonard A. Valentino.
© 2011 John Wiley & Sons, Ltd. Published 2011 by Blackwell Publishing Ltd.

disadvantage for particular tissues like liver. In order to increase the number of cells in division, several strategies have been used, for example partial hepatectomy, gene transfer into neonatal hosts whose hepatocytes are replicating, or transfer into livers of adult animals stimulated by growth factors. Another disadvantage of these viruses is the potential random insertion, so it could integrate in a tumor suppressor gene and subsequently cause oncogene activation as was observed in a gene therapy trial for X-linked severe combined immunodeficiency [4–6].

Lentiviruses

Vectors derived from lentiviruses have been developed recently. These vectors are able to transduce dividing and non-dividing cells. In addition, lentiviruses show a random integration pattern into open-reading frames of genes which seems to reduce the risk of insertional mutagenesis.

The first report using neonatal gene therapy to achieve long-term correction of hemophilia B in either mice or dogs was reported by Xu et al. in 2003. Hemophilia B dogs injected intravenously with retroviruses achieved 12–36% of normal canine FIX antigen levels, which correlated with improved coagulation tests results and a reduction in bleeding in 14 months of follow-up [7].

One trial with retrovirus vector in humans has been completed in hemophilia A. It's an open-label, multicenter, single-dose, dose escalation, phase I study. Thirteen subjects with hemophilia A received, by peripheral intravenous infusion, a retroviral vector (type C retrovirus, MoMLV) carrying a B-domain-deleted human factor 8 (hF8) gene. The results of this study showed clinical and biologic safety but, even though vector has been detected in peripheral blood mononuclear cells by PCR, FVIII activity unrelated to exogenous treatment was low and transient [8].

Adenovirus vectors

Adenoviruses can infect a wide variety of human cells, both dividing and non-dividing, such as hepatocytes, which they transduce efficiently. There are a number of trials demonstrating that gene transfer with adenovirus has achieved therapeutic levels of expression after delivery to liver or muscle. Nevertheless, expression usually falls over time, due to immunomediated destruction of the transduced cells.

One difference compared with retroviruses is that adenoviruses don't integrate into the chromosomes of the host cell, they act as an extra chromosomal or an episomal template and are lost during cell division, avoiding the risk of insertional mutagenesis. But as a result, these vectors have less durable effects than vectors integrated in DNA, like retrovirus vectors.

Another disadvantage of adenoviral vectors is that they characteristically cause an intense inflammatory response due to capsid protein. Inflammatory responses were greater with early-generation adenoviral vectors, because these vectors still contain most viral genes. This immune response contributes both to the toxicity (hepatotoxicity and thrombocytopenia), and to the short-term transgene expression. A serious and fatal toxicity has been reported in a recent trial, directly attributable to gene transfer with an adenoviral vector in an 18-year-old subject with ornithine transcarbamylase (OTC) deficiency who died after intrahepatic artery injection of an early-generation E1/E3/E4-deleted vector [9].

Now novel adenoviral vectors have been developed and designated as high-capacity adenoviral vectors (HC-Ad), devoid of all adenoviral genes ("gutless", helper-dependent or "mini-Ad" vectors). Production of such vectors requires a helper plasmid that supplies necessary adenoviral coding sequences. Three recent studies using fully deleted adenoviral vectors in hemophilia A and B dog models, suggest that the toxicity profile is dose-dependent and that adenoviral gene deletion reduces, but does not eliminate, vector toxicity. Future studies may be improved by minimizing the interaction between HC-Ad vector and the innate immune system, utilizing gamma globulins or targeted HC-Ad vectors that selectively transduce into hepatocytes and bypass the immune response [10,11].

Adeno-associated virus vectors

The genome of adeno-associated viruses (AAV) consists of two inverted terminal repeats (ITRs) and two open reading frames that code for the rep and cap proteins. Rep proteins that regulate AAV replication, and cap protein, form the protein coat of the virus. AAV are capable of infecting both dividing and non-dividing cells. In the absence of a helper virus, AAV integrate into a specific point of the host genome 19q 13-qter (AAVS1), persisting in the host cell in a latent state. This is an important advantage because AAV genome avoids retrovirus random incorporations into the genome, eliminating the risk of mutagenesis. These features make AAV a very attractive candidate for creating viral vectors.

Different serotypes of AAV have been identified, each one with distinct differences in tissue tropism. AAV2 is the most common serotype used for gene transfer studies and its cellular receptor is present on most cells surface. In 2002, Gao et al. reported two new serotypes (AAV7 and AAV8), with a great divergence in capsid proteins compared with AAV2, causing lower neutralizing antibodies than AAV2 and a higher activity. Another advantage of AAV8 is that they efficiently transduce following infusion into a peripheral vein [12].

AAV vectors are generated by retaining ITRs and removing the rest of the viral sequence (96%), including the rep gene. This improved efficiency correlated with increased persistence of vector DNA and higher number of transduced hepatocytes. None of serotypes have shown immunogenicity or hepatotoxicity.

The AAV expression cassette is approximately 5 kb, too small to accommodate the whole F8 cDNA. However, several groups have separately packaged F8 light-and-heavy-chain sequences because they are so big that they cannot be used together.

In preclinical studies, AAV has been well-tolerated with no effects on hematopoiesis, liver function, or other organs. Only in trials of patients with hemophilia B transient liver enzyme did abnormalities occur [13].

Numerous studies have been reported in different animal models using AAV vector-mediated gene transfer for treatment of hemophilia. Therapeutic levels of human Factor IX could be expressed and sustained in mice, dogs and non-human primates. None of these studies reported liver toxicities or abnormalities in serum chemistries [2].

Non-viral vectors

Because of the potential safety issues associated with viral vectors, an alternate approach is to use naked plasmid DNA. It is relatively simple and inexpensive to produce, and does not engender cell-mediated immune responses against the DNA vehicle that would limit the opportunity for repeated delivery [14].

There have been in recent years relevant advances in non-viral transfection that raise hope for considering this possibility. Several research groups are opting for this experimental alternative. There are at least three essential requirements for establishing an effective method of non-viral transduction of a DNA particle: protection against cell nucleases, nuclear location and very low toxicity [15].

A single clinical trial in humans using non-viral vectors has been conducted to date [16]. The study was designed as a single institution, open label phase I trial in which autologous fibroblasts that carried the gene that encodes FVIII protein were administered to six patients with severe hemophilia A. After isolation from a skin biopsy, patient cells were transfected with a plasmid encoding a human F8 cDNA ex vivo and selection for stable transfection was carried out. The transfected cells were then reimplanted into the peritoneal cavity of the patients by laparoscopy.

Although animal model studies using this approach were promising, data acquired from this phase I clinical trial showed only a modest and temporary indication of positive effects. Levels of FVIII activity increased in four of the six patients but sharply declined at 10 months. The treatment was, however, well-tolerated and leaves open the possibility of future attempts using more potent expression systems for the ex vivo transduction and selection process. An important step in advancing this treatment modality will be the determination of the cause for the apparent loss of expression over time. Possible obstacles to durable transgene expression include: senescence of the implanted cells, promoter inactivation, fibrosis around the transplanted cells and immune responses to the gene-modified cells.

Liras et al. have now initiated a preclinical gene therapy project using non-viral ex vivo transfection based on cationic liposomes carrying the F8 or 9 genes delivered into mesenchymal stem cells [17]. This particular strategy, and other non-viral gene therapy approaches in general, may represent an intermediate approach in which the levels and times of expression obtained are lower and shorter respectively as compared to viral vectors, but which provide a potential greater patient safety [15].

Future approaches

Nowadays, there are four active hemophilia gene therapy trials. Two trials using F9-containing AAV vectors for hemophilia B are enrolling subjects. The first one, with government identifier

NCT00515710, is a phase I trial in which patients are injected an AAV human F9 vector into the liver using a catheter inserted into the right hepatic artery. The second clinical trial, with government identifier NCT00979238, is a phase I–II trial in which patients over 18 years of age are injected an AAV vector into a peripheral vein (gene transfer). The third trial using F9-containing AAV vectors for hemophilia B is already terminated (phase I–II trial). Its identifier is NCT00076557, and also injects an AAV human F9 vector into the liver. The fourth trial, which is still recruiting participants, is a phase IIa trial using oral treatment with PTC 124 (Ataluren). The trial is investigating whether Ataluren can safely increase FVIII/FIX activity levels. Ataluren is used in 28-day treatment periods. The drug is orally taken three times per day with meals for 14 days at a dose of 10 mg/kg (morning), 10 mg/kg (midday) and 20 mg/kg (evening). Then, 14 days are without treatment. PTC 124 has demonstrated the ability to read through stop codons in animals. The clinical trials government identifier of this fourth trial is NCT00947193.

There are a variety of new strategies for delivering the missing clotting factor through ectopic expression of the deficient protein. One approach uses hematopoietic stem cells using either a non-specific promoter or using a lineage-specific promoter. The use of hematopoietic stem cells provides an alternative strategy to deliver the therapeutic coagulation factor. More recently, the generation of induced pluripotent stem cells from somatic cells holds the possibility of an alternative source of cells that can be genetically modified for the treatment of hemophilia [18]. An additional approach includes the expression of FVIII or FIX intra-articularly to mitigate the intra-articular bleeding that causes much of the disability for hemophilia patients.

Because activated factor VII can be used to treat patients with inhibitory antibodies to replacement clotting factors, preclinical gene therapy has been performed using platelet or liver targeted FVIIa expression. All of these newer approaches are just beginning to be explored in large animal models [19]. A safe cure of hemophilia is still the desired goal, but many barriers must still be overcome.

Conclusions

Hemophilia is an X-chromosome-linked recessive bleeding disorder resulting from an F8 gene abnormality in hemophilia A and an F9 gene abnormality in hemophilia B. Current products used to replace FVIII or FIX are effective and safe. Nevertheless, gene therapy offers these patients the possibility of achieving a sustained correction of the coagulation defect for their lifetime. Hemophilia has been considered one of the best candidates for a variety of novel gene therapies due to four main factors: (1) It is a monogenic disease involving a single protein. (2) Small increments of clotting factor levels (2–3%) have shown a substantial reduction in the clinical manifestations of the disease. (3) It is easy to measure the efficacy of clotting factor delivery through well-defined coagulation assays. (4) There are excellent animal models available. These four factors make hemophilia an excellent disease to investigate for gene therapy. One clinical trial of gene transfer in hemophilia has been completed (PTC 124) while others are still recruiting participants. Although these trials have demonstrated that gene therapy is feasible, there are still some obstacles to their clinical application.

References

1. Lillicrap D, Vandendriessche T, High K. Cellular and genetic therapies for haemophilia. Haemophilia 2006;12 (Suppl. 3):36–4.

2. Murphy S, High K. Gene therapy for haemophilia. Br J Haematol 2008;140:479–87.

3. Kay MA, Glorioso JC, Naldini L. Viral vectors for gene therapy: the art of turning infectious agents into vehicle of therapeutics. Nat Med 2001;7:33–40.

4. Van Damme A, Chuah MKL, Collen D, Vandendriessche T. Oncoretroviral and lentiviral based gene therapy for hemophilia: preclinical studies. Sem Thromb Hemost 2004;30:185–195.

5. Mitchell RS, Beitzel BF, Schroeder AR, et al. Retroviral DNA integration: ASLV, HIV, and MLV show distinct target site preferences. PLoS Biology 2004;2:E234.

6. Hacein-Bey-Abina S, Von Kalle C, Schmidt M, et al. LMO2-associated clonal T cell proliferation in two patients after gene therapy for SCID-X1. Science 2003;302:415–9.

7. Xu L, Gao C, Sands MS, et al. Neonatal or hepatocyte growth factor-potentiated adult gene therapy with a retroviral vector result in therapeutic levels of canine factor IX for hemophilia B. Blood 2003;101:3924–32.

8. Powel JS, Ragni MV, White GC 2nd, et al. Phase 1 trial of FVIII gene transfer for severe hemophilia A using a retroviral construct administered by peripheral intravenous infusion. Blood 2003;102:2038–45.

9. Raper SE, Yudkoff M, Chirmule N, et al. A pilot study of in vivo liver-directed gene transfer with an adenoviral vector in partial ornithine transcarbamylase deficiency. Hum Gene Ther 2002;13:163–175.

10. Chuah MK, Schiedner G, Thorrez L, et al. Therapeutic factor VIII levels and negligible toxicity in mouse and dog models of hemophilia A following gene therapy with high-capacity adenoviral vectors. Blood 2003;101:1734–43.

11. High K. Gutted adenoviral vectors in hemophilia A. Blood 2004; 103:751–752.

12. Gao GP, Alvira MR, Wang L, Calcedo R, Johnston J, Wilson JM. Novel adeno-associated viruses from rhesus monkeys as vectors for human gene therapy. Proc Natl Acad Sci USA 2002;99:11854–59.

13. Manno CS, Pierce GF, Arruda VR, et al. Successful transduction of liver in hemophilia by AAV-Factor IX and limitations imposed by the host immune response. Nat Med 2006;12:342–47.

14. Rick ME, Walsh CE, Key NS. Congenital bleeding disorders. Hematology Am Soc Hematol Educ Program 2003;559–74.

15. Liras A, Olmedillas S. Gene therapy for haemophilia. . .yes, but. . .with non-viral vectors? Haemophilia 2009;15:811–6.

16. Roth DA, Tawa NE, Jr., O'Brien JM, Treco DA, Selden RF. Non-viral transfer of the gene encoding coagulation factor VIII in patients with severe hemophilia A. N Engl J Med 2001;344(23):1735–42.

17. Picinich SC, Mishra PJ, Glod J, Banerjee D. The therapeutic potential of mesenchymal stem cells. Cell- and tissue-based therapy. Expert Opin Biol Ther 2007;7(7):965–73.

18. Takahashi K, Yamanaka S. Induction of pluripotent stem cells from mouse embryonic and adult fibroblast cultures by defined factors. Cell 2006;126:663–76.

19. Montgomery RR, Monahan PE, Ozelo MC. Unique strategies for therapeutic gene transfer in haemophilia A and haemophilia BWFH State-of-the-Art Session on Therapeutic Gene Transfer Buenos Aires, Argentina. Haemophilia; 2010;16 (Suppl. 5):29–34.

29 New Developments in Hemophilic Arthropathy

Emérito-Carlos Rodríguez-Merchán[1] and Leonard A. Valentino[2]
[1] La Paz University Hospital, Madrid, Spain
[2] Rush University Medical Center, Chicago, IL, USA

Introduction

Hemophilia is a congenital disorder due to the deficiency of clotting factors VIII or IX in hemophilia A or B, respectively that commonly results in musculoskeletal bleeding and orthopedic complications. With repeated bleeding, a target joint develops which is characterized by painless swelling and limited motion. Blood in the joint space provokes a proliferative disorder known as hemophilic synovitis. Overgrowth of the synovial membrane causes mechanical dysfunction and eventually destruction of the articular surface and underlying bone.

In patients with severe hemophilia, bleeding into the joints results in blood-induced synovitis, characterized by inflammation and proliferation of synovial cells which line the joint space. It has been suspected that one or more of the many components of blood, and/or in particular iron, are responsible for initiating and sustaining the inflammatory and synovial cell proliferation response associated with recurrent joint bleeds. Erythrocytes account for roughly 40% of the composition of whole blood and contain approximately 70% hemoglobin, an iron containing protein well known for its role in oxygen transport.

Hemophilia is a debilitating chronic disease with complications including bleeding episodes, hemophilic arthropathy, and hospitalization. Improving the circulating plasma coagulation factor activity is the mainstay of treatment. Adjunctive therapies directed to the joint itself may include joint aspiration or intra-articular corticosteroids, radiation, or sclerosing agents. Little is known about quality of life (QoL) in patients with hemophilia and whether there are differences based on hemophilia type and severity. A major goal in treatment of hemophilia is the avoidance of hemophilic arthropathy secondary to recurrent hemarthroses and chronic synovitis which decrease QoL. Recent studies indicate that only early prophylaxis can prevent arthropathy and improve QoL.

Bymans et al. analysed the baseline QoL in hemophilia patients receiving care at US centers [1]. Their preliminary data indicate reduced baseline QoL in hemophilia patients (HA more than HB) compared to healthy US males. Masurat et al. studied the physical findings of patients with severe hemophilia who received prophylactic treatment in order to investigate the efficacy of a long-term prophylaxis initiated early in life [2]. They found, consistent with previous studies, that early long-term prophylaxis prevents bleeding and should be strongly recommended in children with severe hemophilia.

Experimental studies on hemophilic synovitis and arthropathy

Valentino et al. investigated the impact of joint bleeding and synovitis on physical ability and joint function [3]. The hypothesis that a minimum number (three) of hemarthrosis negatively impacts on joint function and that this would be reflected in a decrease in physical performance of experimental animals was tested. Their results support the following conclusions: (1) hemophilic mice can be trained to ambulate; (2) acute hemarthrosis temporarily impairs their ability to ambulate; and (3) following recovery from acute injury, mice developing synovitis demonstrated inferior physical ability and joint function compared to mice not developing synovitis.

It has been shown that factor IX concentrate injected directly into the joint space protects hemophilia B mice from bleeding-induced joint deterioration in the absence of circulating factor IX [4]. The mechanism by which factor IX in extravascular sites contributes to coagulation is unknown but is currently under study. Protein and gene-based therapies taking advantage of factor IX local hemostasis may have an adjuvant role in avoiding blood-induced joint destruction. Sun et al. demonstrated that local intra-articular expression of factor IX from adeno-associated virus (AVV) vectors prevents the development of hemophilic arthropathy [5]. Intra-articular hemostasis and joint-directed gene therapy may ameliorate the events that lead to hemophilic joint destruction [6].

Clinical studies on hemarthrosis, hemophilic synovitis and hemophilic arthropathy

Klamroth et al. reported a successful angiographic embolization of recurrent elbow joint bleeds in five patients with severe hemophilia A [7]. Spontaneous joint bleeding leads to cartilage destruction and secondary arthrosis. In joints with high-grade arthropathy bleeding may not respond to replacement therapy. The reason may be the development of pathological reactive angiogenesis in the synovium. Bleeding from these vessels typically show a sudden onset of symptoms with massive soft swelling of the joint. Patients often perceive the bleeding as atypical. In joint bleeds not responding to replacement of factor VIII to normal levels, angiographic embolization might be considered as an option.

In a recent publication we stated that prophylaxis is an excellent method to control articular bleeding in hemophilia. However, some patients on prophylaxis still have articular hemorrhages and need radiosynoviorthesis (RS) [8]. We concluded that prophylaxis in severe hemophilia does not avoid articular complications. In our series 12% of patients on prophylaxis required radiosynoviorthesis versus 4% of patients treated on demand.

Inhibitors

Donfield et al. investigated the association between a history of inhibitors and delays in skeletal maturation in adolescents with hemophilia [9]. They have reported their results of an evaluation of skeletal maturation, pubertal progression and serum testosterone levels among participants in the Hemophilia Growth and Development Study (HGDS). The HGDS is a longitudinal study of 333 children and adolescents (mean age 12) enrolled from 1989–90 and followed 7 years. Eighteen percent (n = 60) had a history of inhibitors. The data indicate disruption of normal development for adolescents with inhibitors. This investigation opens an avenue of inquiry into another dimension of hemophilia-related morbidity, and underscores the importance of monitoring the growth and maturation of children and adolescents, particularly those with a history of inhibitors.

Marqués-Verdier et al. performed secondary prophylaxis with rFVIIa in a severe hemophilia A patient with anti-factor VIII inhibitors [10]. A 40-year-old severe hemophilia A patient with inhibitors had hemophilic arthropathy of the right knee and both

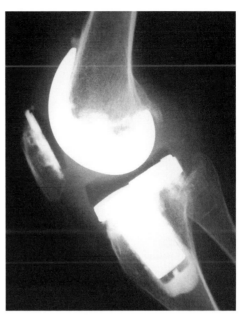

Figure 29.1 Total knee arthroplasty in a hemophilia patient with inhibitor due to severe hemophilic arthropathy. We used a posterior stabilized cemented autoplastic (cement with antibiotics) with a satisfactory result.

elbows. This case report indicates the benefit of secondary prophylaxis with rFVIIa in a patient with severe hemophilia A and inhibitors.

The development of factor eight inhibitor bypassing activity (FEIBA) and recombinant factor VIIa (rFVIIa) now allow for successful surgeries. Multiple surgical procedures were recently evaluated to identify current treatment strategies, clinical outcomes, and factors affecting success. Ninety patients with severe hemophilia and inhibitors underwent a total of 91 surgical procedures [11]. We performed 80 minor procedures and 11 major procedures. Minor procedures included 40 central catheter placements, 23 radiosynoviortheses, 12 dental extractions, two repairs of inguinal hernias, one lipoma removal and one cataract extraction. Twenty-seven of the 80 minor procedures were done with FEIBA and 53 with rFVIIa. Major procedures included three total knee arthroplasties (one bilateral) (Figure 29.1), one knee arthrodesis, one total hip arthroplasty (Figure 29.2), one ankle arthrodesis (Figure 29.3), one internal fixation of a femoral neck fracture (Figure 29.4), one appendicectomy, one craniotomy, one piloroplasty and one corneal transplant. Four of the 11 major procedures were done with FEIBA and seven with rFVIIa. FEIBA monotherapy was used in 31 surgeries; rFVIIa was used alone in 60 surgeries. Change from one bypassing agent to the other was used in one procedure. Eventual hemostatic control was achieved in all cases. One patient with inhibitor treated with rFVIIa had an arterial pseudoaneurysm after a total knee arthroplasty which was solved by arterial embolization, with an eventual fair result. We concluded that surgical procedures in hemophilia patients with factor inhibitors can be accomplished safely and effectively with

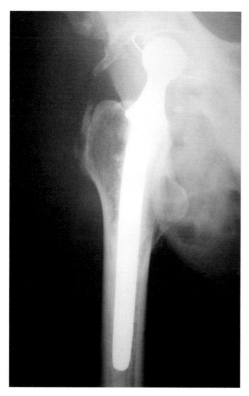

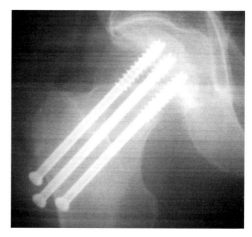

Figure 29.4 Bone fixation of an undisplaced fracture of the femoral neck in a hemophilia patient with inhibitor. Bone fixation was achieved by means of three cannulated screws implanted percutaneously, with an excellent result.

Figure 29.2 Total hip arthroplasty in a hemophilia patient with inhibitor. We used a Charnley cemented prosthesis (cement with antibiotics) with an excellent result.

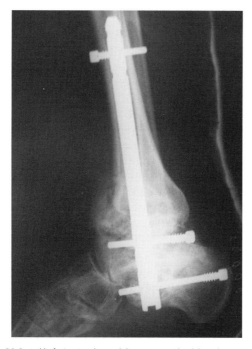

Figure 29.3 Ankle fusion in a hemophilia patient with inhibitor by means of a retrograde locked intramedullary nail. The result was satisfactory.

FEIBA and/or rFVIIa, although the risk of complications is higher than in hemophilia patients without inhibitors.

Negrier et al. reported on the use of FEIBA during surgeries in hemophilia patients with inhibitors to factor VIII and IX [12]. The purpose of their analysis was to evaluate various surgical cases for which FEIBA was used as primary hemostatic cover and to describe the treatment regimens employed in these surgeries. Data were collected from retrospective chart reviews and from previously published cases of perioperative FEIBA use in Europe and the United States. Data were collected for 102 procedures; in 95% of these cases, patients experienced excellent or good hemostatic efficacy. FEIBA was well-tolerated; thrombotic adverse events were reported in two cases and excessive bleeding in eight cases. The cases presented demonstrate that FEIBA is efficacious as a first-line hemostatic agent for surgical procedures. With FEIBA, a wide variety of major and minor surgeries are possible in patients with hemophilia and inhibitors. To further improve the knowledge on the use of FEIBA during surgery, an open label, prospective, non-interventional surveillance (SURF) was conducted through an internet-based data collection system. This international registry will provide a robust body of data for assessing safety and success rates of FEIBA during surgery. Additionally, the best practices in hemostatic management of hemophiliacs with inhibitors undergoing surgery should be progressively captured, as well as the surrogate laboratory markers which may correlate with clinical outcomes.

The economic benefits of knee surgery with rFVIIa in hemophilia patients with inhibitors have also been studied [13]. The goal of the research was to estimate from a US payer perspective the lifetime economic costs and benefits of different elective knee surgeries (total knee replacement – TKR, knee synovectomy, knee arthrodesis – KA, proximal tibial osteotomy and distal femoral osteotomy) with recombinant activated factor VII (rFVIIa) coverage in hemophilia patients with inhibitors. A literature-based Markov model was developed to compare the direct medical costs of two hypothetical cohorts of hemophiliacs with inhibitors and frequent bleeding episodes, one undergoing elective surgery and the other receiving non-operative care. Based on published evidence, surgery reduced the annual number of bleeding episodes at the affected joint from 11.9 to 1.6. Surgery costs included perioperative rFVIIa costs, inpatient and rehabilitation care, and repeat procedures. The cost of managing a bleeding episode was estimated at $15,298, based on the literature. The total cost of surgery is predicted to range from a low of $668,000 for KA to a high of $825,000 for TKR. However, it also reduced the lifetime number of bleeding episodes from 475 to 62 and resultant costs. Specifically, the cost savings due to the avoidance of bleeding episodes over the remaining patient's life varied from $3,462,000 for TKR to $3,489,000 for KA. Therefore, compared to usual care, surgery resulted in net lifetime savings (i.e., cost of surgery minus savings from bleeds avoided) ranging from $2,637,000 per patient for TKR to $2,821,000 for KA. The initial cost of surgery was offset in 5 to 7 years. Changes in assumptions regarding prophylaxis regimen, survival, baseline bleeding frequency, patient weight, HIV seropositivity, and rate of repeat surgery affected the results to various degrees. Despite high up-front costs, knee surgery with rFVIIa in hemophiliacs with inhibitors may be cost saving in just a few years. Future research should examine patient outcomes such as improved quality of life post-surgery.

A multicenter study (EUREKA) on primary total knee arthroplasty (TKA) using rFVIIa as first-line therapy in hemophilia patients with high responding inhibitors has been reported [14]. To date, 27 TKAs (13 right, 14 left) have been performed in 25 patients (21 severe hemophilia A, three severe hemophilia B, one mild hemophilia A) with an average age of 37 years (17–70 years) from 12 European hemophilia centers. Prior to TKA, inhibitor titers were 0–400 BU (median: 5 BU); in two cases titer was <1 BU, in 12 between 1 and 5 BU, and in 12 cases >5 BU. rFVIIa was used as bolus injections (BI) only in 12 cases or as continuous infusion after an initial BI in 15 cases. Antifibrinolytic drugs were used in 24 cases. Red blood cell (RBC) transfusion was required in 15 cases. More than 4 U RBCs were required in six patients including a bilateral TKA. Five bleeding complications were observed in the post-operative period; in one patient, high dose FVIII rescue treatment was used. Global assessment of hemostasis was excellent or good in 23 cases, fair in two cases and worse in two cases (one TKA infection requiring TKA revision; one arthrodesis for a post-traumatic fracture above TKA). Collection of additional cases from Europe is required to obtain a global view of TKAs performed with rFVIIa in inhibitor patients and will allow the comparison of primary KA in inhibitor patients versus non-inhibitor patients as well as of the two treatment regimens used.

Bonnet et al. performed an analysis of aPCC and rFVIIa in hemophilia patients with inhibitors undergoing major orthopedic surgeries [15]. A cost-minimization model was developed after review of published literature describing the recommended dosing regimens and doses used during major surgeries for FEIBA (preop: 75–100 U/kg; postop: 75–100 U/kg q8–12 h day 1–5, and 75–100 U/kg q12 h day 6–14) and rFVIIa (preop: 90 mg/kg; in-

traop: 90 mg/kg q2 h; postop: 90 mg/kg q2 to 4 h day 1–5, and 90 mg/kg q6 h day 6–14). Total drug cost was calculated under three different scenarios: use of FEIBA alone, use of rFVIIa alone and for a third case combining the use of rFVIIa pre- and intraop and FEIBA throughout a 14-day postop period. A typical 75 kg patient and US prices (AWP) were used for the calculations (FEIBA: $1.73/U; rFVIIa: $1.54/mg). The amounts of bypassing agents modeled were similar to cases described in the literature. Using FEIBA instead of rFVIIa would decrease total drug cost by more than 50% and generate savings of over $400,000 per major surgery. The sequential use of both bypassing agents would increase total drug cost by 9% when compared to FEIBA alone, but would remain more than 40% lower than rFVIIa alone. Univariate sensitivity analyses confirmed the robustness of the results. Due to the amount of drug used during major surgeries, cost remains a factor to be taken into consideration. The use of FEIBA alone or in an appropriate combination with rFVIIa emerged as cost-saving approaches.

The cost-effectiveness (CE) of aPCC versus rFVIIa in prophylaxis in hemophilia patients with inhibitors has also been investigated [16]. The safety and efficacy of prophylaxis in inhibitor patients has been reported in the literature. The objective of the study was to assess the CE of FEIBA (APCC) and rFVIIa when used in prophylaxis in inhibitor patients. The analysis assessing the CE of FEIBA and rFVIIa in prophylaxis was conducted from a payer's perspective, using data derived from the literature. Cost included prophylaxis drug cost, and effectiveness was measured by the reduction in number of bleeds/month. Prophylaxis regimens using FEIBA 75 U/kg every-other-day and rFVIIa 90 mg/kg daily were compared. Incremental CE ratios were calculated by dividing the difference in cost between the two prophylaxis regimens by the difference in their respective number of bleeds avoided/month. A 51 kg patient and US prices (2006 AWP) were used for the calculations (FEIBA: $1.73/U; rFVIIa: $1.54/mg). Based on the literature, the estimated numbers of bleeds avoided/month by switching patients experiencing 5.6 bleeds/month on average, to a prophylaxis regimen were 2.8 and 2.5 for FEIBA 75 U/kg every other day and rFVIIa 90mg/kg daily, respectively. The use of FEIBA 75 U/kg every other day as opposed to rFVIIa 90 mg/kg daily would generate savings of $49,082 per bleed avoided/month. Incremental CE ratios indicated that the prevention of bleeding episodes with FEIBA is a dominant strategy and is cost saving relative to rFVIIa. One-way sensitivity analyses confirmed the robustness of the results. The findings suggest that the prophylactic use of FEIBA is a cost-saving strategy relative to rFVIIa in the prevention bleeds in inhibitor patients.

Hemophilic arthropathy in the elderly patient

Over the last few years a progressive increase of life-expectancy, at least in high-income countries, has been observed in patients with hemophilia. However, elderly hemophiliacs have a lower health-related quality of life than that of the general male population.

Most common co-morbidities in the ageing hemophiliac are: cardiovascular diseases, HCV and HIV infection, cancer, arthropathy, inhibitors, and acute and chronic renal failure [17].

In a study performed in 45 Italian Centres, 6.4% of patients (210) were >65 years. Most of these elderly hemophiliacs (208/210) had arthropathy. They also had poorer physical functioning and reported lower health-related quality of life. Hemophiliacs had higher pain and higher orthopedic scores than that of the general male population. Forty-six per cent of hemophiliacs underwent total joint arthroplasty (versus 7% in general population) [18].

Miesbach et al. have analysed 29 patients age 55 and older (mean age 64). HIV infections were more frequent in the elderly hemophilic population (69% versus 0.6%). The prevalence of cancer was 28% (versus 5.2%) [19].

Definitions of elderly vary by country. In Europe elderly patients are those age of 75 years and older. However, in some special cases (HIV infection, hemophilia), elderly patients are those age 55 years and older. In Madrid we have 513 people with hemophilia (PWH) registered (2526 in Spain); 5.2% of them (27 patients) are of an age of 55 and older. The oldest patient in our center is 75 years old and underwent successful TKA at age 73 years.

In the elderly hemophilic with arthropathy we recommend the following sequential analgesia: paracetamol, COX-2 inhibitors, paracetamol plus codeine (or paracetamol plus tramadol), and morphine. Other conservative measures include rehabilitation and physical therapy; secondary prophylaxis; control of balance dysfunctions and risk of falls (adaptation at home). Management of osteoporosis (present in 25% of patients) is also important by means of physical activity, and supplements of calcium and vitamin D.

Hemophilic arthropathy in elderly patients eventually may require an orthopedic intervention. The most frequent are: arthroscopic joint debridement, total knee arthroplasty (TKA), ankle arthrodesis, total hip arthroplasty (THA), and fixation of fractures. Thromboembolic prophylaxis is performed in major orthopedic surgery in patients without inhibitors by means of subcutaneous LMWH 40 mg/24 h, after complete clotting factor correction (for 4–6 weeks). In major orthopedic surgery in patients with inhibitors (treated with bypassing agents) we use mechanical methods (intermittent pneumatic compression for 1 month). In minor surgery (arthroscopy) we only use early mobilization.

In persons with hemophilia, life expectancy is now approaching that of the general male population, at least in countries that can afford regular replacement therapy with coagulation factor concentrates. The new challenges are to provide optimal health care for this aging population of patients, who often present not only with the comorbidities typically associated with hemophilia, but also with common age-related illnesses such as cardiovascular disease and cancer [20].

There are no evidence-based guidelines for the management of common age-related conditions, which often require drugs that interfere with hemostasis, enhance the bleeding tendency, and warrant more intensive replacement therapy. Elderly patients with hemophilia affected by other diseases should be managed like their age-group peers without hemophilia [20].

Our recommended approach is to treat the diseases occurring in the elderly PWH as they would be treated in age-group peers without a bleeding disorder. Co-morbidity in hemophilia patients may lead to complex treatment. Coordinating care for these patients is paramount in Hemophilia Centers [21].

Conclusions

In this chapter the most recent developments on arthropathy in hemophilia patients with and without inhibitors are reviewed. Early long-term prophylaxis is strongly recommended in children with severe hemophilia. In joint bleeds not responding to substitution of factor VIII to normal levels, angiographic embolization might be considered as a promising therapeutic option. Recent data indicate disruption of normal development for adolescents with inhibitors. Some case reports indicate the benefit of secondary prophylaxis with rFVIIa in a patient with severe hemophilia A and inhibitors. Surgical procedures in hemophilia patients with factor inhibitors can be accomplished safely and effectively with FEIBA and/or rFVIIa, although the risk of complications is higher than in hemophilia patients without inhibitors. In elderly hemophilic patients with arthropathy, quality of life can be improved by adequate pain medication, rehabilitation, orthopedic interventions and adaptation at home. Little is known regarding the management of arthropathy in elderly patients, and hence further studies are warranted.

References

1. Byams VR, Soucie JM, Owens S, U.D.C. Project Investigators. Baseline quality of life (QoL) in hemophilia patients receiving care at U.S. Centers. J Thromb Haemost 2007;5 Supplement 2: P-S-142.
2. Masurat S, Weidenhammer A, Christensen K, Spranger T, Takla A, Auerswald G. Physical examination in patients with severe hemophilia under prophylactic treatment – efficacy of an early long-term prophylaxis ?. J Thromb Haemost 2007;5 Supplement 2: P-T-140.
3. Valentino LA, Mejia-Carvajal C, Hakobyan N. The impact of joint bleeding and synovitis on physical ability and joint function. J Thromb Haemost 2007;5 Supplement 2: P-W-107.
4. Sun J, Hakobyan N, Valentino LA, Monahan PE. Factor IX concentrated in the joint space protects hemophilia B mice from bleeding-induced joint deterioration in the absence of circulating factor. J Thromb Haemost 2007;5 Supplement 2: O-M-0135.
5. Sun J, Hakobyan N, Valentino LA, Monahan PE. Local intra-articular expression of factor IX from adeno-associated virus (AAV) vectors prevents development of hemophilic arthropathy. J Thromb Haemost 2007;5 Supplement 2: P-W-233.
6. Valentino LA. Blood-induced joint disease: the pathophysiology of hemophilic arthropathy. J Thromb Haemost 2010;8(9):1895–902.

7. Klamroth R, Essers E, Gottstein S, Wilaschek M, Oldenburg J. Successful angiographic embolization of recurrent elbow joint bleeds in five patients with severe haemophilia A. J Thromb Haemost 2007;5 Supplement 2: P-M-151.

8. Rodriguez-Merchan EC, de la Corte-Rodriguez H, Romero-Garrido JA et al. Radiosynoviorthesis is necessary in haemophilic patients despite prophylaxis. J Thromb Haemost 2007;5 Supplement 2: P-W-126.

9. Donfield SM, Lail AE, Gomperts ED, Hoots W, Berntorp E, Lynn HS. Association between a history of inhibitors and delays in skeletal maturation in adolescents with hemophilia. J Thromb Haemost 2007;5 Supplement 2: O-S-066.

10. Marquès-Verdier A, Chaleteix C, Soulié B, Bay JO. Secondary prophylaxis with recombinant activated factor VII (rFVIIa) in a severe haemophilia A patient with anti-factor VIII inhibitors. J Thromb Haemost 2007;5 Supplement 2: P-T-168.

11. Rodriguez-Merchan EC, Quintana-Molina M, Jiménez-Yuste V, de la Corte-Rodriguez H, Hernández-Navarro F. Surgery in hemophilia patients with inhibitors: results of 91 surgical cases. J Thromb Haemost 2007;5 Supplement 2: P-W-128.

12. Negrier C, Fleury R, Hoots KW, Gajek H, Berg R, Stephens D, Skvortsova E. The use of FEIBA during surgeries in haemophilia patients with inhibitors to factor VIII and IX. J Thromb Haemost 2007;5 Supplement 2: P-T-172.

13. Botteman MF, Ballal R, Joshi A. Economic benefits of knee surgery with recombinant activated factor VII in hemophilia patients with inhibitors. J Thromb Haemost 2007;5 Supplement 2: P-M-171.

14. Laurian YD, Tagariello G, Jimenez Yuste V, Kurth A, Lambert T, Nunez R, Goddard N, Morfini M. Primary knee arthroplasty using recombinant factor VII a (rFVIIa) as first-line therapy in haemophilia patients with high responding inhibitors. J Thromb Haemost 2007;5 Supplement 2: P-M-140.

15. Bonnet P, Yoon B, Ewenstein B, Wong W. Hemophilia patients with inhibitors undergoing major orthopaedic procedures: cost-minimization analysis of activated prothrombin complex concentrate (aPCC) and recombinant FVIIa. J Thromb Haemost 2007;5 Supplement 2:P-M-169.

16. Bonnet P, Yoon B, Ewenstein B, Wong W. Cost-effectiveness (CE) of activated prothrombin complex concentrate (aPCC) vs. recombinant FVIIa in prophylaxis in hemophilia patients with inhibitors. J Thromb Haemost 2007;5 Supplement 2:P-M-168.

17. Franchini M, Manucci PM. Co-morbidities and quality of life in elderly patients with haemophilia. Br J Haematol 2009;148:522–533.

18. Siboni SM, Manucci PB, Gringeri A, et al. Health status and quality of life of elderly persons with severe hemophilia born before the advent of modern replacement therapy. J Thromb Haemost. 2009;7:780–786.

19. Miesbach W, Alesci S, Krekeler S, Seifried E. Comorbidities and bleeding pattern in elderly haemophilia A patients. Haemophilia 2009;15:894–899.

20. Manucci PM, Schutgens REG, Santagostino E, Mauser-Bunschoten EP. How I treat age-related morbidities in elderly persons with hemophilia. Blood. 2009;114:5256–5263.

21. Mauser-Bunschoten EP, Fransen van de Pute DE, Schutgens REG. Co-morbidity in the ageing haemophilia patient: the down side of increase life expectancy. Haemophilia 2009;15:853–863.

30 Physiotherapy Evaluation and Intervention in the Acute Hemarthrosis: Challenging the Paradigm

Nichan Zourikian[1] and Angela L. Forsyth[2]

[1] Sainte-Justine University Hospital Center, Montreal, QC, Canada
[2] Hospital of the University of Pennsylvania, Philadelphia, PA, USA

Introduction

Physiotherapists are essential members of the comprehensive care team who focus on the musculoskeletal system and maximizing function in everyday life, work and play for persons with hemophilia (pwh). Over the years, the physiotherapist's role in hemophilia treatment has expanded [1] and all aspects of care continue to evolve over time. Both clinical and scientific research influences the decision-making in the care of our patients and as the body of evidence has grown, so has physiotherapy practice. It is no longer acceptable to rely solely on anecdotal evidence or to strictly follow the same physiotherapy methods from the past. Therefore, we must continually challenge the paradigm in order to achieve the most beneficial outcome with our patients. As we make clinical decisions, we must be mindful of the risk versus benefit model, always remembering to follow the advice of Hippocrates to, "first, do no harm." Thus, the current and future trend is to engage in evidence based practice thereby improving the quality of services that physiotherapists can offer the pwh. Because there is extremely limited, specific human research combining hemophilia and physiotherapy, the authors will cautiously attempt to extrapolate ideas, using our hemophilia expertise, from general literature, basic science, animal models and clinical observations.

This chapter will discuss several such instances, where physiotherapy practice in the care of the pwh is evolving, over time. While there are numerous noteworthy areas regarding physiotherapy and hemophilia that deserve attention, the authors have chosen to focus the concepts on topics surrounding the promotion of joint health. We will address key points in the physiotherapy evaluation and treatment of acute joint bleeding episodes, relating the current research to clinical practice. While much of this material may be deemed more helpful in the younger pwh, we are confident that this information may also be applied to those patients who are older and may already have some level of joint involvement. These are current issues that deserve consideration and development as we move toward future care standards. We can look back at past physiotherapy models and learn from them, but we must also evaluate practice strategies in the present and continually strive to improve the care provided to our patients.

Key concepts regarding the physiotherapy evaluation

As discussed by Beeton and Ryder [2], a comprehensive physiotherapy evaluation is crucial to guide treatment recommendations. There are several key components which include a subjective history, objective tests and measures, followed by assimilation of the information collected in these sections to help identify the key problems and set measurable goals. Finally, the development of a treatment plan that includes continual re-evaluation and modification of interventions based on patient response.

Although the subjective portion of the evaluation may intuitively seem elementary, in fact, obtaining a thorough, detailed patient history is irreplaceable. It is our role as the team member with musculoskeletal expertise to elucidate the potential causes of hemarthrosis and resultant synovitis. Although this concept has been mentioned in the past, as part of a comprehensive care team (CCT) approach [3], the authors feel that the physiotherapist must take a primary responsibility in this area. We should attempt to identify any causative factors present in the patient's daily life that are contributing to musculoskeletal complications. Only by asking focused questions of the patient regarding his daily routine, can we begin to understand the possible mechanisms that may initiate bleeding and perpetuate synovitis. Our goal is to be proactive, and to prevent or decrease future bleeding episodes.

Just as the subjective portion is important, it must be combined with the use of objective tests and measures. Physiotherapists as CCT members, are trained and should possess the necessary expertise to use multiple anthropometric measures such as postural and gait assessment, palpation, manual muscle testing and goniometry. In addition, there are validated scoring instruments, such as the Hemophilia Joint Health Score (HJHS) [4] and the Functional Independence Score in Haemophilia (FISH) [5]. During subsequent visits, these measures and scores may be used to track changes over time and help guide modifications in treatment.

Only through systematic completion and documentation in the medical record of these components, can physiotherapists create a comprehensive view of the patient's joint health and overall situation. This not only allows the physiotherapist to focus on treatment, but also on prevention of future complications.

Physiotherapy intervention for the acute joint bleed

Physiotherapy intervention during the acute bleeding episode is crucial. It is imperative however, as practice evolves over time, that physiotherapists look toward the available research to gain an understanding of what the best practices may be and the rationale behind them. The physiotherapist should understand the principles, pros and cons behind a chosen intervention and should also transfer this knowledge to the patient.

Initially, as the practice of physiotherapy in hemophilia treatment emerged, there was little if any direct hemophilia evidence upon which to make clinical decisions. Therefore, the practice of "cut and paste" from other medical conditions was often employed to provide intervention strategies. This was the starting point, in developing treatment for people with hemophilia; for instance, the recommendation of RICE (Rest, Ice, Compression, Elevation). This adjunct treatment was borrowed from the sports medicine field and first aid guidelines as a conservative treatment, carrying minimal risk, that is widely proposed following an acute musculoskeletal injury [6–14]. It was then incorporated into the standard of care in hemophilia for treatment of acute bleeding episodes. This is evident in many of the hemophilia publications that are commonly used today [15–19]. However, considering the current research and looking forward, we must ask ourselves if this borrowed, "as is," recommendation is in the best interest of our patients. When we extrapolate information available from other conditions, we should use our hemophilia expertise, weigh and tailor the information, to ensure that we are providing a greater benefit than risk to our patients. In this section, we will address the current and future recommendations on the use of ice and rest for acute hemarthroses in the pwh.

The use of ice in the acute bleeding episode

Factor concentrate infusion is the primary treatment for joint bleeding when it is available, while RICE is an adjunct treatment.

However, what happens in situations when factor is unavailable, infusion is delayed, or if a person has an inhibitor? Let us first address the use of ice (the "I" in RICE) in the acute bleeding episode. In the absence of clotting factor, is our traditional recommendation to use ice an appropriate initial treatment? To answer this question, let us consider some basic information regarding the typical use of ice following acute musculoskeletal injury to help address swelling, inflammation and pain.

It is essential to recognize that swelling and edema are two terms often used interchangeably. Practitioners may state their intent to address both with the use of ice. However, swelling is the general term, and can be caused by a variety of conditions such as infection, lymphatic obstruction, bursitis, hemarthrosis and edema. Following acute soft tissue injury, edema may be caused by the release of pro-inflammatory mediators such as histamine and prostagladins, which can increase permeability of the capillary walls and leakage of protein-rich fluid into the interstitial tissue space [20–22]. According to Knight, the majority of swelling following musculoskeletal injury occurs due to this extracellular edema and secondary injury, rather than hemorrhaging [20].

Secondary injury refers to collateral tissue damage following tissue injury, and is believed to be associated with the acute inflammatory response, hemostasis and local ischemia. Local ischemia is related to reduced blood flow as a result of the inflammation-induced blood viscosity increase and mechanical pressure from an expanding hematoma or edema [20,22–24].

Prompt application of ice following a soft tissue injury is believed to help reduce swelling due to edema formation by: lessening the pro-inflammatory response and by limiting secondary injury by reducing metabolic demands [20,22,23,25,26]. One must be aware that if protein leakage into the interstitial spaces and secondary injury has already occurred, ice will likely have little or no effect on edema reduction [20]. Furthermore, certain authors have concluded ice application can lead to increased edema in the injured and uninjured animal models [27–29].

However, is edema the predominant type of swelling present with a typical joint hemorrhage? A hemarthosis in pwh, without concomitant soft tissue injury, is believed to be caused by a lesion to the capillary rich lining of the synovial membrane [30]. This leads to an acute joint swelling, predominantly due to blood influx into the intra-articular space and to a lesser extent, associated acute synovial membrane inflammation which presumably may also lead to increased synovial fluid production. Therefore, this type of swelling is not primarily due to interstitial tissue edema, nor secondary injury to tissues and will not likely reap the similar, presumed swelling-reduction benefits from the use of ice.

Continuing to focus on the use of ice to control swelling, certain practitioners feel that ice causes vasoconstriction, thereby decreasing local blood flow to the injured tissue. However, there is no definite consensus within the literature regarding vasoconstriction, vasodilatation and blood flow changes in response to ice application. Depending on the author it may decrease [20,31,32], increase [32–36] or cause no effect [37].

Physiotherapists sometimes recommend ice application as a conservative, temporary pain-management modality for musculoskeletal injuries. In this situation, ice has been shown to be effective, partly due to a temporary decrease in nerve conduction velocity [38,39].

Although ice is commonly used in the non-bleeding disorders population to manage acute soft-tissue injury, does it have an effect on overall clinical outcome? Three review studies, published in the general literature, in 2004 [40,41] and 2008 [42], concluded there was insufficient evidence to suggest cryotherapy improved clinical outcome.

Notwithstanding the traditional use of ice for swelling, inflammation and pain, as hemophilia treaters, we must also consider the effects of cold on hemostasis. Localized cold application has been shown by numerous sources to impair in vivo and/or in vitro coagulation in both human and animal models, through a combination of prolonged bleeding time, decreased platelet aggregation, and impaired pro-coagulant enzyme activity [43–50].

We must therefore weigh the evidence-based benefits attributed to ice application against the potential short and long term risks to our patients with bleeding disorders. In a person with normal coagulation, the use of ice following an acute musculoskeletal injury may neither cause harm nor significant additional benefits over and above recommendations of **R**est, **C**ompression and **E**levation. Conversely, in the person with a coagulation disorder without factor or delayed access to factor replacement, ice application in the acute injury may potentially have deleterious effects. These effects may be manifested by a prolonged bleeding time, thereby leading to increased blood in the joint. As demonstrated by the literature, in human and animal models, blood exposure causes negative consequences on the cartilage and synovium [30,51–59,62,66].

What strategies can we employ in the acute bleeding episode to offer benefits while minimizing risk? In consideration of the above findings, instead of ice application to reduce acute intra-articular swelling, we can use a compressive wrap. The addition of ice to compression has not been shown to provide any additional effects over compression alone [40,41]. We can also combine compression with rest and possibly elevation to potentiate management of acute swelling. To treat the acute pain associated with a distended joint capsule, we can similarly use rest, compression, and elevation. Alternately, we might try safe modalities such as TENS (Transcutaneous Electrical Nerve Stimulation) or we could consult the hematologist for pharmaceutical management.

This idea of suspending the use of ice as described, prior to hemostasis being ensured, may be controversial. Nevertheless in this particular situation, the authors feel that the use of ice carries more potential risks overall, versus questionable benefits and therefore warrants additional consideration.

The rationale and advice on rest in the acute bleeding episode

If we address the "R" that stands for Rest in RICE, we may also need to re-evaluate the typical treatment pattern. There has been a shift in the pendulum regarding rest following an acute bleeding

episode. In the past, it was not uncommon for a child or adult, for example, to be hospitalized and confined to bedrest for weeks following a bleed. Movement and activity were severely curtailed, which led to a host of concomitant complications such as muscle atrophy and contractures. Currently, the trend regarding rest following a hemarthrosis seems to have moved to the other extreme. In an attempt to prevent these undesirable complications, early mobilization and return to pre-bleed activity frequently occurs very quickly. For example, the initial treatment of a hemarthrosis often follows this progression: factor, RICE and then return to physical activity, including full weight-bearing. This progression, with a significantly diminished rest period, is often completed as soon as hours following a bleed. The authors surmise that pwh may feel they are protected from further damage after they have received factor. However, is this progression appropriate for a person with hemophilia? Does a diminished rest period and early return to activity perpetuate acute and chronic synovitis, cartilage injury, re-bleeding, and ultimately lead to earlier development of hemophilic arthropathy?

If we examine the rationale behind this idea of adequate rest in prevention of re-bleeding, it leads us to both in vivo and in vitro research, in both human and animal models, examining the detrimental effect of blood in the joint and precarious wound healing in hemophilia. We can attempt to extrapolate these scientific research findings into our clinical practice and consider modifying our rest and return to activity recommendations to maximize the benefits while minimizing potential risks to our patients.

As illustrated in a review by Jansen et al., it should be noted that blood present in the joint is potentially destructive, and sets forth a chain of events whereby there are direct and indirect effects on both the synovial membrane and the cartilage, and whereby these processes influence each other [30]. When focusing on the effects of blood on the synovial membrane, it has been demonstrated, in the canine model, that once the intra-articular space is initially exposed to blood, acute synovitis occurs and can persist at least 16 days [55]. Similarly, in the murine mode, subacute and chronic synovitis has been shown to persist from 3 weeks to 17 months [54]. The acute, inflammatory phase following an injury, in this case post-hemarthrotic synovial inflammation, is a normal step necessary to begin the healing process [64]. However for various physiologic [52,65] and mechanical [54,58,66] reasons, the acutely inflamed synovium may develop into a chronic synovitis. This chronic synovitis is often a painless condition, and may occur as a progression from only one or several joint hemorrhages [51,52,54,58,66]. It has been shown that persistent synovitis, regardless of the presence of coagulopathy, will eventually lead to joint deterioration [30,51–54,58,65–71].

In addition to the link between blood exposure and synovitis, there are also damaging effects on the cartilage [54–59,66,72]. Blood exposure to cartilage causes the cartilage matrix to degrade and chondrocyte cells to die as demonstrated in canine, murine, rabbit and human models [30,55,56,59,66]. It has also been shown, in animal models, that there may be additional damaging effects observed in younger cartilage exposed to blood [57] or when weight-bearing occurs in the presence of intra-articular blood [54,58,59,66]. Furthermore, according to an in vitro human study on cartilage, the amount of blood present may be irrelevant, with even lower concentrations triggering damaging effects [62]. Additionally, even rapid clearance of blood from the joint, as shown in a canine model, cannot prevent negative effects on both the cartilage and synovial tissue [63]. Therefore, in addition to the effects of synovitis, direct damage to the cartilage also leads to joint destruction, and lasting damage may occur after only a single exposure to blood [56].

Impaired wound healing in hemophilia also impacts the synovium [60,61]. When hemostasis is impaired, synovial tissue may be predisposed to re-bleeding during the relatively fragile, wound healing phases of angiogenesis and fibroblast proliferation [73]. This re-bleeding may then cause more inflammation, thus risking perpetuation of chronic synovitis and joint destruction.

As we shape future practice, we must look to the research and achieve a balance between rest and return to activity. The goal is to prevent unwanted complications associated with rest, while minimizing re-bleeding, synovitis and cartilage damage. As physiotherapists, we cannot remove the blood, nor erase the damage it has already caused. However, we can intervene in several ways. For example, we can recommend activity modification and supervised, range-limiting bracing to minimize or prevent biomechanical microtrauma of inflamed or hypertrophied synovial tissue, thereby lessening the chance of re-bleeding. We could also try to protect the cartilage from further damage by limiting premature weight-bearing until clinical signs of synovitis have resolved. Patient education is a key component of physiotherapy intervention as we advise our patients on the rationale behind appropriate return and modification of activity. Using the evaluation methods previously described, the physiotherapist can continually monitor and modify treatment according to the patient's response.

Conclusions

Key concepts in the areas of physiotherapy evaluation and intervention in the acute bleeding episode have been addressed in this chapter. Using our clinical expertise in combination with extrapolation from the body of evidence, we are challenged to question and improve our current practice standards. As we look back at past physiotherapy models and learn from them, we must continually evaluate practice strategies in the present and look to the future with the goal of improving the services we deliver to our patients.

References

1. Brenda Buzzard B, Beeton K. (Editors). Physiotherapy Management of Haemophilia. London. Blackwell Science LTD; 2000.
2. Beeton K, Ryder D. Principles of assessment in haemophilia. In: Brenda Buzzard B, Beeton K. (Editors). Physiotherapy Management of Haemophilia. London: Blackwell Science, 2000; p. 1–13.
3. Ribbans WJ, Giangrande P, Beeton K. Conservative treatment of hemarthrosis for prevention of hemophilic synovitis. Clin Orthop Relat Res. 1997;(343):12–8.
4. Feldman BM, Funk S, Lundin B, Doria AS, Ljung B, Blanchette V. Musculoskeletal measurement tools from the International Prophylaxis Study Group (IPSG). Haemophilia 2008;14(Suppl. 3): 162–9.
5. Poonnoose PM, Thomas R, Keshava SN, Cherian RS, Padankatti S, Pazani D, et al. Psychometric analysis of the Functional Independence Score in Haemophilia (FISH). Haemophilia. 2007;13(5):620–6.
6. Järvinen TA, Järvinen TL, Kääriäinen M, Äärimaa V, Vaittinen S, Kalimo H, et al. Muscle injuries: optimising recovery. Best Pract Res Clin Rheumatol. 2007;21(2):317–31.
7. Ivins D. Acute ankle sprain: an update. Am Fam Physician. 2006;74(10):1714–20.
8. Lynch SA, Renström PA. Treatment of acute lateral ankle ligament rupture in the athlete. Conservative versus surgical treatment. Sports Med. 1999;27(1):61–71.
9. Schneider RC, Kennedy JC, Plant ML. Sports Injuries: Mechanisms, Prevention and Treatment. Baltimore: Williams & Wilkens 1985.
10. Southmayd W, Hoffman M. Sports health: The complete book of athletic injuries. New York: Quick Fox. 1981.
11. Kerr KM, Daily L, Booth L. Guidelines for the management of soft tissue (musculoskeletal) injury with Protection, Rest, Ice, Compression and Elevation (PRICE) during the First 72 Hours. London, Chartered Society of Physiotherapy, 1999. http://www.csp.org.uk/uploads/documents/ACPSMgl.pdf Accessed September 2020.
12. Sprains, strains and other soft-tissue injuries. American Academy of Orthopedic Surgeons website. Patient information library. http://orthoinfo.aaos.org/topic.cfm?topic=A00304 July 2007. Accessed August 2010.
13. Sprains, strains and tears. What they are and what to do about them. ACSM website. Public information brochure. http://www.acsm.org/AM/Template.cfm?Section=Brochures2&Template=/CM/ContentDisplay.cfm&ContentID=1541 Accessed August 2010.
14. Sprain: First aid. Mayo clinic website. Health information. http://www.mayoclinic.com/health/first-aid-sprain/FA00016 January 2010. Accessed September 2010.
15. Hemophilia in pictures. Educator's Guide. World Federation of Hemophilia publication, 2008, p 23.
16. Guidelines for the management of hemophilia. World Federation of Hemophilia publication, 2005, p 8.
17. Chandy M. Treatment options in the management of hemophilia in developing countries. World Federation of Hemophilia Publication, 2005, p 3.
18. All about hemophilia: A guide for families. Canadian Hemophilia Society publication, 2010, Ch 4.
19. Physical therapy in bleeding disorders. National Hemophilia Society publication, 2000
20. Knight KL. Cryotherapy in sport injury management. Champaign, IL. Human Kinetics, 1995.
21. Guyton AC, Hall JE. Textbook of Medical Physiology, 10th edn. Philadelphia. W.B. Saunders Company, 2000, p 397–98, 877.
22. Deal DN, Tipton J, Rosencrance E, Curl WW, Smith TL. Ice reduces edema. A study of microvascular permeability in rats. J Bone Joint Surg Am. 2002;84–A(9):1573–8.
23. Schaser KD, Vollmar B, Menger MD, Schewior L, Kroppenstedt SN, Raschke MJ, et al. In vivo analysis of microcirculation following closed soft-tissue injury. Orthop Res. 1999;17(5):678–85.

24. Merrick MA. Secondary Injury After Musculoskeletal Trauma: A review and update. J Athl Train. 2002;37(2):209–217.

25. McMaster WC, Liddle S. Cryotherapy influence on post traumatic limb oedema. Clin Orthop 1980;150:283–87.

26. Merrick MA, Rankin JM, Andres FA, Hinman CL. A preliminary examination of cryotherapy and secondary injury in skeletal muscle. Med Sci Sports Exerc. 1999;31(11):1516–21.

27. Farry PJ, Prentice NG, Hunter AC, Wakelin CA. Ice treatment of injured ligaments: an experimental model. NZ Med J. 1980;91:12–14.

28. Matsen FA, Questad K, Matsen AL. The effect of local cooling on postfracture swelling. Clin Orthop. 1975;109:201–6.

29. Lievens P, Leduc A. Cryotherapy and sports. Int J Sports Med 1984;5(suppl):37–9.

30. Jansen NWD, Roosendaal G, Lafeber FPJG. Understanding haemophilia arthropathy: an exploration of current open issues. Br J Haematol. 2008;143:632–40.

31. Ho SSW, Coel MN, Kagawa R, Richardson AB. The effects of ice on blood flow and bone metabolism in knees. Am J Sports Med 1994;22:537–40.

32. Meeusen R, Lievens P. The use of cryotherapy in sports injuries. Sports Med. 1986;3(6):398–414.

33. Lewis T. Observations upon the reaction of the vessels of the human skin to cold. Heart. 1929;15:177–208.

34. Clarke RSJ, Hellom RF, Lind AR. Vascular reactions of the human forearm to cold. Clin Sci 1958;17:165–79.

35. Fox RH, Wyatt HT. Cold-induced vasodilatation in various areas of the body surface of man. J Physiol. 1962;162(2):289–97.

36. Baker RJ, Bell GW. The effect of therapeutic modalities on blood flow in the human calf. J Orthop Sports Phys Ther. 1991;13(1):23–27.

37. Lee H, Natsui H, Akimoto T, Yanagi K, Ohshima N, Kono I. Effects of cryotherapy after contusion using real–time intravital microscopy. Med Sci Sports Exerc. 2005;37(7):1093–8.

38. Algafly AA, George KP. The effect of cryotherapy on nerve conduction velocity, pain threshold and pain tolerance. Br J Sports Med 2007;41:365–9.

39. Ernst E, Fialka V. Ice freezes pain? A review of the clinical effectiveness of analgesic cold therapy. J Pain Symptom Manage. 1994;9(1):56–9.

40. Bleakley C, McDonough S, MacAuley D. The use of ice in the treatment of acute soft–tissue injury: a systematic review of randomized controlled trials. Am J Sport Med. 2004;32:251–61.

41. Hubbard TJ, Denegar CR. Does Cryotherapy Improve Outcomes With Soft Tissue Injury? J Athl Train. 2004 Sep;39(3):278–9.

42. Collins NC. Is ice right? Does cryotherapy improve outcome for acute soft tissue injury? Emerg Med J. 2008;25:65–8.

43. Sutor AH, Bowie EJW, Owen CA Jr. Effect of cold on bleeding: Hippocrates vindicated. Lancet. 1970;2(7682):1084.

44. Bahn SL, Mursch PI. The effects of cold on hemostasis. Oral Surg. 1980;49(4) 294–300.

45. Kattlove H, Alexander B. Effect of cold on bleeding. The Lancet. 1970;2(7687):1359.

46. Wolberg AS, Meng ZH, Monroe DM 3rd, Hoffman M. A systematic evaluation of the effect of temperature on coagulation enzyme activity and platelet function. J Trauma. 2004;56(6):1221–8.

47. Copley AL, Lalich JJ. Bleeding time, Lymph time, and clot resistance in men. J Clin Invest. 1942;21:145.

48. Rundgren M, Engstrom M. A thromboelastometric evaluation of the effects of hypothermia on the coagulation system. Anesthes Analg. 2008;107:1465–8.

49. Valeri CR, MacGregor H, Cassidy G, Tinney R, Pompei F. Effects of temperature on bleeding and clotting time in normal male and female volunteers. Crit Care Med. 1995;4:698–704.

50. Niemczura RT, DePalma RG. Optimum compress temperature for wound hemostasis. J Surg Res. 1979;26(5):570–73.

51. Valentino LA, Hakobyan N, Kazarian T, Jabbar KJ, Jabbar AA. Experimental haemophilic synovitis: rationale and development of a murine model of human factor VIII deficiency. Haemophilia. 2004;10:280–87.

52. Rodriguez-Merchan EC. Haemophilic synovitis: basic concepts. Haemophilia, 2007;13(Suppl. 3):1–3.

53. Hoots WK, Rodriguez N, Boggio L, Valentino LA. Pathogenesis of haemophilia synovitis: clinical aspects. Haemophilia. 2007;13(Suppl 3):4–9.

54. Hakobyan N, Kazarian T, Valentino LA. Synovitis in a murine model of human factor VIII deficiency. Haemophilia. 2005;11:227–32.

55. Roosendaal G, Tekoppele JM, Vianen ME, et al. Blood-induced joint damage: a canine in vivo study. Arthrit Rheum. 1999;42:1033–9.

56. Roosendaal G, Vianen ME, Marx JJ, van den Berg HM, Lafeber FP, Bijlsma JW. Blood-induced joint damage: a human in vitro study. Arthrit Rheum. 1999;42:1025–32.

57. Hooiveld, MJ, Roosendaal G, Vianen ME, et al. (2003) Immature articular cartilage is more susceptible to blood-induced damage than mature articular cartilage: an in vivo animal study. Arthrit Rheum. 2003;48:396–403.

58. Hooiveld MJ, Roosendaal G, Jacobs KM, et al. Initiation of degenerative joint damage by experimental bleeding combined with loading of the joint: a possible mechanism of hemophilic arthropathy. Arthrit Rheum. 2004;50:2024–31.

59. Ravanbod A, Torkman G, Esteki A. Biotribological and biomechanical changes after experimental haemarthrosis in the rabbit knee. Haemophilia. Online article. 2010;1–10. Accessed September 2010.

60. Hoffman M and Monroe DM. Wound healing in haemophilia, breaking the vicious cycle. Haemophilia 2010;16(suppl 3):13–18.

61. Monroe DM, Mackman N, Hoffman M. Wound healing in hemophilia B mice and low tissue factor mice. Thromb Res. 2010;125 Suppl 1:S74–7. Epub 2010 Feb 19.

62. Jansen NW, Roosendaal G, Bijlsma JW, DeGroot J, Lafeber FP. Exposure of human cartilage tissue to low concentrations of blood for a short period of time leads to prolonged cartilage damage: an in vitro study. Arthrit Rheum. 2007;56:199–207.

63. Jansen NWD, Roosendaal G, Wenting MJG, et al. Very rapid clearance after a joint bleed in the canine knee can not prevent adverse effects on cartilage and synovial tissue. Osteoarthrit Cartil. 2009;17(4):433–40.

64. Schmidt, CW. Critical care – applying genomics to inflammation outcomes. Environ Health Perspect 2005;(113) 12; 817–21.

65. Valentino LA, Hakobyan N, Rodriguez N, Hoots WK. Pathogenesis of haemophilic synovitis: experimental studies on blood-induced joint damage. Haemophilia. 2007;13(Suppl. 3):10–13.

66. Mejia-Carvajal C, Hakobyan N, Enockson C, Valentino LA. The impact of joint bleeding and synovitis on physical ability and joint function in a murine model of haemophilic synovitis. Haemophilia. 2008;14(1):119–26.

67. Clement JP 4th, Kassarjian A, Palmer WE. Synovial inflammatory processes in the hand. Eur J Radiol. 2005;56(3):307–18.

68. Ehrlich GE Osteoarthritis beginning with inflammation. Definitions and correlations. JAMA. 1975;232(2):157–9.

69. Shay AK, Bliven ML, Scampoli DN, Otterness IG, Milici AJ. Effects of exercise on synovium and cartilage from normal and inflamed knees. Rheumatol Int. 1995;14(5):183–9.

70. Kim DH, Gambardella RA, Elattrache NS, Yocum LA, Jobe FW. Arthroscopic treatment of posterolateral elbow impingement from lateral synovial plicae in throwing athletes and golfers. Am J Sports Med. 2006;34(3):438–44. Epub 2005 Dec 19.

71. Robinson P, White LM. Soft-tissue and osseous impingement syndromes of the ankle: role of imaging in diagnosis and management. Radiographics. 2002;22(6):1457–69.

72. Hooiveld M, Roosendaal G, Vianen M, van den BM, Bijlsma J, Lafeber F. Blood-induced joint damage: long-term effects in vitro and in vivo. J Rheumatol 2003;30:339–44.

73. Hoffman M. Animal models of bleeding and tissue repair. Haemophilia. State of the Art. Vol 14. July 2008.

31 Laboratory Assays to Predict Response to Bypassing Agents

Benny Sørensen[1] and Claude Negrier[2]

[1] Haemostasis Research Unit, Guy's and St Thomas' NHS Foundation Trust, London, UK
[2] Edouard Herriot University Hospital, Lyon, France

Introduction

As of today, development of high titer inhibitors may be considered the most serious complication of hemophilia treatment. The presence of neutralizing antibodies increases the risk of serious and potential hazardous bleeding events, such as intracranial hemorrhage. Furthermore, patients with persistent inhibitors are prone to develop more pronounced joint damage and long-term debilitation. Finally, the need for elective or acute surgery requires special attention to prevent potentially life-threatening hemostatic imbalance. Arrest of bleeding, prophylaxis and maintaining hemostasis require prompt and correct use of bypassing agents, such as plasma-derived activated prothrombin complex concentrate (FEIBA™, Baxter, Vienna, Austria) or recombinant factor VIIa (NOVOSEVEN®, Novo Nordisk, Bagsvaerd, Denmark). Although currently available bypassing agents have roughly comparable overall hemostatic efficacy of 85–90%, prospective studies have suggested that efficacy between the available bypassing agents may change over time [1].

The need for theranostic guidance in management of hemophilia patients with inhibitors

The mechanism of action of recombinant factor VIIa is partly based on TF-dependent activation of factor X, and is more predominantly dependent on direct attachment to the surface of activated platelets and conversion of factor X to Xa facilitated by factor Va. In contrast, plasma-derived prothrombin complex concentrate drives thrombin generation by containing a concentrated form of non-activated and activated coagulation factors II, VII/VIIa, IX, and X/Xa.

In conclusion, timely and optimal management of bleeding patients with severe hemophilia and inhibitors requires an individualized theranostic approach (definition: term used to describe the proposed process of diagnostic therapy for individual patients – to test them for possible reaction to taking a new medication and to tailor a treatment for them based on the test results). Theranostic strategy can be defined by use of a global laboratory assay to tailor choice of the most suitable bypassing agent as well as guide selection of effective dosages.

An ideal global assay would be one that provides information on the dynamics of thrombin generation, includes all components involved in the mode of action of bypassing agents, such as coagulation proteins, natural anticoagulants, blood cells, platelets, endothelium, and flow. Moreover, the ideal global assay should provide a visual assessment of whole blood clot formation and/or fibrin formation, and evaluate the structure and stability of the formed clot. Finally, it should be easy to operate, give rapid and reproducible results and be inexpensive. Most importantly, the ideal global assay should correlate to clinical baseline phenotype and aid in predicting severity of the bleeding pattern. Finally, the assay should be useful for monitoring hemostatic interventions and guide the selection of the most optimal hemostatic drug and necessary dosage to achieve hemostasis.

Standard laboratory tests such as the prothrombin time (PT) and activated partial thromboplastin time (APTT) do not reach any of the listed criteria for the ideal global assay. Unfortunately, the ideal global assay does not exist. There are several attractive candidates including measurement of thrombin generation, thromboelastometry, APTT waveform [2–4]. This chapter gives a description of methods for measuring thrombin generation and whole blood coagulation with thromboelastography/thromboelastometry and focuses on the use of these assays for predicting the response to bypassing agents. We also aim to report on translational clinical application and finally, to discuss future perspectives.

Current and Future Issues in Hemophilia Care, First Edition. Edited by Emérito-Carlos Rodríguez-Merchán and Leonard A. Valentino.
© 2011 John Wiley & Sons, Ltd. Published 2011 by Blackwell Publishing Ltd.

Calibrated automated thrombin generation

The method

The concept of the calibrated automated thrombin generation method was pioneered by H.C. Hemker and S. Béguin [5]. The purpose has been to develop a simple method of quantifying the dynamics of thrombin generation. The method is based on the use of plasma and a fluorogenic thrombin substrate as well as a 96-well microplate fluorometer. Systematic studies of pre-analytical and analytical variables have demonstrated that fluorescence measurements are associated with a high degree of inconsistency caused by non-linearity of the fluorescence intensity. Furthermore, a fluorescence signal depends upon the quenching properties of the medium, and plasma samples differ widely, even samples of the same person obtained on the same day. Thus, in order to quantify thrombin concentrations derived from the fluorescence signal, each sample has to be run in parallel with a calibrator (in the model described by H.C. Hemker, alpha2-macroglobulin-thrombin complexes are used as calibrator). In practice, citrated platelet-poor plasma or platelet-rich plasma is added to the wells of the microplate. The fluorogenic thrombin substrate is then added and coagulation is activated by tissue factor. Following re-calcification, automated continuous measurements of fluorescence are started. A simple computer program converts the fluorescence readings into a quantitative dynamic profile of thrombin generation and several dynamic parameters are derived (Figure 31.1).

Table 31.1 lists currently recommended pre-analytical and analytical procedures for performing thrombin generation measurements for theranostic guidance of bypassing agents [6–9].

The classical thrombin generation curve has a waveform from which several quantifiable parameters can be measured (lag time, time to peak thrombin, and endogenous thrombin potential) (Figure 31.1). The entire course of thrombin generation is usually separated into an initiation phase corresponding to the lag time before the earliest measurable thrombin. This is followed by the amplification phase which likely represents the assembling of the intrinsic tenase (FIXa and FVIIIa) and the prothrombinase complex (FXa and FVa) during which the maximum rate of thrombin generation occurs. Eventually, thrombin generation reaches a peak and the time required to reach this point is described as time-to-peak thrombin. The total amount of thrombin generation (= area under the curve) is frequently called the endogenous thrombin potential (ETP).

In principle, abnormal thrombin generation curves are characterized by (1) a prolonged or shortened lag time; (2) reduced or increased peak thrombin; or (3) reduced or elevated ETP.

The interpretation of the thrombin generation profile includes several variables. The lag time of thrombin is primarily determined by: levels of free tissue factor, tissue factor pathway inhibitor (TFPI), factor VII, factor IX, and fibrinogen. The propagation phase of thrombin is highly dependent on the number and function of platelets. Hence, the higher the platelet count the higher the maximum rate and acceleration of thrombin generation. Other main determinants of the propagation phase of thrombin generation depend on the intensity of activation with tissue factor. Following activation with low levels of tissue factor, fibrinogen, factor XII, free TFPI, antithrombin, and prothrombin are important determinants of thrombin generation. Following stimulation with a high level of tissue factor, prothrombin, antithrombin, fibrinogen, free TFPI, and factor V becomes the predominant determinants of thrombin generation.

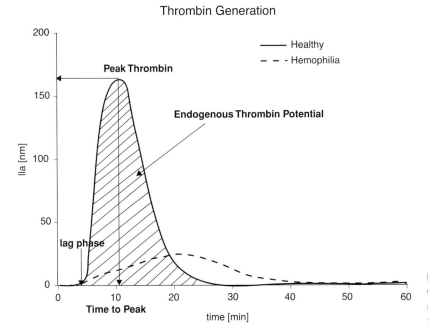

Figure 31.1 The classical thrombin generation curve has a waveform from which several quantifiable parameters can be measured (lag time, time to peak thrombin, and endogenous thrombin potential).

Table 31.1 Currently recommended pre-analytical and analytical procedures for performing thrombin generation measurements for theranostic guidance of bypassing agents [3–6]

	Calibrated automated thrombin generation	Whole blood thromboelastometry
Pre-analytical considerations	Use corn trypsin inhibitor (final concentration minimum 18.3 μg/ml) stabilized citrated (3.2%) blood tubes	Use corn trypsin inhibitor (final concentration minimum 18.3 μg/ml) stabilized citrated (3.2%) blood tubes
	Smooth venipuncture employing minimum stasis is crucial	Smooth venipuncture employing minimum stasis is crucial
	Double centrifugation prior to freezing	Tube size minimum 3 mL
		Run samples after 30 minutes and no later than 2 hours
Analytical considerations	Low tissue factor 1pM preferred for assaying hemophilia and hemostatic intervention with bypassing agents	Low tissue factor (Innovin, final dilution 1:50000) preferred for assaying hemophilia and hemostatic intervention with bypassing agents
		Low tissue factor (Innovin, final dilution 1:50000) and t-PA (1.8 nM) for investigating clot stability
	Platelet rich plasma should be used for monitoring rFVIIa	Whole blood is best medium, however platelet rich plasma can be used
Signal processing	Thrombinoscope software: lag time, peak thrombin, time to peak thrombin, endogenous thrombin potential	Standard parameters: clotting time (CT/r), clot formation time (CFT/k), maximum clot firmness (MCF/MA). Dynamic parameters: maximum velocity (MaxVel), time to maximum velocity (t, MaxVel)

Translation of laboratory results to clinical practice

Correlation of thrombin generation with clinical phenotype

Thrombin generation has been used for laboratory phenotyping a variety of bleeding disorders. The best-characterized hemostatic dysfunction described by thrombin generation profiles is hemophilia A. In contrast to the categorical distinction between mild, moderate, and severe based on assessment of functional levels of factor VIII, the rate specific characteristics of thrombin generation have been reported to illustrate and reflect the clinical heterogeneity of hemophilia [6]. In particular, thrombin generation has been documented as predictive in distinguishing milder phenotypes of severe hemophilia despite similar low levels of factor VIII (e.g. less than 1% of normal).

Prediction of response to bypassing agents

Thrombin generation profiles have also been used for monitoring the hemostatic response to various types of hemostatic treatment. Severe hemophilia is usually managed by substitution with a factor VIII concentrate. A considerable proportion of patients develop allogeneic inhibitory antibodies toward the substitution therapy. These patients require so-called bypassing agents, such as recombinant factor VIIa or plasma-derived activated prothrombin complex concentrates. Thrombin generation measurement has been used to monitor substitution with such bypassing agents [7,8]. The overall experience with thrombin measurements as a surrogate parameter of hemostatic effect is still rather limited; however, the preliminary results appear promising.

Individualized dose tailoring of bypassing agents during orthopedic surgery

During recent years, extensive and systematic research has investigated the use of thrombin generation for tailoring bypassing agents during surgery. Prospective assessment of thrombin generation test for dose monitoring of bypassing therapy in a case series of hemophilia patients with inhibitors undergoing elective surgery was reported by Dargaud et al. [9]. Dose tailoring of bypassing agents was performed using a standardized three-step protocol including (1) in vitro spiking experiments evaluating the thrombin generation ability of increasing concentrations of recombinant factor VIIa (0–90–180–200–240–270 μg/kg) and plasma derived activated prothrombin complex concentrate (0–75–100 U/kg) in order to determine the minimal dose of each bypassing agent that normalizes thrombin generation capacity; (2) an ex vivo confirmation step where thrombin generation is measured before and after the administration of the bypassing agent which gave the best hemostatic profile in the previous in vitro spiking experiment using the dose which fully normalized in vitro thrombin generation; and (3) monitoring of the chosen dose of the bypassing agent during surgery and the postoperative period. As recombinant factor VIIa predominantly induces FXa and FIXa generation on activated platelets, the hemostatic efficacy of recombinant factor VIIa was evaluated using platelet rich plasma (PRP). Plasma-derived activated prothrombin complex concentrate, having a different mechanism of action, was evaluated using platelet-poor plasma (PPP). Preliminary results show a good correlation between in vivo clinical response to bypassing agents and thrombin generating capacity. Furthermore, data suggest that thrombin generation may represent a surrogate marker for monitoring bypassing therapies in surgical situations.

Whole blood thromboelastometry

The method

The thrombelastographic principle introduced by Hartert [10] has been adopted in the computerized version of TEG® apparatus manufactured by Haemoscope®. In 1996 Calatzis et al. invented another principle of thrombelastography, today named thromboelastometry (ROTEM®) [11] in which the pin oscillates instead of the cup. A ball bearing focusing the pin apparently makes the ROTEM® less sensitive to movements.

Both the TEG® and the ROTEM® provide a digital signal allowing for additional computation of the continuous coagulation signal leading to the derivation of several quantifiable parameters (Figure 31.2, Panels a & b).

The underlying principle of the TEG and ROTEM is the continuous assessment of the elastic properties of a forming clot. Both devices consist of a cup into which the sample (whole blood, platelet-rich or platelet-poor plasma) and reagents are placed and

a pin which sits in the center of the cup when the device is running. Once the sample is in place and the cup is pushed up into the pin, the pin ROTEM® or cup TEG® begins to oscillate. Reduced movement of the pin during formation of strands of fibrin that attach the pin to the wall of the cup is registered with specialized computer software and visualized on a computer providing a coagulation signal similar to that of the traditional thrombelastography (Figure 31.2, Panel a).

Complementary additional information on overall hemostatic capacity

Demonstrating abnormalities in clot stability and effect of clot stabilizing intervention

Thromboelastometry complements thrombin generation measurements by being able to provide information about clot firmness and clot stability. Clot stability and resistance toward facilitated fibrinolysis can be investigated in assays containing TF and tissue plasminogen activator. Adopting such assays, thromboelastometry studies have shown effect of tranexamic acid [12] and also recently factor XIII supplementation [13].

Correlation of thrombelastography with clinical phenotype

A number of studies have demonstrated considerable heterogeneity in the baseline whole blood coagulation patterns amongst patients with verified factor VIII levels <1% [14]. Furthermore, data have illustrated that patients diagnosed with severe hemophilia A (FVIII:C <1%) but having unusually good whole blood clotting profiles are associated with a less severe bleeding phenotype [15].

Prediction of response to bypassing agents

The low tissue factor assay has also been used to illustrate different response patterns to various levels of coagulation factor VIII concentrate. In addition, both in vitro and in vivo studies have demonstrated the ability of thromboelastography to predict the clinical response to bypassing agents in patients with inhibitors [16–18]. A small clinical study has shown that thromboelastography may be used to individualize therapy and provide more judicious use of bypassing agents as well as more convenient treatment regimens [19]. Recently, thromboelastometry has been utilized to correct the hemostatic performance of recombinant factor VIIa during surgery by showing need for fresh platelet concentrate to secure effect of recombinant factor VIIa [20].

Conclusions

Ongoing scientific activities aim to further standardize the use of thrombin generation and thromboelastometry for use in hemophilia. Important future questions will include source and concentration of tissue factor for the global assays.

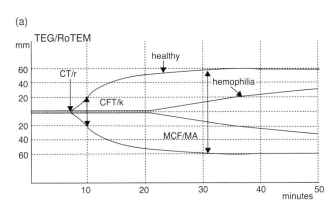

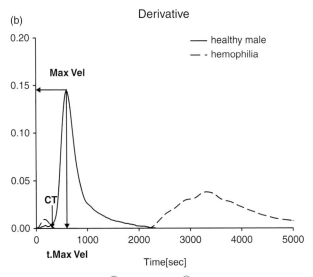

Figure 31.2 Both the TEG® and the ROTEM® (a) provide a digital signal allowing for additional computation of the continuous coagulation signal leading to the derivation of several quantifiable parameters (b).

A series of additional bypassing agents are in development [21], thus further emphasizing the need for global assay to monitoring and provide theranostic guidance.

References

1. Astermark, J., et al., A randomized comparison of bypassing agents in hemophilia complicated by an inhibitor: the FEIBA NovoSeven Comparative (FENOC) Study. Blood, 2007;109(2):546–51.

2. Shima, M., Matsumoto, T., Fukuda, K., et al. The utility of activated partial thromboplastin time (aPTT) clot waveform analysis in the investigation of hemophilia A patients with very low levels of factor VIII activity (FVIII:C). Thromb. Haemost. 2002;87(3): 436–41.

3. Carr, M.E. Measurement of platelet force: the Hemodyne hemostasis analyzer. Clin Lab Manage Rev. 1995 Jul–Aug;9(4):312-4, 316–8, 320.

4. Goldenberg, N.A., Hathaway, W.E., Jacobson, L., Manco-Johnson, M.J. CLOFAL assay: A new global assay of coagulation and fibrinolysis. Thromb Res. 2005;116(4):345–56.

5. Hemker, H.C., et al., Continuous registration of thrombin generation in plasma, its use for the determination of the thrombin potential. Thromb. Haemost. 1993;70(4):617–24.

6. Dargaud, Y., et al., Evaluation of thrombin generating capacity in plasma from patients with haemophilia A and B. Thromb. Haemost. 2005;93(3):475–80.

7. Dargaud, Y., et al., Use of the thrombin generation test to evaluate response to treatment with recombinant activated factor VII. Semin. Hematol. 2008;45(2 Suppl 1):S72–S73.

8. Dargaud, Y., et al., Major surgery in a severe haemophilia A patient with high titre inhibitor: use of the thrombin generation test in the therapeutic decision. Haemophilia. 2005;11(5):552–8.

9. Dargaud Y, et al., Prospective assessment of thrombin generation test for dose monitoring of bypassing therapy in hemophilia patients with inhibitors undergoing elective surgery. Blood 2010;116(25): 5734–7.

10. Hartert, H., Blutgerinnungsstudien mit der thrombelastographie, einem neuen untersuchungsverfahren. Klinische Wochenschrift. 1948;26: 577–83.

11. Calatzis, A., et al., A comparison of the technical principle of the roTEG coagulation analyser and conventional thrombelastographic systems. Ann.Haematol. 1996;72 (Suppl. 1): p. P90 (abstract).

12. Hvas, A.M., et al., Tranexamic acid combined with recombinant factor VIII increases clot resistance to accelerated fibrinolysis in severe hemophilia A. J. Thromb. Haemost. 2007;5(12): p. 2408–14.

13. Rea, C.J., et al., Factor XIII combined with recombinant factor VIIa: a new means of treating severe haemophilia A. J Thromb Haemost. 2011 Mar;9(3):510–6.

14. Ingerslev, J., L.H. Poulsen, and B. Sorensen, Potential role of the dynamic properties of whole blood coagulation in assessment of dosage requirements in haemophilia. Haemophilia. 2003;9(4):348–52.

15. Chitlur, M., et al., Thromboelastography in children with coagulation factor deficiencies. Br. J. Haematol. 2008 Jun;142(2):250–6.

16. Sorensen, B., Ingerslev, J. Whole blood clot formation phenotypes in hemophilia A and rare coagulation disorders. Patterns of response to recombinant factor VIIa. J. Thromb. Haemost. 2004;2(2):102–110.

17. Sorensen, B., Ingerslev, J. Thromboelastography and recombinant factor VIIa-hemophilia and beyond. Semin. Hematol. 2004;41 (Suppl 1):140–44.

18. Sorensen, B., Persson, E., Ingerslev, J. Factor VIIa analogue (V158D/E296V/M298Q-FVIIa) normalises clot formation in whole blood from patients with severe haemophilia A. Br. J. Haematol. 2007;137(2):158–65.

19. Young, G., et al., Individualization of bypassing agent treatment for haemophilic patients with inhibitors utilizing thromboelastography. Haemophilia. 2006;12(6):598–604.

20. Sorensen, B., Ingerslev, J. Platelet infusion supports recombinant factor VIIa in a patient with severe haemophilia A and inhibitor – clinical outcome and laboratory observations. Thromb. Haemost. 2010;103(6):1275–6.

21. Sorensen, B. Future pharmacological strategies in management of haemophilia. Thromb. Res., 2010 Oct;126(4):259–61.

32 Combination/Sequential Use of Bypassing Agents

Alessandro Gringeri

Ospedale Maggiore Policlinico and University of Milan, Milan, Italy

Introduction

The development of inhibitors to factor VIII (FVIII) is the most common, severe, challenging and expensive complication of the treatment of patients with hemophilia [1,2]. In particular, the presence of high level inhibitors renders replacement therapy completely ineffective, so that bypassing agents are required to induce clot formation [3,4].

Two bypassing agents are currently available and have been shown to be safe and efficacious in the treatment of bleeding episodes in patients with inhibitors [5]: the anti-inhibitor coagulant complex FEIBA (factor eight inhibitor bypassing activity) (Baxter AG, Vienna, Austria), which is an activated prothrombin complex concentrate (aPCC) [6,7], and recombinant activated factor VII (rFVIIa; NovoSeven®, Novo Nordisk A/S, Bagsvaerd, Denmark) [8,9]. Unfortunately, whichever treatment is used initially, 10–20% of bleeding events in hemophilia patients with high-responding inhibitors cannot be controlled by bypassing agents [10,11].

Once a lack of a hemostatic response has been observed, a decision needs to be made whether to continue the same treatment, to increase the dose, to shorten the intervals between doses, or to change product. A poor response to one or both of these agents leads to a potentially very dangerous situation for the patient and requires the use of huge amounts of human and economic resources [2,10]. There is no recognized or standard way out of this dilemma, particularly for life- and limb-threatening bleeding. An international panel of physicians therefore applied their collective knowledge of problem hemorrhage associated with hemophilia and inhibitors and suggested a consensus algorithm that would aid physicians in dealing with unresponsive bleeding [10]. This algorithm included sequential use of both bypassing agents when the bleed was unresponsive to each of these agents used singly and at high dosage.

In fact, a synergistic effect of these two bypassing agents has been reported in vitro and in vivo.

In vitro findings

In 2002, Key and colleagues reported for the first time the successful use of a sequential regimen with the alternate administration of rFVIIa and aPCC in a patient with a suboptimal response to rFVIIa [12]. Additionally, these authors showed an exceptionally strong response to rFVIIa in vitro when it was added to whole blood after the patient received PCC therapy, as shown by a whole blood clotting time assay.

These in vitro findings were subsequently confirmed by Tomokiyo et al. [13], who found that the addition of FX to rFVIIa dramatically enhanced the thrombin generation rate in an in vitro coagulation model and corrected the prolonged aPTTs of FVIII- and FIX-depleted plasmas. In addition, the co-administration of rFVIIa and FX in a hemophilia B monkey model resulted in a more robust and persistent hemostatic effect on the secondary bleeding time and whole-blood clotting time of thromboelastography than that of rFVIIa alone.

Subsequently, Allen et al. [14] showed that at all concentrations of rFVIIa, increased prothrombin concentrations led to increases in the peak and rate of thrombin generation. The authors concluded that manipulation of the prothrombin level may influence the response of bleeding patients to rFVIIa.

Nakatomi et al. [15] have very recently reported the in vitro efficacy of a virus-inactivated and nano-filtrated plasma-derived FVIIa/FX concentrate prepared by assembling plasma-derived FVIIa and FX at a weight ratio of 1:10. The FVIIa/FX mixture

Current and Future Issues in Hemophilia Care, First Edition. Edited by Emérito-Carlos Rodríguez-Merchán and Leonard A. Valentino.
© 2011 John Wiley & Sons, Ltd. Published 2011 by Blackwell Publishing Ltd.

proved superior to rFVIIa with regards to shortening the APTT and accelerating the thrombin generation ex vivo in hemophilic plasma.

All these findings indicate that the increase of FX and/or of prothrombin levels by means of a prothrombin complex concentrate might improve the hemostatic efficacy of rFVIIa in controlling the bleeding in patients with hemophilia and inhibitors.

In vivo findings

A more extensive report on the use of sequential combination of bypassing agents was made by Schneiderman and colleagues [16,17]. These authors reported their experience in five hospitalized children with severe hemophilia and inhibitors treated with sequential doses of aPCC and rFVIIa for unresponsive bleeding. The regimen, which included 1 to 3 doses of rFVIIa given at 2-hour intervals between aPCC doses given every 12 hours (Table 32.1), was found to be safe and effective, and no clinical or laboratory evidence of thrombosis, thrombocytopenia, or disseminated intravascular coagulation (DIC) was observed.

An update by the investigators, published in 2007 [17], described further sequential bypassing treatment in four of these five patients for 206 cumulative days. Bleeding that had failed to respond to a median of 3 days of monotherapy resolved after a median of 3 days of sequential therapy, suggesting that the treatment regimen was safe and efficacious in the cases reported. No patient developed thrombosis or overt DIC, but elevations in the D-dimer above 5000 ng/mL were noted in 42% of the courses that extended beyond 3 days.

In the report of surgical interventions in a cohort of patients with hemophilia A and inhibitors, Kraut et al. [18] described three patients (two children and one adult) treated sequentially

Table 32.1 Regimens used for sequential therapy. (Reproduced from Schneiderman J, Nugent DJ, Young G. Sequential therapy with activated prothrombin complex concentrate and recombinant factor VIIa in patients with severe haemophilia and inhibitors. Haemophilia, 2004;10:347–351.)

Hour	Regimen 1*	Regimen 2	Regimen 3
0	aPCC	aPCC	aPCC
2			
4			
6	rFVIIa	rFVIIa	rFVIIa
8		rFVIIa	rFVIIa
10			rFVIIa
12	aPCC	aPCC	aPCC
14			
16			
18	rFVIIa	rFVIIa	rFVIIa
20		rFVIIa	rFVIIa
22			rFVIIa
24	aPCC	aPCC	aPCC

*Used most commonly.

with rFVIIa and FEIBA with effective bleeding control and no adverse events.

Another child was reported to have undergone combination therapy [19]: he was a 13-year-old boy with severe hemophilia A unresponsive to treatment with rFVII 90 µg/kg every 2 hours administered for 10 days to try to stop a bleeding in the chest (hemothorax), around the liver and spleen, in the small pelvis, in the small and large intestine, in the left kidney and the right perinephral area, occurred after surgery for abdominal pain, with a possible diagnosis of acute appendicitis. A combined bypassing agent therapy was consequently prescribed at a regimen consisting of 90 µg/kg rFVIIa given every two hours and 50 U/Kg FEIBA given every third rFVIIa dose, i.e. every six hours. The authors asserted that this rescue treatment regimen proved effective and safe, as the bleed was finally controlled with no systemic reaction, anamnesis of inhibitor titer or thrombosis.

Recently, Gringeri and colleagues described their experience with sequential therapy in two children with refractory joint bleeding and two adults with refractory postoperative bleeding following orthopedic surgery [20]. aPCC and rFVIIa were administered in alternating fashion every 8 to 12 hours, and complete bleeding control was achieved within 24 to 48 hours. Doses ranged from 90 to 270 µg/kg rFVIIa and from 50 to 100 U/kg FEIBA. No clinical adverse events occurred, although a rise in D-dimer levels was noted in two of the four patients. D-dimers levels decreased as soon as the combination therapy was discontinued by stopping the administration of rFVIIa.

Martinowitz et al. have suggested the possibility of co-administration of low doses of rFVIIa with FEIBA in hemophilia A patients with high responding inhibitors [21]. The authors reported efficacy and safety of this co-administration in five of these patients to treat overall 400 bleeding events. The dosing of rFVIIa and FEIBA was chosen on the basis of results of thrombin generation assays after addition ex vivo of increasing doses of the products to platelet-rich and platelet-poor plasma samples of each single patient. The doses eventually administered were ranging from 30 to 70 µg/kg rFVIIa and 20–30 U/kg FEIBA. This combination treatment was effective in controlling most bleeding episodes, most commonly joint hemorrhage, but also muscle bleeding, recurrent hematuria and one surgery (gallbladder stent insertion) were efficaciously treated. No adverse vents were reported by the authors.

A survey undertaken in 2010 by the European Haemophilia Treatment Standardisation Board (EHTSB) [22] collected by a retrospective medical record review 11 sequential bypassing therapy courses in nine patients, aged 9–73 years (median 24 years) with hemophilia A and two with hemophilia B with unresponsive bleeds to single therapy with one or both bypassing agents, including 5 major surgeries. By-passing agents were sequentially administered by alternating one APCC dose (20–80 U kg^{-1} every 8–12 h) to 1–3 rFVIIa doses (90–270 µg kg^{-1} every 3–12 h). Bleeding control was achieved in 12–24 h in all patients. Sequential combination of bypassing agents was discontinued after 1–15 days. No clinical adverse events were observed, but a significant increase in D-dimer levels was seen in three of five patients who were assessed.

Discussion

No clear-cut and definite evidence is available yet on safety and efficacy of SCBT in the treatment of unresponsive hemorrhage in children and adults, particularly in those with unresponsive bleeding after major surgery.

Preliminary in vitro findings suggest a potential synergistic effect of the use of a combination of the two major bypassing agents, namely rFVIIa and APCC.

Overall 18 patients were reported in the literature to have received a combination therapy with the two major bypassing agents. All of them were efficaciously treated, also when a previous monotherapy had failed.

Various regimens were administered: in general, when high doses of rFVIIa were prescribed, they were associated with lower doses of aPCC. Combined bypassing therapy was shown to be well-tolerated by children and adults, who showed no clinical signs and symptoms of thrombosis or DIC during and after treatment. On the other hand, some patients showed a significant and progressive increase of D-dimer values, although without a decreased fibrinogen and platelet count below critical values for DIC definition [23]. These findings indicate that this form of aggressive therapy be limited to the inpatient setting and include close clinical monitoring and frequent laboratory screening to assess for thrombosis and disseminated intravascular coagulopathy (DIC).

Conclusions

In conclusion, combined bypassing therapy seems efficacious in children and in adults without clinical adverse events; nevertheless it remains a salvage treatment due to its potential risks. Nevertheless, the very limited evidence available may represent a sound background for planning a prospective clinical trial that is needed to confirm these findings, and provide more solid evidence and guidelines for its use.

References

1. Lloyd-Jones M, Wight J, Paisley S, Knight C. Control of bleeding in patients with haemophilia A with inhibitors: a systematic review. Haemophilia, 2003;9:464–520.
2. Gringeri A, Mantovani LG, Scalone, Mannucci PM COCIS Study Group. Cost of care and quality of life for patients with hemophilia complicated by inhibitors: the COCIS Study Group. Blood, 2003;102:2358–2363.
3. Gringeri A, Mannucci PM: Italian Association of Haemophilia Centres. Italian guidelines for the diagnosis and treatment of patients with haemophilia and inhibitors. Haemophilia, 2005;11:611–619.
4. Hay CR, Brown, S., Collins PW, Keeling DM, Liesner R. The diagnosis and management of factor VIII and IX inhibitors: a guideline from the United Kingdom Haemophilia Centre Doctors' Organisation. Br J Haematol, 2006;133:591–605.
5. Astermark J, Donfield SM, DiMichele DM, Gringeri A, Gilbert SA, Waters J, Berntorp E. For the FENOC Study Group. A randomized comparison of bypassing agents in hemophilia complicated by an inhibitor: the FEIBA NovoSeven Comparative (FENOC) Study. Blood, 2007;109:546–551.
6. FEIBA. VH Anti-Inhibitor Coagulant Complex package insert. Westlake Village, CA: Baxter Healthcare Corporation, 2005.
7. Hilgartner M, Aledort L, Andes A, Gill J. Efficacy and safety of vapor-heated anti-inhibitor coagulant complex in hemophilia patients. FEIBA Study Group. Transfusion, 1990;30:626–630.
8. Novo Nordisk A/S. NovoSeven package insert. Princeton, NJ: Novo Nordisk A/S, 2005.
9. Macik BG, Lindley CM, Lusher J, Sawyer WT, Bloom AL, Harrison JF, et al. Safety and initial clinical efficacy of three dose levels of recombinant activated factor VII (rFVIIa): results of a phase I study. Blood Coag Fibrinol, 1993;4:521–527.
10. Teitel J, Berntorp E, Collins P, D'Oiron R, Ewenstein B, Gomperts E, et al. A systematic approach to controlling problem bleeds in patients with severe congenital haemophilia A and high-titer inhibitors. Haemophilia, 2007;13:256–263.
11. Berntorp E. Differential response to bypassing agents complicates treatment in patients with haemophilia and inhibitors. Haemophilia, 2009;15:3–10.
12. Key NS, Christie B, Henderson N, Nelsestuen GL. Possible synergy between recombinant factor VIIa and prothrombin complex concentrate in hemophilia therapy. Haemophilia, 2002;88:60–65.
13. Tomokiyo K, Nakatomi Y, Araki T, Teshima K, Nakano H, Nakagaki T, et al. A novel therapeutic approach combining human plasma-derived Factors VIIa and X for haemophiliacs with inhibitors: evidence of a higher thrombin generation rate in vitro and more sustained haemostatic activity in vivo than obtained with Factor VIIa alone. Vox Sanguinis, 2003;85:290–299.
14. Allen GA, Hoffman M, Roberts HR, Monroe DM. Manipulation of prothrombin concentration improves response to high-dose factor VIIa in a cell-based model of haemophilia. B J Haematol, 2006;134:314–319.
15. Nakatomi Y, Nakashima T, Gokudan S, Miyazaki H, Tsuji M, Hanada-Dateki T, Araki T, Tomokiyo K, Hamamoto T, Ogata Y. Combining FVIIa and FX into a mixture which imparts a unique thrombin generation potential to hemophilic plasma: an in vitro assessment of FVIIa/FX mixture as an alternative bypassing agent. Thromb Res 2010;125:457–463.
16. Schneiderman J, Nugent DJ, Young G. Sequential therapy with activated prothrombin complex concentrate and recombinant factor VIIa in patients with severe haemophilia and inhibitors. Haemophilia, 2004;10:347–351.
17. Schneiderman J, Rubin E, Nugent DJ, Young G. Sequential therapy with activated prothrombin complex concentrates and recombinant FVIIa in patients with severe haemophilia and inhibitors: update of our previous experience. Haemophilia, 2007;13:244–248.
18. Kraut EH, Aledort LM, Arkin S, Stine KC, Wong WY. Surgical interventions in a cohort of patients with haemophilia A and inhibitors: an experiential retrospective chart review. Haemophilia, 2007;13:508–517.

19. Economou M, Teli A, Tzantzaroudi A, Tsatra I, Zavitsanakis A, Athanassiou-Metaxa M. Sequential therapy with activated prothrombin complex concentrate (FEIBA) and recombinant factor VIIa in a patient with severe haemophilia A, inhibitor presence and refractory bleeding. Haemophilia 2008;14:390–1.

20. Gringeri A, Santagostino E, Mancuso A, et al. Sequential combined bypassing therapy: a rescue option in refractory bleeds – the Italian experience. Haemophilia. 2008;14:49 (abstract 08 PO 42).

21. Martinowitz U, Livnat T, Zivelin A, Kenet G. Concomitant infusion of low doses of rFVIIa and FEIBA in haemophilia patients with inhibitors. Haemophilia, 2009;15:904–910.

22. Gringeri A, Fischer K, Karafoulidou A, Klamroth R, Lopez-Fernandez MF, Mancuso E, on behalf of the European Haemophilia Treatment Standardisation Board (EHTSB). Sequential combined bypassing therapy is safe and effective in the treatment of unresponsive bleeding in adults and children with haemophilia and inhibitors. Haemophilia, 2010 (in press).

23. Toh CH, Hoots WK. The scoring system of the Scientific and Standardisation Committee on Disseminated Intravascular Coagulation of the International Society on Thrombosis and Haemostasis: a 5-year overview. Thromb Haemost 2007;5:604–606.

Index

Note: Page numbers with italicized *f*'s and *t*'s refer to figures and tables, respectively.

Current and Future Issues in Hemophilia Care, First Edition. Edited by Emérito-Carlos Rodríguez-Merchán and Leonard A. Valentino.
© 2011 John Wiley & Sons, Ltd. Published 2011 by Blackwell Publishing Ltd.